Radiation Response Biomarkers for Individualised Cancer Treatments

Radiation Response Biomarkers for Individualised Cancer Treatments

Editors

Eric Andreas Rutten
Christophe Badie

MDPI • Basel • Beijing • Wuhan • Barcelona • Belgrade • Manchester • Tokyo • Cluj • Tianjin

MDPI

Editors
Eric Andreas Rutten
Department of Oncology
University of Oxford
Oxford
United Kingdom

Christophe Badie
Cancer Mechanisms and
Biomarkers, Radiation Effects
Department
Public Health England
Harwell
United Kingdom

Editorial Office
MDPI
St. Alban-Anlage 66
4052 Basel, Switzerland

This is a reprint of articles from the Special Issue published online in the open access journal *Journal of Personalized Medicine* (ISSN 2075-4426) (available at: www.mdpi.com/journal/jpm/special_issues/radiation_cancer).

For citation purposes, cite each article independently as indicated on the article page online and as indicated below:

LastName, A.A.; LastName, B.B.; LastName, C.C. Article Title. *Journal Name* **Year**, *Volume Number*, Page Range.

ISBN 978-3-0365-1684-4 (Hbk)
ISBN 978-3-0365-1683-7 (PDF)

Contents

Eric Andreas Rutten and Christophe Badie
Radiation Biomarkers: Silver Bullet, or Wild Goose Chase?
Reprinted from: *Journal of Personalized Medicine* **2021**, *11*, 603, doi:10.3390/jpm11070603 . . . . . . **1**

Jared J. Luxton, Miles J. McKenna, Aidan M. Lewis, Lynn E. Taylor, Sameer G. Jhavar, Gregory P. Swanson and Susan M. Bailey
Telomere Length Dynamics and Chromosomal Instability for Predicting Individual Radiosensitivity and Risk via Machine Learning
Reprinted from: *Journal of Personalized Medicine* **2021**, *11*, 188, doi:10.3390/jpm11030188 . . . . . . **7**

Volodymyr Vinnikov, Manoor Prakash Hande, Ruth Wilkins, Andrzej Wojcik, Eduardo Zubizarreta and Oleg Belyakov
Prediction of the Acute or Late Radiation Toxicity Effects in Radiotherapy Patients Using Ex Vivo Induced Biodosimetric Markers: A Review
Reprinted from: *Journal of Personalized Medicine* **2020**, *10*, 285, doi:10.3390/jpm10040285 . . . . . . **29**

Jayne Moquet, Kai Rothkamm, Stephen Barnard and Elizabeth Ainsbury
Radiation Biomarkers in Large Scale Human Health Effects Studies
Reprinted from: *Journal of Personalized Medicine* **2020**, *10*, 155, doi:10.3390/jpm10040155 . . . . . . **65**

Anne Dietz, Maria Gomolka, Simone Moertl and Prabal Subedi
Ionizing Radiation Protein Biomarkers in Normal Tissue and Their Correlation to Radiosensitivity: Protocol for a Systematic Review
Reprinted from: *Journal of Personalized Medicine* **2020**, *11*, 3, doi:10.3390/jpm11010003 . . . . **79**

Prabal Subedi, Maria Gomolka, Simone Moertl and Anne Dietz
Ionizing Radiation Protein Biomarkers in Normal Tissue and Their Correlation to Radiosensitivity: A Systematic Review
Reprinted from: *Journal of Personalized Medicine* **2021**, *11*, 140, doi:10.3390/jpm11020140 . . . . . . **89**

Mariola Śliwińska-Mossoń, Katarzyna Wadowska, Łukasz Trembecki and Iwona Bil-Lula
Markers Useful in Monitoring Radiation-Induced Lung Injury in Lung Cancer Patients: A Review
Reprinted from: *Journal of Personalized Medicine* **2020**, *10*, 72, doi:10.3390/jpm10030072 . . . . . . **115**

Katalin Balázs, Lilla Antal, Géza Sáfrány and Katalin Lumniczky
Blood-Derived Biomarkers of Diagnosis, Prognosis and Therapy Response in Prostate Cancer Patients
Reprinted from: *Journal of Personalized Medicine* **2021**, *11*, 296, doi:10.3390/jpm11040296 . . . . . . **131**

Niall M. Byrne, Prajakta Tambe and Jonathan A. Coulter
Radiation Response in the Tumour Microenvironment: Predictive Biomarkers and Future Perspectives
Reprinted from: *Journal of Personalized Medicine* **2021**, *11*, 53, doi:10.3390/jpm11010053 . . . . . . **163**

Naoto Osu, Daijiro Kobayashi, Katsuyuki Shirai, Atsushi Musha, Hiro Sato, Yuka Hirota, Atsushi Shibata, Takahiro Oike and Tatsuya Ohno
Relative Biological Effectiveness of Carbon Ions for Head-and-Neck Squamous Cell Carcinomas According to Human Papillomavirus Status
Reprinted from: *Journal of Personalized Medicine* **2020**, *10*, 71, doi:10.3390/jpm10030071 . . . . . . **179**

Anna Wojakowska, Aneta Zebrowska, Agata Skowronek, Tomasz Rutkowski, Krzysztof Polanski, Piotr Widlak, Lukasz Marczak and Monika Pietrowska
Metabolic Profiles of Whole Serum and Serum-Derived Exosomes Are Different in Head and Neck Cancer Patients Treated by Radiotherapy
Reprinted from: *Journal of Personalized Medicine* **2020**, *10*, 229, doi:10.3390/jpm10040229 . . . . . . **187**

Daijiro Kobayashi, Takahiro Oike, Kazutoshi Murata, Daisuke Irie, Yuka Hirota, Hiro Sato, Atsushi Shibata and Tatsuya Ohno
Induction of Micronuclei in Cervical Cancer Treated with Radiotherapy
Reprinted from: *Journal of Personalized Medicine* **2020**, *10*, 110, doi:10.3390/jpm10030110 . . . . . . **201**

Simon Sioen, Karlien Cloet, Anne Vral and Ans Baeyens
The Cytokinesis-Block Micronucleus Assay on Human Isolated Fresh and Cryopreserved Peripheral Blood Mononuclear Cells
Reprinted from: *Journal of Personalized Medicine* **2020**, *10*, 125, doi:10.3390/jpm10030125 . . . . . . **209**

Takahiro Oike, Yuka Hirota, Narisa Dewi Maulany Darwis, Atsushi Shibata and Tatsuya Ohno
Comparison of Clonogenic Survival Data Obtained by Pre- and Post-Irradiation Methods
Reprinted from: *Journal of Personalized Medicine* **2020**, *10*, 171, doi:10.3390/jpm10040171 . . . . . . **221**

Journal of *Personalized Medicine*

MDPI

Editorial

Radiation Biomarkers: Silver Bullet, or Wild Goose Chase?

Eric Andreas Rutten [1,2,*] and Christophe Badie [1]

1 Cancer Mechanisms and Biomarkers Group, Radiation Effects Department, Centre for Radiation, Chemical & Environmental Hazards Public Health England Chilton, Didcot OX11 0RQ, UK; Christophe.badie@phe.gov.uk
2 Department of Oncology, University of Oxford, Oxford OX1 4BH, UK
* Correspondence: eric.andreasrutten@phe.gov.uk

Humans have learned to harness the power of radiation for therapeutic ends, with 50% of all patients diagnosed with cancer undergoing radiotherapy as part of their treatment [1], second only to surgery, with technical progress evident with new machines such as Cyberknife, MR-Linac, proton or carbon ion [2] therapy and the highly promising flash irradiation [3]. Radiotherapy is an important and effective therapy in the arsenal to treat numerous solid tumours. Improving the precision of radiotherapy has long been the quest of cancer scientists and clinicians. Recent improvements in its precision have helped to deliver most of the dose to the tumour, sparing the surrounding healthy tissues, hence limiting radiation toxicity and long-term effects, such as therapy-related cancer caused by, amongst others, a combination of radiation-induced somatic mutations, modifications of the microenvironment, and inflammation.

However, therapeutic radiation can still potentially lead to harmful secondary effects on patients. Humans exhibit much variability, with unique disease pathologies, especially concerning cancers [4]. The need for medicine to treat patients as individuals, rather than a general "one size fits all" method, is needed. Despite recent significant advances in this field of personalized medicine, the 5-year survival rate of certain cancers, such as lung cancers, remains dismally low, without much improvement, due to a dearth of biomarkers for individual radiosensitivity. However, even with precise planning, radiotherapy treatment outcome depends on multiple factors and can, in the process, damage healthy tissue with a degree of severity that is, until now, exceedingly difficult to predict. Moreover, radiotherapy induces cancer cell death by damaging their DNA and can also trigger the release of pro- and anti-inflammatory mediators. As such, biomarkers are needed to inform and guide the clinicians (external beam and molecular radiation therapy) for them to identify ideal treatment, total dose and fractionation regime as well as assess the toxicity and long-term risks on an individual basis.

Biomarkers for cancer fall into two primary categories: diagnostic and predictive. In the case of radiotherapy for cancers, there is a need for both: (1) diagnosis of radiation response and subsequent effect on the cancer and (2) prediction of possible secondary cancers arising in the long term because of radiotherapy, e.g., acute myeloid leukaemia and sarcomas. Radiation biomarkers are thus necessary, not only for understanding the actual effects of treatment on a tumour, but also for monitoring the most effective total dose to the tumour and identifying mechanisms that may allow a tumour to resist radiation therapy, as well as identifying the risks to the patient stemming from the therapy. Ever-evolving technologies should allow the detection and validation of emerging or new radiation biomarkers, whether genetic, epigenetic, cell-based or cell-free.

In terms of personalised medicine, biomarkers are especially important for tailoring cancer treatment purposes. This refers to a twofold issue: First, we are all different. Not two cancers are alike, with a multitude of unique factors amongst them genetic, epigenetic and inflammatory at play within each tumour. To effectively tailor a cancer therapy regimen for a patient, one must ideally know the radiosensitivity of the tumour. Moreover,

Citation: Rutten, E.A.; Badie, C. Radiation Biomarkers: Silver Bullet, or Wild Goose Chase? *J. Pers. Med.* **2021**, *11*, 603. https://doi.org/10.3390/jpm11070603

Received: 14 June 2021
Accepted: 23 June 2021
Published: 25 June 2021

studies focusing on tumour microenvironment have provided a better understanding of the effects of clinical radiation therapy and how it is influenced by the famous R's (Repair, Redistribution, Reoxygenation, Repopulation, Radiosensitivity and Reactivation of an anti-tumour response in the case of combination of immunotherapy/radiotherapy. Importantly for radiation protection purposes, the identification of the patient's individual susceptibility to radiation would be valuable perhaps especially for paediatric radiotherapy.

Biomarkers are essential for predicting and/or monitoring radiation exposure-associated effects. They take on many forms. In this Special Issue alone, multiple different kinds of biomarkers are explored and reviewed, from proteins such as TGF-β to miRNAs, and more classic methods based on cytogenetics or cytogenetic assays. Currently, there is much argument in the field as to the reliability and clinical application of different biomarker methods, which require professional researcher oversight and assessment, meaning that widescale processing of samples, necessary for true implementation of personalised medicine, remains difficult. As such, the push for biomarkers which lend themselves to upscaled processing methods, or even automated assays, is of vital importance. A question though thus remains: are radiation biomarkers a proverbial silver bullet for personalised treatment of cancers and an essential step towards the improvement of treatment? Or is there simply too much variability and biological noise to integrate and ever achieve, with confidence, a biomarker panel allowing for a holistic insight allowing for individualised courses of radiotherapy?

Overall, the aim of this Special Issue is to present an insight into some of the ongoing research in the oncology radiation response biomarker field and its applications in the ever-evolving field of personalised medicine.

Understanding of the relative biological effectiveness (RBE) of new radiotherapy techniques on cancers and biological states is critical, and a field in which new biomarkers of radiosensitivity and biological effect are indispensable. Naoto Osu et al. [5] demonstrated that carbon ion radiotherapy is more effective in HPV-negative head-and-neck squamous cell carcinomas than in HPV-positive carcinomas, indicating that HPV status is an important prognostic factor for patients. Daijiro Kobayashi et al. [6], in turn, have shown that micronuclei can be detected in solid tumours treated by radiotherapy; they are most likely signalling the activation of antitumour immune responses, showing that micronuclei formation could be an important indicator of radiotherapy effectivity. Niall M. Byrne et al. [7] discussed mechanisms of radioresistance in the tumour microenvironment, including predictive biomarkers for tumour fate post-radiotherapy. Studies such as these demonstrate the vital interplay between radiotherapy and biomarkers, whether they are biomarkers of RBE, or biomarkers demonstrating the opposite in the form of radioresistance within the tumour.

As shown by Mariola Śliwińska-Mossoń et al. [8] in their review, despite advances in understanding the molecular biology of lung cancer and the development of new therapeutic agents, the 5-year overall survival rate of non-small cell lung carcinoma (NSCLC) patients has remained largely the same for decades, at sub-16%. This is a powerful demonstrator of how, despite significant advances in the science of understanding NSCLC and how to treat it, general treatment schedules can only go so far and a deeper look into individuals is required. The review indicates that pre-clinical data supports the idea of miRNA being one such factor to consider.

Interestingly, Jared Luxton et al. [9] proposed to use telomere length and chromosomal instability to predict individual radiosensitivity, using a machine learning model trained on clinical data to predict post-therapy outcomes. Their method shows incredible promise: based on mean telomere length (MTL), the type of long-term secondary effect can be distinguished. Lower MTLs post radiation indicates a propensity for degenerative radiation disease, while higher MTLs demonstrate a predilection towards proliferative cancers. However, the authors themselves are quick to point out that while their machine learning model was effective under their conditions, there is no guarantee that it would also yield comparable results when used on data sets derived under different clinical parameters.

Nevertheless, especially given the development of machine learning models and their ever-increasing computational power, this is but a temporary hurdle.

Tools for developing and assessing the viability of such biomarkers panels are already being developed, with one such example within this Special Issue. In their protocol, Anne Dietz et al. [10] outline a procedure by which the effects of ionizing radiation on the human proteome can be determined, with a focus on radiosensitivity. Their method allows for a comprehensive insight into biomarker databases and the generation of a confidence rating, allowing for the development of a panel pooling many different studies and publications, ranked by reliability. Protocols such as this are probably vital for the development of personalized medicine and will doubtless prove highly useful to researchers in the future for biomarker development.

Questions arise as to the source of biomarkers with most promises: what is best? One specific biological sample being sufficient or a combination of them? While messengers such as extracellular vesicles (EVs) seem like promising mines of biomarkers, with Katalin Balázs et al. reporting on a blood-derived panel for prostate cancer utilising EV-miRNA [11], nevertheless doubts can be cast as to their ability to demonstrate radiation-specific markers, as shown in Anna Wojakowska et al. [12], with their pilot study into metabolic profiles of whole serum and serum-derived EVs in head and neck cancer (HNC). While radiation therapy displayed a clear pattern of changes on the serum metabolome, the same could not be said for EVs, which failed to reveal a specific pattern of metabolite changes. However, other sources of research indicate that EVs are a rich source of miRNAs, which have been shown on multiple occasions to have the potential to be powerful indicators of radiation exposure, sensitivity, disease presence and progression.

Furthermore, questions regarding methodology remain, as shown by Takahiro Oike et al. [13] in their paper on clonogenic assays to assess in vitro radiosensitivity, in which they compare whether pre- or post-IR plating has an impact on the outcome, concluding that there is a negligible difference. Simon Sioen et al. [14] continue this vein of standardizing methodology by investigating whether the cytokinesis-block micronucleus assay works on both fresh and cryopreserved PBMCs, ultimately developing a standardized assay useable on both. Work such as this is important in not only establishing a consensus, but also allowing for inter-study comparison.

Despite the optimism transpiring from the findings described above it remains important to realize that the actual application of biomarkers remains limited, and as such they are, as of yet, wishful thinking. Without actual widescale clinical application methods, their impact and relevance to personalized medicine remains theoretical. The limitations of current methods are outlined by Volodymyr Vinnikov et al.'s [15] insightful review on ex vivo cytogenetic radiation biomarkers, and logistical issues dealing with large scale studies are shown in Jayne Moquet et al.'s [16] RENEB report, detailing the problems faced by undertaking a large scale human health effect study; this same logistical issue could be faced when dealing with a large cohort of patients and an individualized care approach to each. Prabal Subedi et al.'s [17] review concludes that while most IR biomarker studies use repair foci as their biomarker of choice, their actual association to final clinical outcomes remains contradictory. However, not all is lost, despite such limitations and issues: both articles contain plans for overcoming such problems, and as such for transforming radiation biomarkers from theoretical marvels into practical, clinical solutions for cancer radiotherapy.

Doubtless, many questions remain regarding the validity and practicality of using a panel of biomarker to drive treatment decision ultimately leading to personalized medicine. However, significant inroads have been made in recent years, elucidating the radiation response of tumours, and biomarkers have been derived therefrom. However, there is undoubtedly much to be discovered, and even more to be optimized—the road from lab result to clinical application is still long and fraught with challenges. As such, one must be forced to conclude that biomarkers are not, in fact, some proverbial silver bullet, at least for now. They are difficult to identify and validate, and, ultimately, possibly too expensive, time consuming or complex to implement. However, biomarkers are not a fool's errand—far from it. In fact, although the knowledge of radiation biomarkers is currently insufficient for widescale implementation of personalized cancer treatments, it does not mean that this will continue to be the case in the near future. In fact, with the expansion of studies as well as the development of ever more sophisticated technologies, one would hope that reliable and useful radiation biomarkers are on the cusp of becoming a silver bullet. Given the articles published in this Special Issue, it is not unwise to be optimistic. The dawn of radiation biomarkers is approaching, bringing with it a new horizon of therapeutic possibilities.

Funding: This research received no external funding.

Institutional Review Board Statement: Not applicable.

Informed Consent Statement: Not applicable.

Data Availability Statement: Not applicable.

Acknowledgments: We would like to thank all the authors for providing excellent papers for this Special Issue of the Journal of Personalised Medicine, and for helping to further understanding and foster discussion within the vital field of radiation biomarkers. We would also like to thank the Journal of Personalised Medicine for the opportunity to edit this Special Issue, and we would in particular like to thank Iris Qiao for her professionalism, help, and kind support. Finally, we would like to offer our sincere gratitude to the expert reviewers for offering fair and constructive criticism and oversight on the papers published in this issue.

Conflicts of Interest: The authors declare no conflict of interest.

References

1. Delaney, G.; Jacob, S.; Featherstone, C.; Barton, M. The role of radiotherapy in cancer treatment: Estimating optimal utilization from a review of evidence-based clinical guidelines. *Cancer Interdiscip. Int. J. Am. Cancer Soc.* **2005**, *104*, 1129–1137. [CrossRef] [PubMed]
2. Loeffler, J.S.; Durante, M. Charged particle therapy—Optimization, challenges and future directions. *Nat. Rev. Clin. Oncol.* **2013**, *10*, 411–424. [CrossRef] [PubMed]
3. Lokody, I. FLASHing tumours. *Nat. Rev. Cancer* **2014**, *14*, 577. [CrossRef]
4. Gomolka, M.; Blyth, B.; Bourguignon, M.; Badie, C.; Schmitz, A.; Talbot, C.; Hoeschen, C.; Salomaa, S. Potential screening assays for individual radiation sensitivity and susceptibility and their current validation state. *Int. J. Radiat. Biol.* **2019**, *96*, 280–296. [CrossRef] [PubMed]
5. Osu, N.; Kobayashi, D.; Shirai, K.; Musha, A.; Sato, H.; Hirota, Y.; Shibata, A.; Oike, T.; Ohno, T. Relative Biological Effectiveness of Carbon Ions for Head-and-Neck Squamous Cell Carcinomas According to Human Papillomavirus Status. *J. Pers. Med.* **2020**, *10*, 71. [CrossRef] [PubMed]
6. Kobayashi, D.; Oike, T.; Murata, K.; Irie, D.; Hirota, Y.; Sato, H.; Shibata, A.; Ohno, T. Induction of Micronuclei in Cervical Cancer Treated with Radiotherapy. *J. Pers. Med.* **2020**, *10*, 110. [CrossRef]
7. Byrne, N.; Tambe, P.; Coulter, J. Radiation Response in the Tumour Microenvironment: Predictive Biomarkers and Future Perspectives. *J. Pers. Med.* **2020**, *11*, 53. [CrossRef] [PubMed]
8. Śliwińska-Mossoń, M.; Wadowska, K.; Trembecki, Ł.; Bil-Lula, I. Markers Useful in Monitoring Radiation-Induced Lung Injury in Lung Cancer Patients: A Review. *J. Pers. Med.* **2020**, *10*, 72. [CrossRef] [PubMed]
9. Luxton, J.; McKenna, M.; Lewis, A.; Taylor, L.; Jhavar, S.; Swanson, G.; Bailey, S. Telomere Length Dynamics and Chromosomal Instability for Predicting Individual Radiosensitivity and Risk via Machine Learning. *J. Pers. Med.* **2020**, *11*, 188. [CrossRef] [PubMed]
10. Dietz, A.; Gomolka, M.; Moertl, S.; Subedi, P. Ionizing Radiation Protein Biomarkers in Normal Tissue and Their Correlation to Radiosensitivity: Protocol for a Systematic Review. *J. Pers. Med.* **2020**, *11*, 3. [CrossRef] [PubMed]
11. Balázs, K.; Antal, L.; Sáfrány, G.; Lumniczky, K. Blood-Derived Biomarkers of Diagnosis, Prognosis and Therapy Response in Prostate Cancer Patients. *J. Pers. Med.* **2021**, *11*, 296. [CrossRef] [PubMed]
12. Wojakowska, A.; Zebrowska, A.; Skowronek, A.; Rutkowski, T.; Polanski, K.; Widlak, P.; Marczak, L.; Pietrowska, M. Metabolic Profiles of Whole Serum and Serum-Derived Exosomes Are Different in Head and Neck Cancer Patients Treated by Radiotherapy. *J. Pers. Med.* **2020**, *10*, 229. [CrossRef] [PubMed]
13. Oike, T.; Hirota, Y.; Darwis, N.D.M.; Shibata, A.; Ohno, T. Comparison of Clonogenic Survival Data Obtained by Pre- and Post-Irradiation Methods. *J. Pers. Med.* **2020**, *10*, 171. [CrossRef] [PubMed]
14. Sioen, S.; Cloet, K.; Vral, A.; Baeyens, A. The Cytokinesis-Block Micronucleus Assay on Human Isolated Fresh and Cryopreserved Peripheral Blood Mononuclear Cells. *J. Pers. Med.* **2020**, *10*, 125. [CrossRef] [PubMed]

15. Vinnikov, V.; Hande, M.P.; Wilkins, R.; Wojcik, A.; Zubizarreta, E.; Belyakov, O. Prediction of the Acute or Late Radiation Toxicity Effects in Radiotherapy Patients Using Ex Vivo Induced Biodosimetric Markers: A Review. *J. Pers. Med.* **2020**, *10*, 285. [CrossRef] [PubMed]
16. Moquet, J.; Rothkamm, K.; Barnard, S.; Ainsbury, E. Radiation Biomarkers in Large Scale Human Health Effects Studies. *J. Pers. Med.* **2020**, *10*, 155. [CrossRef] [PubMed]
17. Subedi, P.; Gomolka, M.; Moertl, S.; Dietz, A. Ionizing Radiation Protein Biomarkers in Normal Tissue and Their Correlation to Radiosensitivity: A Systematic Review. *J. Pers. Med.* **2020**, *11*, 140. [CrossRef] [PubMed]

Journal of *Personalized Medicine*

MDPI

Article

Telomere Length Dynamics and Chromosomal Instability for Predicting Individual Radiosensitivity and Risk via Machine Learning

Jared J. Luxton [1,2], Miles J. McKenna [1,2], Aidan M. Lewis [1], Lynn E. Taylor [1], Sameer G. Jhavar [3], Gregory P. Swanson [3] and Susan M. Bailey [1,2,*]

1 Department of Environmental and Radiological Health Sciences, Colorado State University, Fort Collins, CO 80523, USA; Jared.Luxton@colostate.edu (J.J.L.); miles.mckenna@gmail.com (M.J.M.); aidanlew@rams.colostate.edu (A.M.L.); Lynn.Taylor@colostate.edu (L.E.T.)
2 Cell and Molecular Biology Program, Colorado State University, Fort Collins, CO 80523, USA
3 Baylor Scott & White Medical Center, Temple, TX 76508, USA; sameer.jhavar@bswhealth.org (S.G.J.); Gregory.Swanson@bswhealth.org (G.P.S.)
* Correspondence: susan.bailey@colostate.edu

Abstract: The ability to predict a cancer patient's response to radiotherapy and risk of developing adverse late health effects would greatly improve personalized treatment regimens and individual outcomes. Telomeres represent a compelling biomarker of individual radiosensitivity and risk, as exposure can result in dysfunctional telomere pathologies that coincidentally overlap with many radiation-induced late effects, ranging from degenerative conditions like fibrosis and cardiovascular disease to proliferative pathologies like cancer. Here, telomere length was longitudinally assessed in a cohort of fifteen prostate cancer patients undergoing Intensity Modulated Radiation Therapy (IMRT) utilizing Telomere Fluorescence in situ Hybridization (Telo-FISH). To evaluate genome instability and enhance predictions for individual patient risk of secondary malignancy, chromosome aberrations were assessed utilizing directional Genomic Hybridization (dGH) for high-resolution inversion detection. We present the first implementation of individual telomere length data in a machine learning model, XGBoost, trained on pre-radiotherapy (baseline) and in vitro exposed (4 Gy γ-rays) telomere length measurements, to predict post radiotherapy telomeric outcomes, which together with chromosomal instability provide insight into individual radiosensitivity and risk for radiation-induced late effects.

Keywords: telomeres; chromosomal instability; inversions; prostate cancer; IMRT; machine learning; individual radiosensitivity; late effects; personalized medicine

Citation: Luxton, J.J.; McKenna, M.J.; Lewis, A.M.; Taylor, L.E.; Jhavar, S.G.; Swanson, G.P.; Bailey, S.M. Telomere Length Dynamics and Chromosomal Instability for Predicting Individual Radiosensitivity and Risk via Machine Learning. *J. Pers. Med.* **2021**, *11*, 188. https://doi.org/10.3390/jpm11030188

Academic Editor: Christophe Badie

Received: 10 February 2021
Accepted: 2 March 2021
Published: 8 March 2021

1. Introduction

Radiation late effects are a broad class of negative and often permanent health effects experienced by cancer patients long after radiation therapy [1,2], which can include cardiovascular disease (CVD) [3], pulmonary and arterial fibrosis [4], cognitive deficits [5], bone fractures [6], and secondary cancers [7]. Such late effects are of particular concern for pediatric patients [8], and risks for radiation late effects are highly dependent on patient-intrinsic factors as well, including genetics, age, sex, and lifestyle [1,2,9]. Therefore, identifying a patient's specific risks for radiation late effects prior to radiotherapy is important for improving individual treatment planning and overall patient outcome. A number of strategies for predicting risk of developing radiation late effects have been employed, which tend to involve irradiating patient-derived samples in vitro and monitoring of biomarker(s) to infer in vivo cellular and normal tissue responses to exposure [10]; e.g., evaluation of γ-H2AX foci kinetics [11,12], apoptosis in normal blood lymphocytes [13], and chromosome aberration frequencies [14–16]. Additionally, Genome Wide Association Studies (GWAS) [17,18], sequencing [19], and imaging studies (i.e., radiogenomics [20]) have revealed promising putative indicators for predicting risks of late effects. However, accurately predicting an individual patient's response to radiotherapy and associated risk of developing adverse late health effects remains challenging in terms of cost-effectiveness, throughput, and predictive power, therefore new approaches are needed.

Telomeres have been proposed as sensitive biomarkers of radiation exposure and a valuable parameter for predicting individual radiosensitivity of patients [21]. Telomeres are protective features of chromosomal termini that guard genome integrity and prevent inappropriate activation of DNA damage responses (DDRs) [22,23]. It is well established that telomeres shorten with cell division, oxidative stress [24], and aging [25]. Telomeres also shorten with a host of lifestyle factors (e.g., nutrition [26], exercise [27], stress [28]) and environmental exposures (e.g., air pollution [29], UV [30]). Telomere length is a highly heritable trait, as is telomere length regulation [31–34], supportive of individual variation in telomeric response to specific stressors. Interestingly, telomeres are regarded as hallmarks of radiosensitivity [35], and ionizing radiation (IR) exposure has been shown to evoke both shortening and lengthening of telomeres [36–38]. A large Mendelian randomization study [39] and recent quantitative estimates have shown that both short and long telomeres are associated with increased disease risk—of approximately equal degree [40,41]. Short telomeres are robust biomarkers and even determinants for a range of aging-related pathologies [42], including dementias, CVD and pulmonary fibrosis [43], and aplastic anemia [44], degenerative conditions also regarded as radiation late effects [45–47]. On the other hand, longer telomeres are associated with increased cancer risk, particularly for leukemias [48], a common cancer following IR-exposure [49]. Thus, telomere length could be used to identify radiosensitive individuals (i.e., those with shorter telomeres before radiotherapy) to better inform personalized treatment regimens. Furthermore, evaluating telomere length dynamics associated with radiotherapy could serve to identify individuals at risk for developing radiation-induced late effects; i.e., patients with shorter telomeres would be at higher risk of degenerative pathologies (fibrosis, CVD), while those with longer telomeres following radiotherapy would be at higher risk for developing proliferative pathologies, namely secondary malignancy.

Given that telomere length is influenced by a variety of genetic factors [31–34], and exposures including IR [36–38,50–52], we reasoned that a patient's telomeric outcome post-radiation therapy, rather than their pre-treatment (baseline) measures, would be most informative for assessing individual risks for radiation late effects and long-term health consequences. Furthermore, since patient-derived pre-radiation therapy samples irradiated in vitro provide an informative proxy for individual patient radiosensitivity and response in vivo [53–56], developing an effective means to accurately predict an individual patient's telomeric outcome post-radiation therapy would serve to improve personalized treatment strategies and individual outcomes.

Chromosome aberrations (CAs) are well-established biomarkers of IR-exposure [57] associated with virtually all cancers [58], and highly informative indicators of risk for radiation late effects, in particular, secondary cancers [14–16]. Ionizing radiation is exceptional in its ability to induce prompt double-strand breaks (DSBs) [59], DNA damage that necessitates a cellular response. Chromosome rearrangements result from the misrepair of such damage, and so provide a quantitative measure of cellular capacity for DNA repair [57]. In general, IR-induced CAs negatively impact cell survival and genome stability, resulting in senescence, apoptosis, and cancer [57]. Notably, chromosomal inversions and deletions have previously been proposed as signatures of radiation-induced secondary cancers [60]. Cytogenetic analysis however, is both time and labor intensive, often requiring that hundreds or even thousands of cells be scored, limiting its clinical utility [61]. We speculated that for this pilot study, inclusion of an additional type of CA, specifically inversions detected by the strand-specific methodology of directional Genome Hybridization (dGH) [62], might serve to reduce the number of cells required, while also better informing individual risk for secondary malignancy.

Significant advancements have also been made in the application of machine learning (ML) to a variety of scenarios, including predictions related to acute radiation toxicity [63], treatment planning [64], and secondary cancer risk post radiation therapy [65]. Extreme Gradient Boosting (XGBoost) is a powerful ML model that uses a gradient boosted ensemble of decision trees to learn complex relationships (linear and nonlinear) within datasets [66]. XGBoost has many translational applications, such as predicting future gastric cancer risk [67], lung cancer detection [68], and radiation-related fibrosis [69]. One potentially limiting caveat to ML is the requirement for extraordinarily large amounts of data to create robust, generalizable models. Telomere Fluorescence in situ Hybridization (Telo-FISH) is a cell-by-cell imaging-based approach for measuring telomere length capable of generating sufficient volumes of data for developing ML models; average experiments generate 200,000–1,000,000 individual telomere length measurements [70]. To date, individual telomere length measurements (Telo-FISH, Q-FISH, flow-FISH, etc.) have not been utilized in ML models for risk predictions, despite the informative nature of such an approach.

Here we provide a proof-of-principle demonstration utilizing longitudinal analysis of telomere length and chromosomal instability in fifteen (15) prostate cancer patients undergoing Intensity Modulated Radiation Therapy (IMRT). We present the first implementation of individual telomere length (Telo-FISH) data in a ML model—XGBoost—and evaluate its ability to predict post-IMRT telomeric outcomes using individual patient's pre-IMRT (baseline) and in vitro irradiated telomere lengths. Overall, our results support use of telomere length dynamics and chromosomal instability for improved prediction of individual radiosensitivity and risk for developing radiation-induced late effects post RT.

2. Materials and Methods

2.1. Patient Consent, IMRT Therapy Information

With informed consent as per the institutional review board, 16 consecutive patients receiving pelvic and prostate or prostate fossa radiation therapy were asked to participate in the study. No patient had received androgen ablation or chemotherapy to avoid confounding factors. One patient was found to have metastatic disease after consent and was removed from further study. A total of 15 patients provided consent and blood was collected pre-IMRT (baseline), immediately post-IMRT (the last week), and 3-months post-IMRT (prior to returning to personal medical oncologist). Blood was subject to complete blood counts, and telomere length and chromosome aberration analyses. Each patient received a radiation regime consisting of 54 Gy to the pelvic lymphatics, with a total of 70 Gy ($n = 11$) or 78 Gy ($n = 3$) to the prostate fossa. One patient underwent brachytherapy boost.

2.2. Sample Collection and Processing for Telo-FISH and dGH

Peripheral blood was drawn and shipped in 10 mL sodium heparin tubes (Becton, Dickinson and Co, Franklin Lakes, NJ, USA; #367874) under ambient conditions to Colorado State University and received within 24 h of blood draw. All heparinized blood samples were cultured in T-25 tissue culture flasks, at 1 parts blood per 9 parts Gibco PB-Max Karyotyping Medium (Thermo Fisher, Waltham, MA, USA; #12557013), with 5.0 mM 5-bromo-deoxyuridine (BrdU) and 1.0 mM 5-bromo-deoxycytidine (BrdC) added to the medium as previously described [62]. Pre-IMRT blood samples were split into two fractions (non-irradiated and in vitro irradiated) with identical culturing conditions as other time point samples; irradiated fraction was exposed in vitro at a dose rate of 2.5 Gy/min for a total dose of 4 Gy (^{137}Cs gamma-ray Mark I irradiator; J.L. Shepherd & Associates, San Fernando, CA USA). Forty-eight hours after stimulation, KaryoMax Colcemid (Thermo Fisher, Waltham, MA, USA; #15210040) was added (0.1 μg per mL of medium) for four hours of incubation, then metaphase chromosome spreads were harvested with standard cytogenetic protocols [71]. Prior to Telo-FISH and dGH, slides with metaphase chromosome spreads were subject to CO-FISH protocol for removal of BrdU/BrdC incorporated DNA as previously described [72].

2.3. Telomere Fluorescence In Situ Hybridization (Telo-FISH), Imaging, Quantifications

Protocol: Slides with metaphase chromosome spreads were prepared and hybridized with a fluorescently labeled telomere probe as previously described [70]. Briefly, slides were washed in 1× PBS for 5 min, dehydrated through an ice-cold ethanol series (75%, 85% and 100%) for 2 min each, air dried, and denatured in 70% formamide in 2× saline sodium citrate (SSC) at 75 °C for 2 min, followed by a second ice-cold ethanol series, and air dried again. Probe hybridization mixture consisted of G-rich (TTAGGG-′3) peptide nucleic acid (PNA) telomere probe labeled with Cyanine-3 (Cy3; Bio-synthesis, Inc., Lewisville, TX USA) at 5 nM concentration in 36 μL of formamide, 12 μL of 0.5 M Tris-HCl, 2.5 μL of 0.1 M KCl, and 0.6 μL of 0.1 M $MgCl_2$. Hybridization mixture was incubated at 75 °C for 5 min and cooled on ice for 10 min, then 50 μL of mix was applied to each slide. Slides were coverslipped and hybridized at 37 °C for 4 h. After hybridization, slides were washed five times at 43.5 °C for three min each: washes one and two: 50% formamide in 2× SSC; washes three and four: 100% 2× SSC; and washes five and six: 2× SSC plus 0.1% Nonidet P-40. After washing, slides were counterstained with DAPI in Prolong Gold Antifade (Thermo Fisher, Waltham, MA, USA; #P36931), coverslipped, and stored at 4 °C for 24 h prior to imaging.

Image acquisition: Metaphase spreads (50 per patient/time point) were imaged at 100× mag on a Zeiss Axio Imager.Z2, Cool SNAP ES2 camera, and X-cite 120 LED lamp light source.

Individual telomere quantifications: Relative fluorescence intensity of individual telomeres was quantified using the ImageJ plugin Telometer [73]. Variation in Telo-FISH was controlled by assigning each patient a pair of slides made from BJ1 and BJ-hTERT fibroblast cell lines (ATCC, Manassas, VA USA). For each patient, slide preparation, Telo-FISH protocol, image acquisition and telomere quantifications were performed on the full time-course of samples and pair of BJ1/BJ-hTERT controls (50 metaphases per control) at the same time and on the same respective days. Mean telomere length was quantified for each pair of control samples yielding a ratio for standardizing patients' telomere values as previously described [74].

2.4. Telo-FISH Data Processing, Feature Engineering of Short and Long Telomeres

Processing individual telomere length data: For each patient, outliers were removed from individual telomere length data per sample by omitting measurements three standard deviations from the mean; between all samples and patients, less than 1% of individual telomere measurements were considered outliers per this approach. For samples with fewer individual telomere length measurements than the theoretical number (human cells, 50 metaphase spreads), missing telomere values were imputed by randomly sampling measurements from the observed distribution of individual telomeres; randomly sampled telomeres were added up to the theoretical number of telomeres per sample.

Feature engineering short and long telomeres: Individual telomeres from the pre-IMRT non-irradiated time point were split into quartiles, designating telomeres in the bottom 25% in yellow, the middle 50% in blue, and top 25% in red. Quartile cut-off values, established by the pre-IMRT non-irradiated sample's distribution (values that separate quartiles), were applied to subsequent time points to feature engineer the relative shortest (yellow), mid-length (blue), and longest (red) individual telomeres per time point.

2.5. Statistical and Clustering Analyses of Telo-FISH Data

Statistical and clustering analyses were conducted with Python in Jupyter notebooks (see Code availability). With the statsmodels library [75], mean telomere length and numbers of short and long telomeres were analyzed with a repeated measures ANOVA and post hoc Tukey's HSD test (two-tailed p values for both tests). Analyses were performed on all patients ($n = 14$, less patient ID 13; 3-month post-IMRT sample failed to culture) and all four time points. A square root transformation was performed on numbers of short and long telomeres prior to statistical analysis. Ordinary least squares linear regression was performed with the scikit-learn LinearRegression tool. Hierarchical clustering analyses were performed on z-score normalized data using the scipy library [76] with a single linkage method and Pearson correlation metric. Pearson correlations between patients' longitudinal measurements of telomere length and complete blood count data was done with Python.

2.6. XGBoost Models with Individual Telomere Length Data, Randomized Hyperparameter Search, Cross Validation

XGBoost models, model hyperparameter tuning, and cross validation tools were performed in Python through the scikit-learn API [77]. XGboost model features were individual telomere length values and sample labels denoted pre-IMRT sample origin (non-irradiated, in vitro irradiated), which were encoded as 0/1. Model hyperparameters were tuned using a randomized search with RandomizedSearchCV. For models predicting mean telomere length at late post-IMRT, final model hyperparameters were modified as follows: n_estimators = 200, max_depth = 7, learning_rate = 0.2, objective = 'reg:squarederror', random_state = 1. For models predicting short and long telomeres at late post-IMRT, final model hyperparameters were similar as for mean telomere length, with max depth = 6. Five-fold cross validation was performed with cross_val_score and a negative mean absolute error metric.

2.7. Directional Genomic Hybridization (dGH), Image Acquisition, Data Processing

High-resolution detection of chromosome aberrations (inversions, translocations) was performed utilizing dGH whole chromosome (Cy3) and sub-telomere (Cy5) paints specific to chromosomes 1, 2, and 3 (KromaTiD Inc., Longmont, CO USA) as previously described [62]. Briefly, slides were stained with Hoechst 33,258 (MilliporeSigma, Burlington, MA USA; #B1155) for 15 min, photolyzed for 35 min using a SpectroLinker UV Crosslinker (365 nm UV), and digested with exonuclease III (New England Biolabs, Ipswich, NA, USA; #M0206L) for 30 min. Paint hybridization mixture was applied to slides, which were then coverslipped, sealed with rubber cement, and denatured at 70 °C for three min. Slides were hybridized for 24 h at 37 °C, followed by five washes in 2× SSC at 43.5 °C. After washing, slides were counterstained with one drop of DAPI in Prolong Gold Antifade (Thermo Fisher, Waltham, MA, USA; #P36931), coverslipped, and stored at 4 °C for 24 h prior to imaging. Metaphase spreads (30 per patient/time point) were imaged/scored at 63× mag on a Zeiss Axio Imager.Z2, Cool SNAP ES2 camera, and X-cite 120 LED lamp light source. Counts of chromosome aberrations were corrected for clonality, where identical aberrations between cells for a patient's given time point were noted but scored only once.

2.8. Statistical and Clustering Analyses of Chromosome Aberrations (dGH)

Statistical and clustering analyses were conducted with Python in Jupyter notebooks (see Code availability). With the statsmodels library, average chromosome aberration frequencies were analyzed with a repeated measures ANOVA and post hoc Tukey's HSD test (two-tailed p values for both tests). Analyses were performed on all patients ($n = 14$, less patient ID 13; 3-month post-IMRT sample failed to culture) and all-time course samples (4). Ordinary least squares linear regression was performed with the scikit-learn LinearRegression tool. Hierarchical clustering analyses were performed on z-score normalized data using the scipy library with a single linkage method and Pearson correlation metric. Pearson correlations between patients' longitudinal measurements of average chromosome aberration frequencies and complete blood count data was done with Python.

2.9. XGBoost Model Design with Chromosome Aberrations

XGBoost models, model hyperparameter tuning, and cross validation were accessed in Python via the same manner as described for Telo-FISH data above. XGboost model features were counts of scored chromosome aberrations per cell, with sample labels denoting pre-IMRT sample origin (non-irradiated, in vitro irradiated; encoded as 0/1). Model hyperparameters were tuned using a randomized search with RandomizedSearchCV;

models were ultimately non-performant. Final model hyperparameters (used with all chromosome aberrations) were: n_estimators = 200, max_depth = 15, learning_rate = 0.1, objective = 'reg:squarederror', random_state = 0. Five-fold cross validation was performed with a negative mean absolute error metric.

3. Results

3.1. Longitudinal Analyses of Telomere Length Associated with Radiation Therapy

Blood was collected from 15 prostate cancer patients undergoing IMRT at baseline (pre-IMRT), immediately post-IMRT (conclusion of treatment regimen), and 3-months post-IMRT. Baseline blood samples were split, half serving as the non-irradiated control (0 Gy), and the other half irradiated in vitro (4 Gy, Cs^{137} γ-rays) as a proxy for individual radiation response [55].The lengths of thousands of individual telomeres (n = 50 cells/patient/time point) were measured on metaphase chromosomes (lymphocytes stimulated from whole blood) by Telo-FISH at all time points [pre-therapy non-irradiated (0 Gy); pre-therapy in vitro irradiated (4 Gy); immediately post-IMRT; and 3-months post-IMRT] (Figure 1A). For the overall cohort, differences in mean telomere length (MTL) between samples approached but did not reach statistical significance ($p = 0.059$, repeated measures ANOVA). Relative to the pre-IMRT non-irradiated samples (0 Gy), overall MTL modestly increased after 4 Gy in vitro irradiation, and showed an even greater increase immediately after completion of the IMRT regimen, suggesting that increased MTL is an overall response to radiation exposure in this cohort. At 3-months post-IMRT, MTL for the cohort approached pre-IMRT levels.

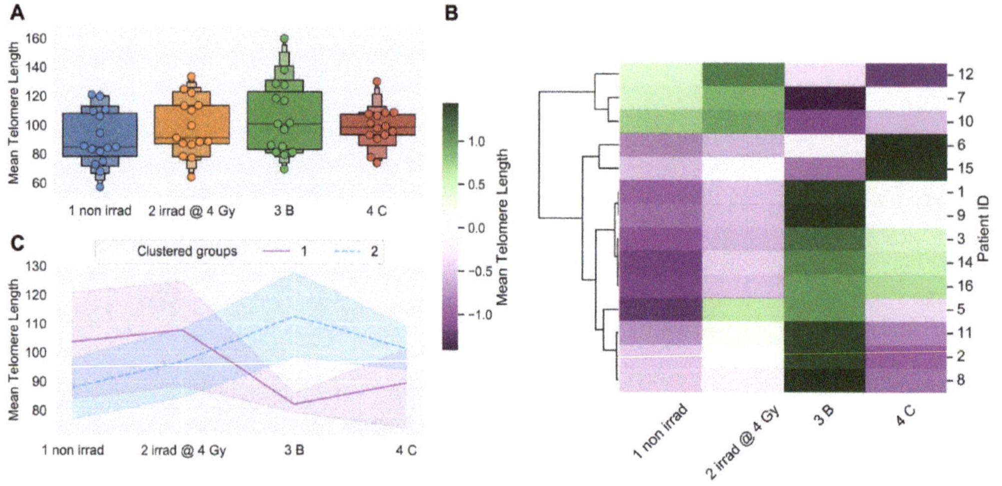

Figure 1. Telomere length dynamics (Telo-FISH). Mean telomere length expressed as relative fluorescence intensity. (**A**) Time-course of blood sample collection for all prostate cancer patients (n = 15; 50 cells/patient/time point scored): 1 non irrad = pre-IMRT non-irradiated (0 Gy); 2 irrad @ 4 Gy: pre-IMRT in vitro irradiated; 3B: immediate post-IMRT; and 4C: 3-months post-IMRT. Boxes denote quantiles, horizontal grey lines denote medians. Telomere length values were standardized using BJ1/BJ-hTERT controls. (**B**) Hierarchical clustering of patients by longitudinal changes in mean telomere length (z-score normalized). (**C**) Time-course for clustered groups of patients (n = 3, purple; n = 11, blue); center lines denote medians, lighter bands denote confidence intervals. Patient ID 13 not clustered (sample failed to culture). Significance was assessed using a repeated measures ANOVA and post hoc Tukey's HSD test.

Complete blood counts (CBC) were evaluated in the same samples, and longitudinal changes in patients' MTL negatively correlated ($R^2 = -0.126$) with total peripheral white blood cell (WBC) counts (Figure S1A). Longitudinal correlations between numbers of WBC types and MTL (all time points, for each patient) revealed a positive relationship with basophils ($R^2 = 0.278$) and a negative relationship with lymphocytes ($R^2 = -0.294$) (Figure S1B). Furthermore, longitudinal correlations between MTL and the proportions of lymphocyte sub-groups (all time points, for each patient) revealed positive relationships with natural killer (NK) and CD4 cells ($R^2 = 0.408, 0.282$), and negative relationships with CD8 and CD19 cells ($R^2 = -0.251, -0.288$) (Figure S1C). These results support the notion that the overall changes in MTL associated with radiation exposure, specifically apparent telomere elongation, could be at least partially due to cell killing and shifts in lymphocyte populations, as previously proposed [78,79].

3.2. Telomere Length Dynamics Revealed Individual Differences in Radiation Response

We hypothesized that groups of patients would cluster based on differential telomeric responses to radiation therapy, with sub-groups displaying either shorter or longer MTL post-IMRT. Clustering patients by longitudinal changes in MTL revealed two broad trends over time (Figure 1B). Patients that clustered in group 1 ($n = 3$) had relatively longer MTL at baseline (pre-IMRT), and showed a dramatic, persistent decrease in MTL post-IMRT (Figure 1C). Those patients that clustered in group 2 ($n = 11$) had relatively shorter MTL at baseline, and showed a dramatic, sustained increase in MTL post-IMRT (Figure 1C). Reduced MTL 3-months post-IMRT suggests increased risks for degenerative radiation late effects [43], while increased MTL suggests increased risks for proliferative secondary cancers [48].

In addition to MTL, Telo-FISH provides measures for many hundreds of individual telomeres, enabling generation of telomere length distributions and longitudinal analysis of shifts in populations of short and long telomeres [70]. For the overall cohort, numbers of short telomeres decreased and numbers of long telomeres dramatically increased 3-months post-IMRT (Figure 2A). When individual telomeres from patients in the MTL clustered group 1 ($n = 3$) were combined, dramatic and persistent increases in the numbers of short telomeres post-IMRT were observed (Figure 2B), while MTL clustered group 2 patients ($n = 11$) showed dramatic and persistent increases in numbers of long telomeres post-IMRT (Figure 2C). Again, patients with increased numbers of short telomeres are presumed to have increased risks for degenerative radiation late effects [43], while those with increased numbers of long telomeres are at increased risk of secondary cancers [48]. Numbers of short and long telomeres were feature engineered (see Materials and Methods) from each patient's individual telomere length data for further analysis.

Differences in the average number of short and long telomeres between samples approached but did not reach statistical significance for the overall cohort ($p < 0.1$; repeated measures ANOVA) (Figure 3A). We speculated that clustering patients by numbers of short or long telomeres would reveal longitudinal trends similar to those observed when clustering patients by MTL (Figure 1B,C). Clustering patients by longitudinal changes in numbers of short or long telomeres (Figure 3B,D) revealed two broad trends over time (Figure 3C,E). Clustered group 1 ($n = 3$) showed a dramatic, sustained increase in numbers of short telomeres post-IMRT, with a corresponding decrease in numbers of long telomeres (Figure 3C,E). Clustered group 2 ($n = 11$) showed a dramatic, nearly uniform decrease in numbers of short telomeres post-IMRT, with a corresponding increase in long telomeres (Figure 3C,E). Importantly, clustering patients either by MTL or by numbers of short or long telomeres post-IMRT identified the same three patients with shorter telomeres, and eleven with longer telomeres (Figures 1B and 3B,D).

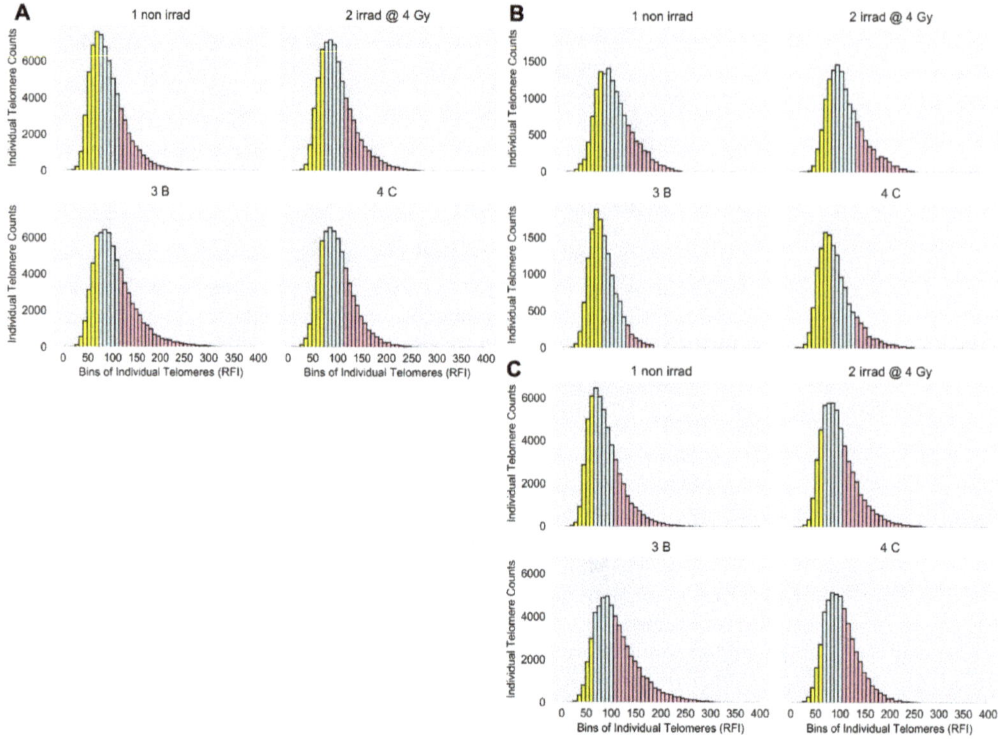

Figure 2. Telomere length distributions (Telo-FISH). Individual telomere length distributions of prostate cancer patients (n = 15): 1 non irrad = pre-IMRT non-irradiated (0 Gy); 2 irrad @ 4 Gy = pre-IMRT in vitro irradiated; 3B = immediate post-IMRT; and 4C = 3-months post-IMRT. RFI: Relative Fluorescence Intensity. Individual telomeres from the pre-therapy non-irradiated time point were split into quartiles, designating telomeres in the bottom 25% (yellow), middle 50% (blue), and top 25% (red). Quartile cut-off values, established by the distribution of the pre-therapy non-irradiated time point, were applied to subsequent time points to feature engineer the relative shortest, mid-length, and longest individual telomeres per time point. (**A**) Individual telomere length distributions for all patients (averaged) per time point. (**B**) Individual telomere length distributions for patients in mean telomere length clustered group 1 (n = 3) and (**C**) group 2 (n = 11).

3.3. Linear Regression Failed to Predict Post-IMRT Telomeric Outcomes

Based on the two distinct groups identified by MTL and numbers of short and long telomeres 3-months post-IMRT (Figures 1 and 3), we hypothesized that pre-IMRT measurements of MTL and numbers of short and long telomeres could predict their respective post-IMRT outcomes using linear regression. For MTL, two linear regression models were created. The first used only MTL from pre-IMRT (baseline) non-irradiated samples as the independent variable, and the second used MTL from both the non-irradiated and in vitro irradiated pre-IMRT samples as independent variables for predicting post-IMRT MTL (Figure 4A). The R^2 values for the two models were 0.161 and 0.165, respectively (Figure 4A), evidence that linear regression poorly captured the relationship between pre- and post-IMRT MTL. For numbers of short and long telomeres, two linear regression models were similarly created. The models for short telomeres yielded R^2 values of 0.433 and 0.554, and the models for long telomeres yielded R^2 values of 0.046 and 0.208 (Figure 4B,C). While the models for numbers of short telomeres had modestly higher R^2 values than those for MTL or long telomeres, all linear regression models performed too poorly to confidently predict telomeric outcomes.

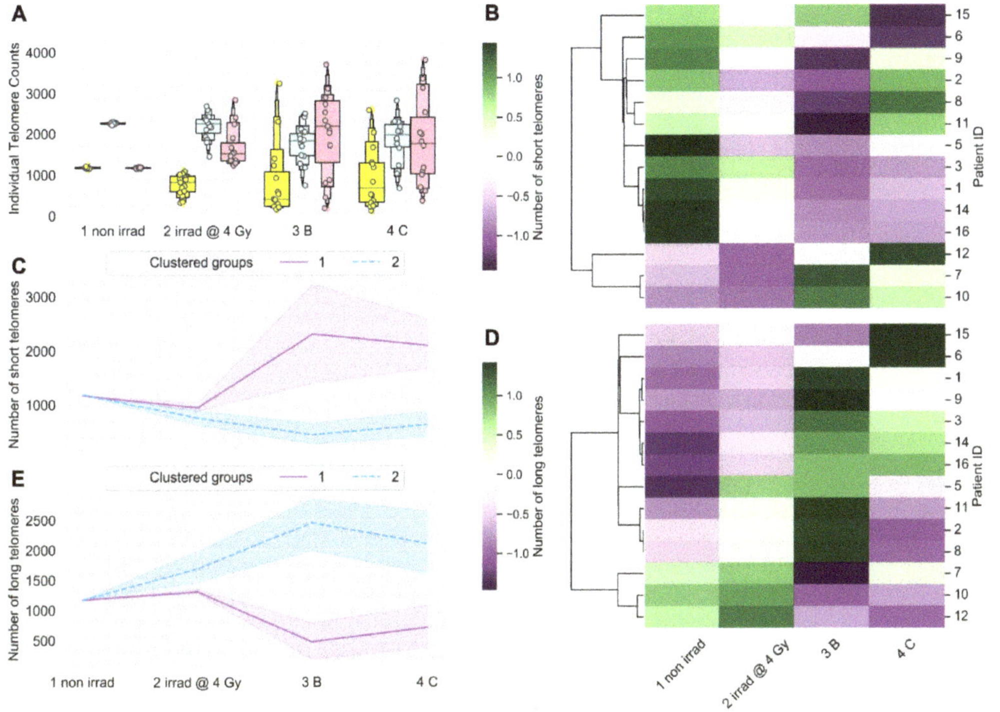

Figure 3. Longitudinal shifts in numbers of short and long telomeres (Telo-FISH). Numbers of short and long telomeres from individual telomere length distributions: 1 non irrad = pre-IMRT non-irradiated (0 Gy); 2 irrad @ 4 Gy = pre-IMRT in vitro irradiated; 3B = immediate post-IMRT; and 4C = 3-months post-IMRT. Shortest (yellow), mid-length (blue), and longest (red) telomeres were feature engineered per patient (n = 15). (**A**) Counts of short, medium, and long telomeres; 4600 individual telomeres per patient per time point. Significance was assessed using a square-root transformation and a repeated measures ANOVA with post hoc Tukey's HSD test. Hierarchical clustering of patients by longitudinal changes in numbers of short (**B**) and long telomeres (**D**) (z-score normalized). Time-courses of patient groups (n = 3, purple; n = 11, blue) clustered by numbers of short (**C**) and long (**E**) telomeres; center lines denote medians and lighter bands denote confidence intervals. Patient ID 13 not clustered (sample failed to culture).

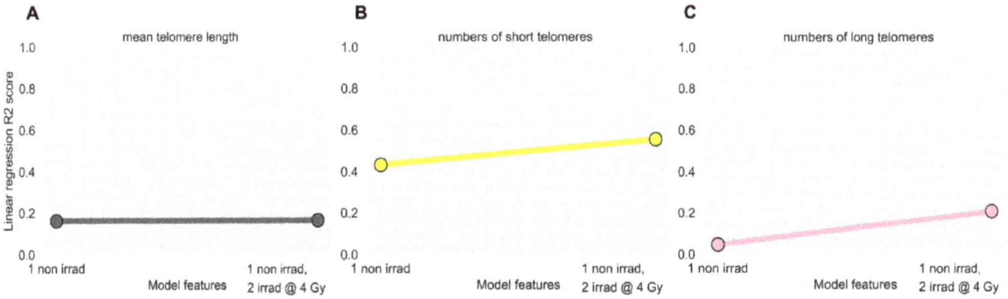

Figure 4. Linear regression models failed to predict post-IMRT telomeric outcomes. Ordinary least squares linear regression models were employed using pre-IMRT telomeric data (Telo-FISH) from the pre-IMRT non-irradiated (0 Gy) or the pre-IMRT in vitro irradiated (4 Gy) samples to predict 3-month post-IMRT telomeric outcomes. Models were made using (**A**) mean telomere length (R^2 = 0.161, 0.165), (**B**) numbers of short (R^2 = 0.433, 0.554), and (**C**) numbers of long (R^2 = 0.046, 0.208) telomeres.

3.4. Development of XGBoost Machine Learning Models for Accurate Prediction of Post-IMRT Telomeric Outcomes

The fact that linear regression poorly predicted post-IMRT telomeric outcomes could be due to the low number of observations ($n = 14$), and/or the nonlinearity of telomere length dynamics (changes over time) in response to radiation exposure (Figures 1–4). We sought an alternative approach that could effectively utilize our vast dataset of pre-IMRT individual telomere length measurements ($n = 128{,}800$), and also capture the nonlinearity of telomeric responses. Considering that XGBoost had recently been used to predict cancer risk and radiation-induced fibrosis using patient data [66–69], we hypothesized that XGBoost models could be trained with pre-IMRT individual telomere length measurements to accurately predict post-IMRT telomeric outcomes.

Pre-IMRT (baseline) telomere length data required extensive processing prior to training the XGBoost model for predicting three-month post-IMRT MTL (Figure 5). Data was reshaped into a matrix consisting of 128,800 rows (one for each individual telomere measurement) and four columns: patient ID, individual telomere length value, label denoting pre-IMRT sample of origin (non-irradiated or in vitro irradiated), and three-month post-IMRT MTL (Table S1A). Reshaped data was randomly shuffled and stratified by patient ID and sample of origin, then split into training (80% of total) and test (20% of total) datasets. Shuffling guarded against order of measurement bias (Telo-FISH image acquisition), while stratifying ensured equivalent numbers of individual telomeres from each patients' pre-IMRT samples (non-irradiated vs. in vitro irradiated) in the training and test datasets. Patient IDs were stripped from the training and test datasets, and individual telomeres from the non-irradiated and in vitro irradiated samples were encoded as 0 and 1 to denote sample origin (Table S1B). XGBoost model hyperparameters were optimized using a randomized hyperparameter search [80].

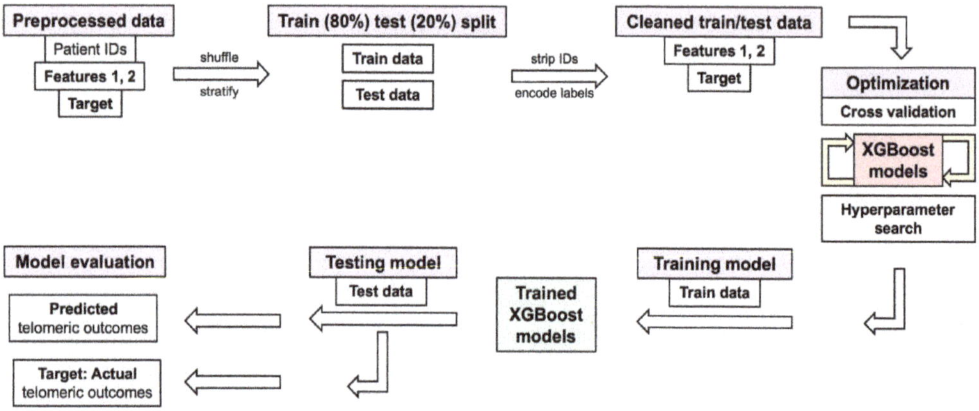

Figure 5. Processing of Telo-FISH data for training and testing XGBoost models. Schematic for machine learning pipeline used for individual telomere length data (Telo-FISH). Preprocessed data: Feature 1: pre-IMRT individual telomere length measurements ($n = 128{,}800$); Feature 2: pre-IMRT sample labels (non-irradiated, in vitro irradiated, encoded as 0/1); Target: 3 months post-IMRT telomeric outcomes (mean telomere length or numbers of short and long telomeres). Data is randomly shuffled and stratified (by patient ID and pre-therapy sample origin) and split into training (80%) and test (20%) datasets; patient IDs are stripped after splitting. Five-fold cross validation was used, and models were evaluated with Mean Absolute Error (MAE) and R^2 scores between predicted and true values in the test set.

XGBoost model performance was evaluated across the training dataset using five-fold cross validation [81]. Mean absolute error (MAE), the mean of all differences between predicted and actual values of mean telomere length, was used to assess the model's performance and ability to generalize to new data (Table S2A). Five-fold cross validation on the full training dataset yielded an average MAE of 3.233 with a standard deviation of 0.052

(Table S2A), suggesting that the model was not overfitting to portions (folds) of the training data and that it could generalize to new data. Model performance was also evaluated when training across variable numbers of individual telomere measurements (n = 100 to 103,040) (Table S2A). After training the XGBoost model on the full training dataset, the model was challenged to predict three-month post-IMRT MTL using new data—the test dataset. The XGBoost model predictions for MTLs in the test set matched the true values with an R^2 value of 0.882 (Figure 6A; Table S2A). Averaging predictions per patient for three-month post-IMRT MTL in the test set increased the R^2 value to 0.931 (Figure 6D).

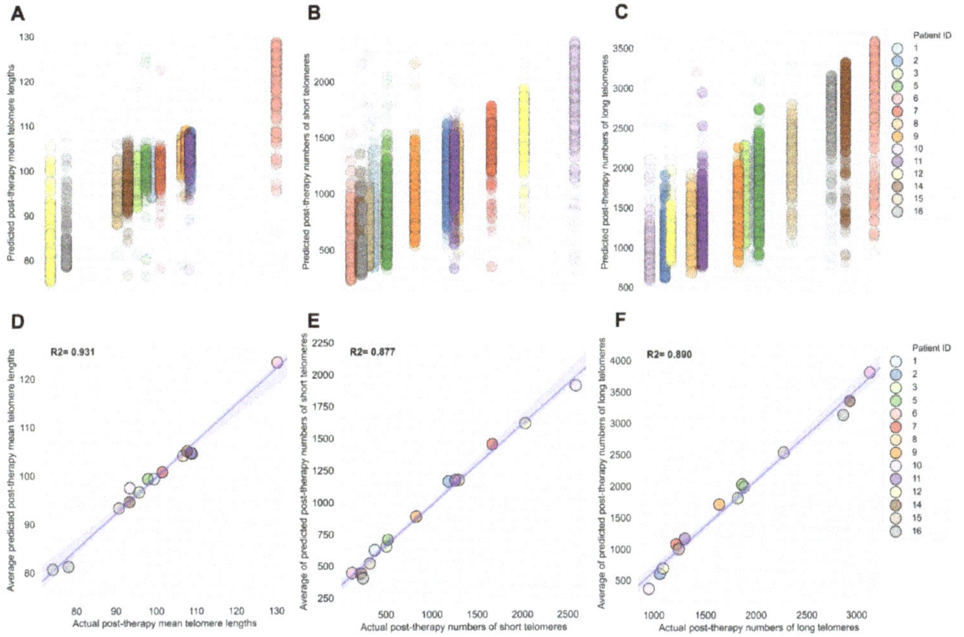

Figure 6. High performance of XGBoost models for predicting post-IMRT telomeric outcomes. Three separate XGBoost models were trained on pre-IMRT individual telomere length measurements (n = 103,040, Telo-FISH) to predict 3-month post-IMRT telomeric outcomes. Trained XGBoost models were challenged with the test set (new data, n = 25,760 individual telomeres) to predict 3-month post-IMRT telomeric outcomes for (**A**) mean telomere length, (**B**) numbers of short, and (**C**) numbers of long telomeres. XGBoost predictions were averaged on a per patient basis for (**D**) mean telomere length, (**E**) numbers of short, and (**F**) numbers of long telomeres; blue line represents a simple regression line (X/Y), lighter bands the 95% confidence interval, R^2 values (coefficient of determination) are noted in bold.

XGBoost models were then challenged to predict post-IMRT telomere length of patients whose pre-IMRT individual telomeres they were not trained on. We iteratively trained 14 XGBoost models, where in each model one patient's individual telomeres were "left out" of the training (i.e., round robin approach), but were included during model testing. Generally speaking, the XGboost models were extremely performant in predicting post-IMRT telomere length on entirely new patients (Figure 7A–N). Some deviations in performance were observed—we attribute these deviations in performance to low sample size. We also attempted a "leave two" and "leave three" patients out training and testing approach to understand the limits of generalizability for our XGBoost models (Figures S2A–M and S3A–L). We again found evidence of strong generalizability of the models to new patients. Together, these results demonstrate that the XGBoost model learned the nonlinear relationships between pre-IMRT individual telomere length data and three-month post-IMRT MTLs (training dataset), and also generalized to new data (test dataset) and new patients with highly accurate predictions.

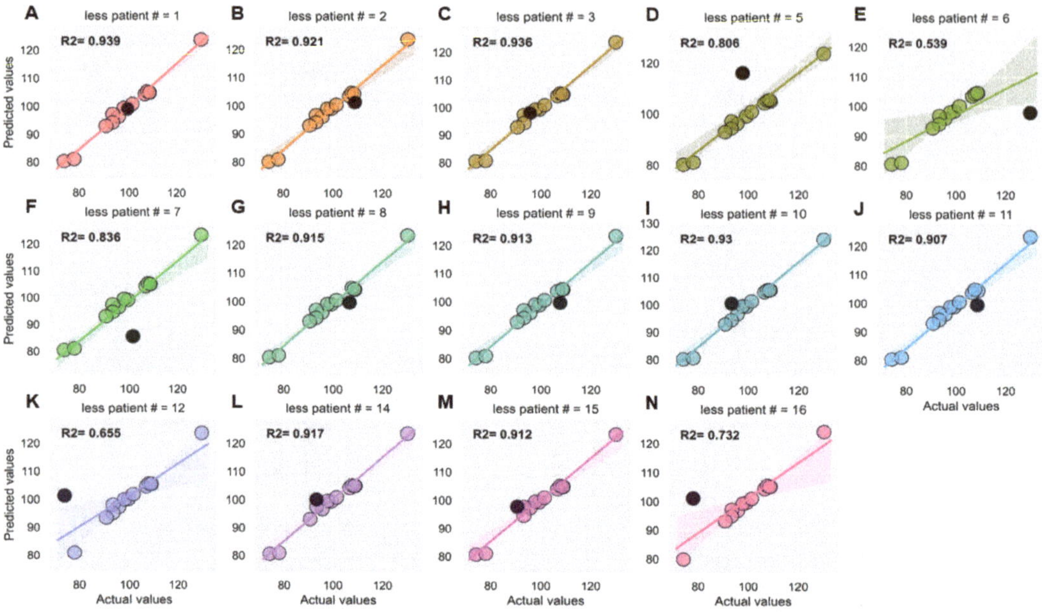

Figure 7. Strong generalizability of XGBoost models to new patient data (leave one out approach). (**A–N**) Fourteen separate XGBoost models were iteratively trained on pre-IMRT individual telomere length measurements (n = 93,840, Telo-FISH) excluding one patient, and tested to predict 3-month post-IMRT mean telomere length, with inclusion of the patient excluded during training. Each panel is one model; patients excluded during training for that model are noted in the panel headers and plotted in black. Lines represent a simple regression line (X/Y), lighter bands the 95% confidence interval, R^2 values (coefficient of determination) are noted in bold.

Pre-IMRT individual telomere length data was also processed and reshaped for training separate XGBoost models to predict numbers of short or long telomeres 3-months post-IMRT (Figure 5, Table S1C,E). Reshaped data was split into training (80%) and test (20%) datasets and shuffled and stratified in an identical manner as described for MTL (Table S1D,F). Hyperparameters of the XGBoost models were optimized using a randomized search [80], and the models performance and generalizability were analyzed using five-fold cross validation [81] with a MAE error metric. For XGBoost models of short telomeres, five-fold cross validation on the full training dataset yielded an average MAE of 236.283 with a standard deviation of 2.059 (Table S2B), while XGBoost models of long telomeres yielded an average MAE of 330.352 and standard deviation of 2.086, suggesting that both models were reasonably good at fitting the data and likely to generalize to new data (Table S2C). Model performance was also evaluated using variable numbers of training data (n = 100 to 103,040). Fully trained XGBoost models were challenged with predicting three-month post-IMRT numbers of short or long telomeres in the test set, and predictions matched the true values with an R^2 value of 0.811 and 0.819, respectively (Figure 6B,C; Table S2B,C). Averaging predictions per patient for post-IMRT numbers of short or long telomeres increased the R^2 value to 0.877 and 0.890, respectively (Figure 6E,F). These results demonstrate that the XGBoost models learned the relationships between pre-IMRT individual telomere length data and three-month post-IMRT numbers of short or long telomeres (training dataset), and effectively generalized to new data (test dataset).

3.5. Longitudinal Analyses of Chromosomal Instability Associated with Radiation Therapy

Directional Genomic Hybridization (dGH) is a cytogenomics-based methodology for high-resolution detection of chromosome aberrations (CAs), including structural variants missed even by sequencing [82], particularly inversions [62,78]. We hypothesized that including inversions would facilitate scoring fewer metaphase spreads (n = 30/time point/patient) [61], while also improving evaluation of individual chromosomal instability, and thus the ability to infer patients at higher risks for secondary cancers. Many significant differences in frequencies of IR-induced rearrangements were observed (Figure 8A–D), with inversions occurring at the highest frequencies, consistent with expectations [62,78]. Interestingly, overall average frequencies of inversions at 3-months post-IMRT were comparable to the in vitro irradiated samples (Figure 8A). Frequencies of translocations, dicentrics, and excess chromosome fragments (deletions) were highest after in vitro irradiation, and were also significantly elevated immediately post-IMRT (Figure 8B–D). Significantly elevated frequencies of translocations, dicentrics, and chromosome fragments persisted 3-months post-IMRT (Figure 8B–D). Frequencies of sister chromatid exchanges (SCE) did not significantly change over time (Figure 8E), consistent with expectation and low linear energy transfer (LET) radiation exposure [83,84]. Taken together, significantly elevated frequencies of CAs 3-months post-IMRT confirmed genomic instability in the cohort [57,58,60].

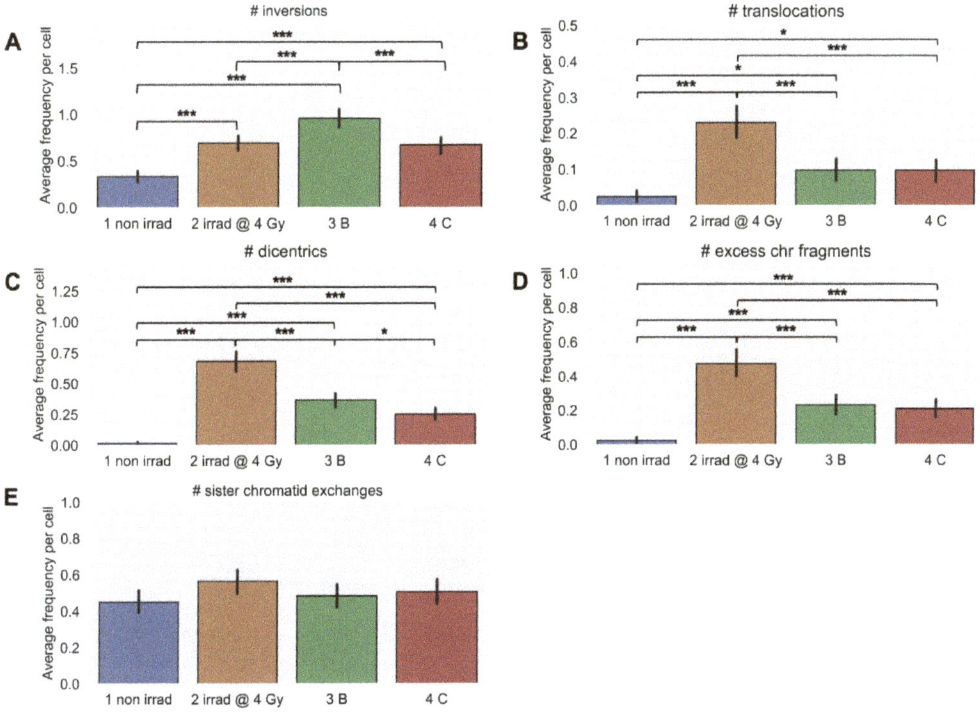

Figure 8. Longitudinal analyses of chromosomal instability. Whole blood was collected from prostate cancer patients undergoing IMRT (n = 15) and chromosome aberrations assessed using directional Genomic Hybridization (dGH) on metaphase spreads (n = 30/patient/timepoint scored): 1 non irrad = pre-IMRT non-irradiated (0 Gy); 2 irrad @ 4 Gy = pre-IMRT in vitro irradiated; 3B = immediate post-IMRT; and 4C = 3-month post-IMRT. Frequencies of (**A**) inversions, (**B**) translocations, (**C**) dicentrics, (**D**) excess chromosome fragments (deletions), and (**E**) sister chromatid exchanges (SCE). Significance was assessed for average aberration frequencies using a repeated measures ANOVA and post hoc Tukey's HSD test. $p < 0.05$ *, $p < 0.01$ **, $p < 0.001$ ***.

Significant changes in frequencies of IR-induced rearrangements also correlated with numbers of peripheral blood lymphocytes. Longitudinal correlations between patients' average frequencies of CAs and numbers of peripheral blood lymphocytes (all time points) revealed strongly negative correlations (Figure S4A–D). Frequencies of inversions and dicentrics had the highest negative correlations (R^2 = −0.752, −0.751), indicating they were highly informative—and similar—markers for cell death. These results suggest that patients demonstrating chromosomal instability (specifically, elevated frequencies of inversions and/or dicentrics), also experience higher levels of cell killing (i.e., greater radiosensitivity) consistent with previous reports [85,86].

Next, we hypothesized that clustering patients by longitudinal changes in CA frequencies (all samples) would reveal groups of patients with lower or higher frequencies of CAs, which would be indicative of individual chromosomal instability and radiosensitivity. When clustering patients by CA type, we observed groups of patients with differential responses only for inversions and excess chromosome fragments (deletions), which displayed increased frequencies immediately post-IMRT (Figure 9A,D, Figure S5A,B). We note that the two patients with the highest post-IMRT frequencies of inversions (ID #16) and chromosome fragments (ID #6), also had very high post-IMRT MTLs, supportive of correlation between these informative biomarkers, and suggestive of increased risks for secondary cancers [14–16,48] (Figures 1C and 9A,D, Figure S5A,B).

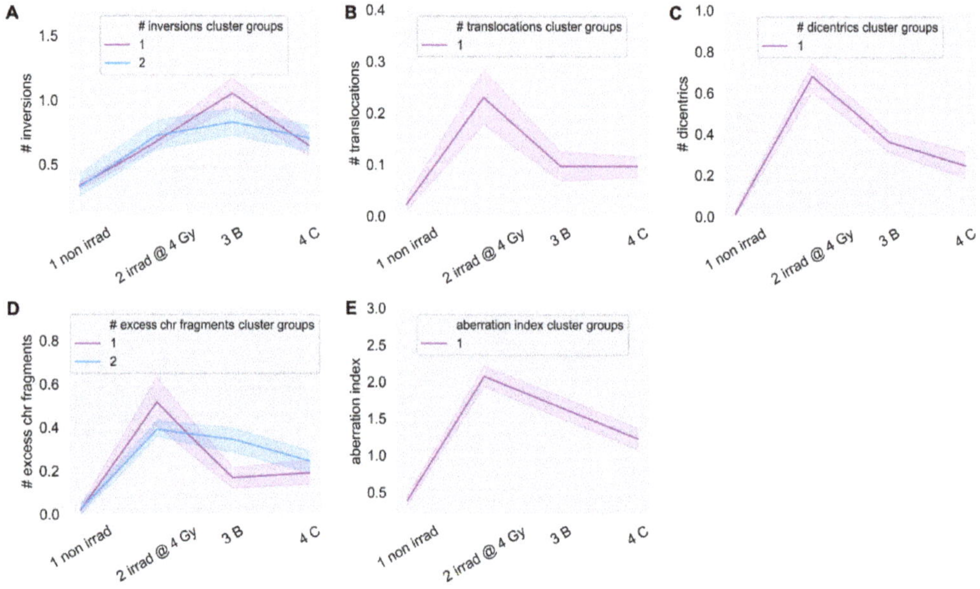

Figure 9. Clustering of patients by chromosome aberration frequencies. Time-courses for groups of patients hierarchically clustered into discrete groups (blue, purple) per aberration type: 1 non irrad = pre-IMRT non-irradiated (0 Gy); 2 irrad @ 4 Gy = pre-IMRT in vitro irradiated; 3B = immediate post-IMRT; and 4C = 3-month post-IMRT. Clustered groups of patients for frequencies of (**A**) inversions, (**B**) translocations, (**C**) dicentrics, (**D**) excess chromosome fragments (deletions), and (**E**) aberration index, which was created by summing all aberration types. Center lines denote medians and lighter bands denote confidence intervals.

Other CA types presented longitudinal responses that were relatively similar between patients and did not cluster patients (Figure 9B,C and Figure S6A,B). We hypothesized that while individual types of CAs failed to cluster patients into groups, individual patients may show lower or higher frequencies of CAs. To determine if some patients showed a general susceptibility to chromosomal instability, we feature engineered an 'aberration index' by summing all types of CAs (less sister chromatid exchanges) (Figure 9A–D) per cell for all time points. As indicated by the aberration index, groups of patients with lower or higher total CA frequencies were not observed (Figure 9E and Figure S6C). These results, together with the telomere length data, identified two patients (ID #s 6, 16) at potentially increased risks for secondary cancers [14–16,48], and are supportive of inversions and deletions being more informative than other CA types for predicting IR-induced secondary cancers, consistent with previous report [60]. While results indicate that the numbers of cells scored were too low ($n = 30$) to detect significant differences in individual patient susceptibility to chromosomal instability in general, including inversions improves power on an individual basis.

3.6. Linear Regression Poorly Predicted Radiation-Induced Chromosomal Instability

We speculated that pre-IMRT CA frequencies could be predictive of post-IMRT frequencies. Two linear regression models were made for each CA type to predict post-IMRT frequencies; the first used only the pre-IMRT (baseline) non-irradiated sample CA frequency, and the second used CA frequencies from both pre-IMRT non-irradiated and in vitro irradiated samples. The models showed poor predictive power overall, and although inclusion of the in vitro irradiated sample data improved performance overall, both models were insufficient for predicting post-IMRT CA frequencies with confidence (Figure 10A–E). The model for dicentrics performed best, with an R^2 score of 0.514 when using data from both irradiated and non-irradiated baseline samples. These results suggest that while in vitro irradiated sample data added predictive power, the number of cells scored per time point/patient ($n = 30$) was too low to enable accurate predictions of individual patient outcomes regarding CAs frequencies post-IMRT using linear regression.

3.7. XGBoost Machine Learning Models Poorly Predicted Radiation-Induced Chromosomal Instability

We attempted training XGBoost models using pre-IMRT (baseline) CA data to predict post-IMRT CA frequencies. Rather than using CA data per patient, which would be insufficient for model training ($n = 15$), we used pre-IMRT CA frequencies on a per cell basis ($n = 840$) to predict three-month post-IMRT average CA frequencies. Pre-IMRT CA frequency data was extensively processed prior to XGBoost model training (Figure S7; Table S3A–D), in a nearly identical manner as described for pre-IMRT telomere length data. The key difference was that CA data was reshaped to train XGBoost models with pre-IMRT CA count data per cell ($n = 672$ cells) in order to predict three-month post-IMRT average CA frequencies. Separate datasets and XGBoost models were created for each type of CA (see Materials and Methods).

XGBoost models for each CA type were evaluated across their respective training sets using five-fold cross validation [81] with a MAE metric. The cross-validation metrics for all XGBoost models with CA data suggested a failure of the models to learn relationships between pre-IMRT CA count data per cell and three-month post-IMRT average CA frequencies (Table S4A). Furthermore, dramatic fluctuations in model performance were noted when running multiple iterations of cross-validation, again suggesting that the models failed to learn the relationships between the pre- and post-IMRT CA frequencies (Table S4A–C). We attempted to improve model performance with many types of feature engineering (e.g., Boolean features), numerical transformations, and adjustments to model hyperparameters, none of which yielded meaningful improvements in any combination (data not shown). Regardless of poor model performance in cross-validation, we challenged the XGBoost models to predict post-IMRT average CA frequencies using pre-IMRT CA count data per cell in the test set ($n = 168$ cells). In XGBoost model predictions for 3-month post-IMRT CA frequencies in the test set, none of the predictions matched the true values, with an R^2 above 0.1 (Figure 10F–J, Table S4A–C). These results indicate that either the amount of data was insufficient for training XGBoost models ($n = 840$ cells at pre-IMRT), or the strategy of predicting post-IMRT average CA frequencies using pre-IMRT CA count data per cell was inherently faulty.

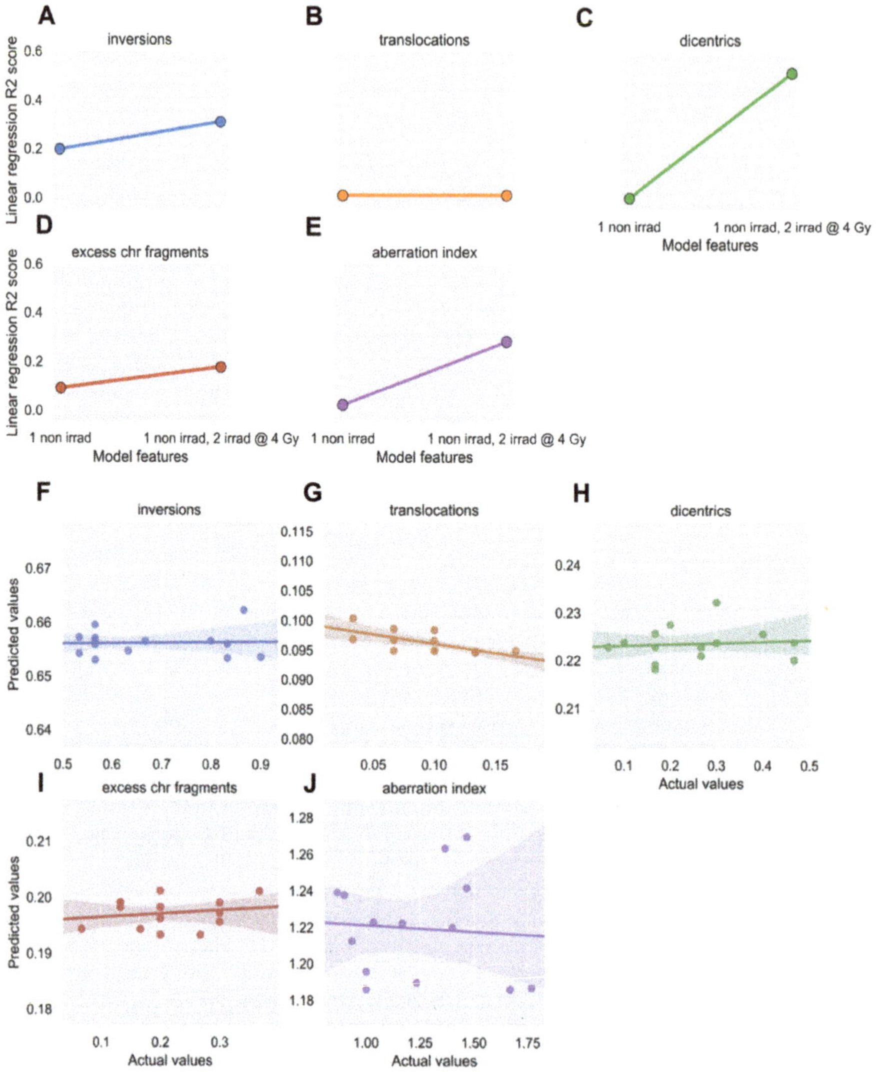

Figure 10. Neither linear regression nor XGBoost models successfully predicted post-IMRT chromosome aberration (CA) frequencies. Ordinary least squares linear regression models were made using pre-IMRT average CA frequencies from the non-irradiated (0 Gy) or in vitro irradiated (4 Gy) samples to predict 3-month post-IMRT average CA frequencies. Models were made for (**A**) inversions, (**B**) translocations, (**C**) dicentrics, (**D**) excess chromosome fragments (deletions), and (**E**) aberration index, which was created by summing all CA per cell. The model for dicentrics performed best, with an $R^2 = 0.514$. XGBoost models were trained on pre-IMRT counts of different CA types per cell ($n = 672$) to predict 3-month post-IMRT average CA frequencies. Trained XGBoost models were challenged with the test set (new data, $n = 168$ cells) to predict 3-month post-IMRT average CA frequencies. XGBoost predictions were averaged on a per patient basis for (**F**) inversions, (**G**) translocations, (**H**) dicentrics, (**I**) excess chromosome fragments (deletions), and (**J**) aberration index. For all models, R^2 values between averaged predictions and actual values did not exceed 0.100.

4. Discussion

The response of patients to radiotherapy varies considerably. Thus, it is important to identify radiosensitive individuals, as well as those most at risk of developing adverse late effects. Better prediction of a cancer patient's individual response to radiation therapy and risk for developing adverse late health effects remains a prime objective for the treatment modality in general [1–7], and particularly in regard to pediatric patients [8]. Over recent years, a variety of approaches for predicting radiation late effects have been developed [10–20], albeit with varying degrees of compromise between cost-effectiveness, throughput, and predictive power. One particularly promising exception is the use of ML models, which can leverage extensive amounts of patient data to make accurate predictions of treatment outcomes [63–65,67–69].

Predicting a patient's telomeric response to radiation therapy is of clinical interest for predicting risks of radiation late effects, as shorter telomeres confer radiosensitivity [35] and increase the risk of degenerative late effects (CVD and pulmonary fibrosis (Martínez and Blasco, 2018), aplastic anemia [44]), while longer telomeres increase risk for secondary cancers, particularly leukemias [48]. Given that telomeric responses to radiation exposure can be highly dynamic [36–38,50–52] and vary between individuals (Figures 1–3), a framework for predicting a patient's particular telomeric responses to radiation therapy is essential for utilizing telomere length as an informative biomarker of radiation late effects and secondary cancers. Here, we demonstrate the feasibility of using ML to accurately predict an individual patient's telomeric response to radiation therapy. We successfully implemented individual telomere length data in a machine learning model, XGBoost, for highly accurate predictions of post-IMRT telomeric outcomes (Figures 5 and 6; Table S3). The ML models and Telo-FISH methods used are fully available, providing a valuable resource for continued research into telomere length as a biomarker for radiation late effects associated with any manner of exposure.

The possibility of improving assessment of chromosomal instability and associated risk for development of secondary cancers following radiation therapy [14–16] was explored utilizing dGH, which facilitated inversion detection at higher resolution than traditional cytogenetic assays [62,78]. Indeed, inversions were observed at higher frequencies than other types of CAs both before and after radiation therapy (Figure 8A), consistent with prior reports [62,78]. Groups of patients with increased frequencies of chromosomal inversions and excess fragments (deletions), previously proposed signatures of radiation-induced cancers [60], were also observed 3-months post-IMRT (Figure 9A,D). Two patients from these groups had very high MTLs 3-months post-IMRT as well, also supportive of increased risks for secondary cancers [14–16,48]. We attempted to derive some predictive value from CA data with linear regression and XGBoost implementations, however, neither approach was successful. Even with the inclusion of inversions, the low numbers of cells scored per patient likely subverted successful predictions from the data.

Although we were unable to predict post-IMRT CA frequencies, the strong correlations between patients' average frequencies of CAs and changes in peripheral blood lymphocyte counts associated with IMRT supported the value of inversions for evaluating chromosomal instability. Inversions and dicentrics in particular had strong, negative correlations with lymphocyte cell counts ($R^2 = -0.752, -0.751$) (Figure S1A,B). Thus, patients with higher levels of radiation therapy-induced chromosomal instability also experienced increased levels of cell death, i.e., they exhibited individual radiosensitivity [85,86].

Relationships between peripheral blood cell count data and MTL were also observed. Counts of peripheral WBCs were negatively correlated with MTL associated with IMRT ($R^2 = -0.126$), supportive of shorter telomeres contributing to cell killing and individual radiosensitivity (Figure S1A). When parsing WBCs by sub-type, a stronger negative relationship between MTL and lymphocyte counts was seen ($R^2 = -0.294$). When parsing lymphocytes by sub-type and correlating MTL with the proportions of cell-types, positive correlations with NK and CD4 cells ($R^2 = 0.408, 0.282$), and negative correlations with CD8 and CD19 cells ($R^2 = -0.251, -0.288$) were observed. These results support our previously proposed supposition that the observed changes in MTL associated with radiation exposure could be at least partially due to cell killing and associated changes in peripheral blood lymphocyte cell populations [78,79].

Longitudinal assessment of individual telomere lengths by Telo-FISH in cancer patients undergoing IMRT facilitated demonstration of XGBoost as the ML model of choice for predicting telomeric outcomes post-IMRT. Given the notion that risks for radiation late effects occur on a spectrum [1–8], and the differential telomeric responses between individuals and radiation modalities, we posit that the true range of telomeric responses for radiation therapy patients in general is much broader than those observed here in this prostate cancer cohort (Figures 1–3). Thus, while our XGBoost models effectively generalized to new data within our experimental design (similar patient sex, radiation modality, cancer type, etc.), it is unlikely that our trained models, in their current iteration, would generalize to data collected under different experimental or clinical parameters. Moreover, with regard to measurement of individual telomere lengths for training XGBoost models, Telo-FISH could readily be interchanged with comparable assays (Q-FISH, flow-FISH), which would provide higher throughput. Additionally, the ML approaches described here were not strictly dependent upon XGBoost, and could be conducted using other machine learning models and frameworks (e.g., random forests, kNN). Our paradigm of training ML models with individual telomere length data for prediction of post-IMRT telomeric outcomes provides improved predictive power and novel insight into individual radiosensitivity and risk of radiation-late effects, as well as a general framework that could be implemented for radiation therapy patients regardless of cancer type, radiation modality, or individual patient sex or genetic susceptibilities.

Supplementary Materials: The following are available online at https://www.mdpi.com/2075-4426/11/3/188/s1, Figure S1. Correlations between telomere length, peripheral white blood cells, and lymphocytes, Figure S2. Strong generalizability of XGBoost models to new patient data (leave one out), Figure S3. Strong generalizability of XGBoost models to new patient data (leave two out), Figure S4. Correlations between chromosome aberrations and lymphocyte cell counts, Figure S5. Clustering of patients by inversions and excess chromosome fragments (deletions), Figure S6. Chromosome aberration frequencies generally failed to cluster patients, Figure S7. Processing of chromosome aberration data for XGBoost models, Table S1. Examples of individual telomere length data matrices used to train XGBoost models, Table S2. Metrics of XGBoost models for predicting post-IMRT telomeric outcomes, Table S3. Examples of chromosome aberration data matrices used to train XGBoost models, Table S4. Metrics of trained XGBoost models for predicting post-IMRT chromosome aberration frequencies.

Author Contributions: Conceptualization, M.J.M., G.P.S. and S.M.B.; Data curation, J.J.L. and L.E.T.; Formal analysis, J.J.L., A.M.L., L.E.T. and S.M.B.; Funding acquisition, G.P.S. and S.M.B.; Investigation, J.J.L., M.J.M., S.G.J., G.P.S. and S.M.B.; Methodology, J.J.L., M.J.M., A.M.L., L.E.T. and G.P.S.; Project administration, G.P.S. and S.M.B.; Resources, L.E.T., G.P.S. and S.M.B.; Software, J.J.L.; Supervision, L.E.T., G.P.S. and S.M.B.; Validation, J.J.L. and S.M.B.; Visualization, J.J.L. and S.G.J.; Writing—original draft, J.J.L. and S.M.B.; Writing—review and editing, J.J.L., M.J.M., A.M.L., L.E.T., G.P.S. and S.M.B. All authors have read and agreed to the published version of the manuscript.

Funding: This research was funded by the Colorado Office of Economic Development and International Trade (OEDIT) Advanced Industry (AI) Bioscience Proof of Concept (POC) award program, Colorado State University (CSU) Ventures. Graduate student fellowships awarded by CSU's Program of Research and Scholarly Excellence (PRSE), and the Cancer Biology and Comparative Oncology (CB&CO) PRSE to support quantitative Cell and Molecular Biology (qCMB) studies, are also gratefully acknowledged.

Institutional Review Board Statement: The study was conducted according to the guidelines of the Declaration of Helsinki, and approved by the Institutional Review Board of Baylor Scott and White Clinic, Temple, Texas, USA (protocol code 170524; date of approval: 03/22/2017).

Informed Consent Statement: Informed consent was obtained from all subjects involved in the study.

Data Availability Statement: Raw and processed individual telomere length (Telo-FISH) data files and chromosome aberration score sheets (dGH) are available for download at https://github.com/Jared-Luxton/. All data processing pipelines and code were written in Python and stored in Jupyter notebooks at https://github.com/Jared-Luxton/. The Jupyter notebooks can be run within a web browser and are available for download.

Conflicts of Interest: S.M.B. is a cofounder and scientific advisory board member of KromaTiD, Inc.

References

1. Barnett, G.C.; West, C.M.L.; Dunning, A.M.; Elliott, R.M.; Coles, C.E.; Pharoah, P.D.P.; Burnet, N.G. Normal Tissue Reactions to Radiotherapy. *Nat. Rev. Cancer* **2009**, *9*, 134–142. [CrossRef]
2. Bentzen, S.M. Preventing or Reducing Late Side Effects of Radiation Therapy: Radiobiology Meets Molecular Pathology. *Nat. Rev. Cancer* **2006**, *6*, 702–713. [CrossRef]
3. Yusuf, S.W.; Venkatesulu, B.P.; Mahadevan, L.S.; Krishnan, S. Radiation-Induced Cardiovascular Disease: A Clinical Perspective. *Front. Cardiovasc. Med.* **2017**, *4*. [CrossRef]
4. Carver, J.R.; Shapiro, C.L.; Ng, A.; Jacobs, L.; Schwartz, C.; Virgo, K.S.; Hagerty, K.L.; Somerfield, M.R.; Vaughn, D.J.; ASCO Cancer Survivorship Expert Panel. American Society of Clinical Oncology Clinical Evidence Review on the Ongoing Care of Adult Cancer Survivors: Cardiac and Pulmonary Late Effects. *J. Clin. Oncol.* **2007**, *25*, 3991–4008. [CrossRef]
5. Greene-Schloesser, D.; Robbins, M.E. Radiation-Induced Cognitive Impairment-from Bench to Bedside. *Neuro Oncol.* **2012**, *14*, iv37–iv44. [CrossRef]
6. Yaprak, G.; Gemici, C.; Temizkan, S.; Ozdemir, S.; Dogan, B.C.; Seseogullari, O.O. Osteoporosis Development and Vertebral Fractures after Abdominal Irradiation in Patients with Gastric Cancer. *BMC Cancer* **2018**, *18*, 972. [CrossRef]
7. Suit, H.; Goldberg, S.; Niemierko, A.; Ancukiewicz, M.; Hall, E.; Goitein, M.; Wong, W.; Paganetti, H. Secondary Carcinogenesis in Patients Treated with Radiation: A Review of Data on Radiation-Induced Cancers in Human, Non-Human Primate, Canine and Rodent Subjects. *Radiat. Res.* **2007**, *167*, 12–42. [CrossRef]
8. Armstrong, G.T.; Stovall, M.; Robison, L.L. Long-Term Effects of Radiation Exposure among Adult Survivors of Childhood Cancer: Results from the Childhood Cancer Survivor Study. *Radiat. Res.* **2010**, *174*, 840–850. [CrossRef]
9. Rajaraman, P.; Hauptmann, M.; Bouffler, S.; Wojcik, A. Human Individual Radiation Sensitivity and Prospects for Prediction. *Ann. ICRP* **2018**, *47*, 126–141. [CrossRef]
10. Habash, M.; Bohorquez, L.C.; Kyriakou, E.; Kron, T.; Martin, O.A.; Blyth, B.J. Clinical and Functional Assays of Radiosensitivity and Radiation-Induced Second Cancer. *Cancers* **2017**, *9*, 147. [CrossRef]
11. Banáth, J.P.; MacPhail, S.H.; Olive, P.L. Radiation Sensitivity, H2AX Phosphorylation, and Kinetics of Repair of DNA Strand Breaks in Irradiated Cervical Cancer Cell Lines. *Cancer Res.* **2004**, *64*, 7144–7149. [CrossRef] [PubMed]
12. Redon, C.E.; Dickey, J.S.; Bonner, W.M.; Sedelnikova, O.A. γ-H2AX as a Biomarker of DNA Damage Induced by Ionizing Radiation in Human Peripheral Blood Lymphocytes and Artificial Skin. *Adv. Space Res.* **2009**, *43*, 1171–1178. [CrossRef]
13. Schmitz, A.; Bayer, J.; Dechamps, N.; Goldin, L.; Thomas, G. Heritability of Susceptibility to Ionizing Radiation-Induced Apoptosis of Human Lymphocyte Subpopulations. *Int. J. Radiat. Oncol. Biol. Phys.* **2007**, *68*, 1169–1177. [CrossRef]
14. Baeyens, A.; Thierens, H.; Claes, K.; Poppe, B.; Messiaen, L.; De Ridder, L.; Vral, A. Chromosomal Radiosensitivity in Breast Cancer Patients with a Known or Putative Genetic Predisposition. *Br. J. Cancer* **2002**, *87*, 1379–1385. [CrossRef] [PubMed]
15. Baria, K.; Warren, C.; Roberts, S.A.; West, C.M.; Scott, D. Chromosomal Radiosensitivity as a Marker of Predisposition to Common Cancers? *Br. J. Cancer* **2001**, *84*, 892–896. [CrossRef] [PubMed]
16. Huber, R.; Braselmann, H.; Geinitz, H.; Jaehnert, I.; Baumgartner, A.; Thamm, R.; Figel, M.; Molls, M.; Zitzelsberger, H. Chromosomal Radiosensitivity and Acute Radiation Side Effects after Radiotherapy in Tumour Patients—A Follow-up Study. *Radiat. Oncol.* **2011**, *6*, 32. [CrossRef]
17. Kerns, S.L.; Dorling, L.; Fachal, L.; Bentzen, S.; Pharoah, P.D.P.; Barnes, D.R.; Gómez-Caamaño, A.; Carballo, A.M.; Dearnaley, D.P.; Peleteiro, P.; et al. Meta-Analysis of Genome Wide Association Studies Identifies Genetic Markers of Late Toxicity Following Radiotherapy for Prostate Cancer. *EBioMedicine* **2016**, *10*, 150–163. [CrossRef]
18. Kerns, S.L.; Ostrer, H.; Stock, R.; Li, W.; Moore, J.; Pearlman, A.; Campbell, C.; Shao, Y.; Stone, N.; Kusnetz, L.; et al. Genome-Wide Association Study to Identify Single Nucleotide Polymorphisms (SNPs) Associated with the Development of Erectile Dysfunction in African-American Men after Radiotherapy for Prostate Cancer. *Int. J. Radiat. Oncol. Biol. Phys.* **2010**, *78*, 1292–1300. [CrossRef]
19. Young, A.; Berry, R.; Holloway, A.F.; Blackburn, N.B.; Dickinson, J.L.; Skala, M.; Phillips, J.L.; Brettingham-Moore, K.H. RNA-Seq Profiling of a Radiation Resistant and Radiation Sensitive Prostate Cancer Cell Line Highlights Opposing Regulation of DNA Repair and Targets for Radiosensitization. *BMC Cancer* **2014**, *14*. [CrossRef]
20. Bodalal, Z.; Trebeschi, S.; Nguyen-Kim, T.D.L.; Schats, W.; Beets-Tan, R. Radiogenomics: Bridging Imaging and Genomics. *Abdom. Radiol.* **2019**, *44*, 1960–1984. [CrossRef]
21. Mirjolet, C.; Boidot, R.; Saliques, S.; Ghiringhelli, F.; Maingon, P.; Créhange, G. The Role of Telomeres in Predicting Individual Radiosensitivity of Patients with Cancer in the Era of Personalized Radiotherapy. *Cancer Treat. Rev.* **2015**, *41*, 354–360. [CrossRef]
22. De Lange, T. How Telomeres Solve the End-Protection Problem. *Science* **2009**, *326*, 948. [CrossRef]

23. Moyzis, R.K.; Buckingham, J.M.; Cram, L.S.; Dani, M.; Deaven, L.L.; Jones, M.D.; Meyne, J.; Ratliff, R.L.; Wu, J.R. A Highly Conserved Repetitive DNA Sequence, (TTAGGG)n, Present at the Telomeres of Human Chromosomes. *Proc. Natl. Acad. Sci. USA* **1988**, *85*, 6622–6626. [CrossRef]
24. Von Zglinicki, T. Role of Oxidative Stress in Telomere Length Regulation and Replicative Senescence. *Ann. N. Y. Acad. Sci.* **2000**, *908*, 99–110. [CrossRef]
25. Aubert, G.; Lansdorp, P.M. Telomeres and Aging. *Physiol. Rev.* **2008**, *88*, 557–579. [CrossRef]
26. Vidaček, N.Š.; Nanić, L.; Ravlić, S.; Sopta, M.; Gerić, M.; Gajski, G.; Garaj-Vrhovac, V.; Rubelj, I. Telomeres, Nutrition, and Longevity: Can We Really Navigate Our Aging? *J. Gerontol. Ser. A* **2017**. [CrossRef]
27. Arsenis, N.C.; You, T.; Ogawa, E.F.; Tinsley, G.M.; Zuo, L. Physical Activity and Telomere Length: Impact of Aging and Potential Mechanisms of Action. *Oncotarget* **2017**, *8*, 45008–45019. [CrossRef] [PubMed]
28. Epel, E.S.; Blackburn, E.H.; Lin, J.; Dhabhar, F.S.; Adler, N.E.; Morrow, J.D.; Cawthon, R.M. Accelerated Telomere Shortening in Response to Life Stress. *Proc. Natl. Acad. Sci. USA* **2004**, *101*, 17312–17315. [CrossRef]
29. Miri, M.; Nazarzadeh, M.; Alahabadi, A.; Ehrampoush, M.H.; Rad, A.; Lotfi, M.H.; Sheikhha, M.H.; Sakhvidi, M.J.Z.; Nawrot, T.S.; Dadvand, P. Air Pollution and Telomere Length in Adults: A Systematic Review and Meta-Analysis of Observational Studies. *Environ. Pollut.* **2019**, *244*, 636–647. [CrossRef]
30. Stout, G.J.; Blasco, M.A. Telomere Length and Telomerase Activity Impact the UV Sensitivity Syndrome Xeroderma Pigmentosum C. *Cancer Res.* **2013**, *73*, 1844–1854. [CrossRef]
31. Broer, L.; Codd, V.; Nyholt, D.R.; Deelen, J.; Mangino, M.; Willemsen, G.; Albrecht, E.; Amin, N.; Beekman, M.; De Geus, E.J.C.; et al. Meta-Analysis of Telomere Length in 19 713 Subjects Reveals High Heritability, Stronger Maternal Inheritance and a Paternal Age Effect. *Eur. J. Hum. Genet.* **2013**, *21*, 1163–1168. [CrossRef]
32. Delgado, D.A.; Zhang, C.; Gleason, K.; Demanelis, K.; Chen, L.S.; Gao, J.; Roy, S.; Shinkle, J.; Sabarinathan, M.; Argos, M.; et al. The Contribution of Parent-to-Offspring Transmission of Telomeres to the Heritability of Telomere Length in Humans. *Hum. Genet.* **2019**, *138*, 49–60. [CrossRef] [PubMed]
33. Honig, L.S.; Kang, M.S.; Cheng, R.; Eckfeldt, J.H.; Thyagarajan, B.; Leiendecker-Foster, C.; Province, M.A.; Sanders, J.L.; Perls, T.; Christensen, K.; et al. Heritability of Telomere Length in a Study of Long-Lived Families. *Neurobiol. Aging* **2015**, *36*, 2785–2790. [CrossRef] [PubMed]
34. Weng, Q.; Du, J.; Yu, F.; Huang, T.; Chen, M.; Lv, H.; Ma, H.; Hu, Z.; Jin, G.; Hu, Y.; et al. The Known Genetic Loci for Telomere Length May Be Involved in the Modification of Telomeres Length after Birth. *Sci. Rep.* **2016**, *6*, 1–7. [CrossRef]
35. Ayouaz, A.; Raynaud, C.; Heride, C.; Revaud, D.; Sabatier, L. Telomeres: Hallmarks of Radiosensitivity. *Biochimie* **2008**, *90*, 60–72. [CrossRef]
36. Berardinelli, F.; Antoccia, A.; Buonsante, R.; Gerardi, S.; Cherubini, R.; Nadal, V.D.; Tanzarella, C.; Sgura, A. The Role of Telomere Length Modulation in Delayed Chromosome Instability Induced by Ionizing Radiation in Human Primary Fibroblasts. *Environ. Mol. Mutagenesis* **2013**, *54*, 172–179. [CrossRef]
37. Maeda, T.; Nakamura, K.; Atsumi, K.; Hirakawa, M.; Ueda, Y.; Makino, N. Radiation-Associated Changes in the Length of Telomeres in Peripheral Leukocytes from Inpatients with Cancer. *Int. J. Radiat. Biol.* **2013**, *89*, 106–109. [CrossRef]
38. Sgura, A.; Antoccia, A.; Berardinelli, F.; Cherubini, R.; Gerardi, S.; Zilio, C.; Tanzarella, C. Telomere Length in Mammalian Cells Exposed to Low- and High-LET Radiations. *Radiat. Prot. Dosim.* **2006**, *122*, 176–179. [CrossRef]
39. Telomeres Mendelian Randomization Collaboration; Haycock, P.C.; Burgess, S.; Nounu, A.; Zheng, J.; Okoli, G.N.; Bowden, J.; Wade, K.H.; Timpson, N.J.; Evans, D.M.; et al. Association Between Telomere Length and Risk of Cancer and Non-Neoplastic Diseases: A Mendelian Randomization Study. *JAMA Oncol.* **2017**, *3*, 636–651. [CrossRef] [PubMed]
40. Protsenko, E.; Rehkopf, D.; Prather, A.A.; Epel, E.; Lin, J. Are Long Telomeres Better than Short? Relative Contributions of Genetically Predicted Telomere Length to Neoplastic and Non-Neoplastic Disease Risk and Population Health Burden. *PLoS ONE* **2020**, *15*, e0240185. [CrossRef] [PubMed]
41. Stone, R.C.; Horvath, K.; Kark, J.D.; Susser, E.; Tishkoff, S.A.; Aviv, A. Telomere Length and the Cancer–Atherosclerosis Trade-Off. *PLoS Genet.* **2016**, *12*, e1006144. [CrossRef]
42. Armanios, M.; Blackburn, E.H. The Telomere Syndromes. *Nat. Rev. Genet.* **2012**, *13*, 693–704. [CrossRef]
43. Martínez, P.; Blasco, M.A. Heart-Breaking Telomeres. *Circ. Res.* **2018**, *123*, 787–802. [CrossRef]
44. Calado, R.T.; Cooper, J.N.; Padilla-Nash, H.M.; Sloand, E.M.; Wu, C.O.; Scheinberg, P.; Ried, T.; Young, N.S. Short Telomeres Result in Chromosomal Instability in Hematopoietic Cells and Precede Malignant Evolution in Human Aplastic Anemia. *Leukemia* **2012**, *26*, 700–707. [CrossRef]
45. Adams, M.J.; Hardenbergh, P.H.; Constine, L.S.; Lipshultz, S.E. Radiation-Associated Cardiovascular Disease. *Crit. Rev. Oncol. Hematol.* **2003**, *45*, 55–75. [CrossRef]
46. Green, D.E.; Rubin, C.T. Consequences of Irradiation on Bone and Marrow Phenotypes, and Its Relation to Disruption of Hematopoietic Precursors. *Bone* **2014**, *0*, 87–94. [CrossRef]
47. Tsoutsou, P.G.; Koukourakis, M.I. Radiation Pneumonitis and Fibrosis: Mechanisms Underlying Its Pathogenesis and Implications for Future Research. *Int. J. Radiation Oncol.* Biol.* Phys.* **2006**, *66*, 1281–1293. [CrossRef]
48. McNally, E.J.; Luncsford, P.J.; Armanios, M. Long Telomeres and Cancer Risk: The Price of Cellular Immortality. *J. Clin. Investig.* **2019**, *129*, 3474–3481. [CrossRef]

49. Dracham, C.B.; Shankar, A.; Madan, R. Radiation Induced Secondary Malignancies: A Review Article. *Radiat. Oncol. J.* **2018**, *36*, 85–94. [CrossRef]
50. Bains, S.K.; Chapman, K.; Bright, S.; Senan, A.; Kadhim, M.; Slijepcevic, P. Effects of Ionizing Radiation on Telomere Length and Telomerase Activity in Cultured Human Lens Epithelium Cells. *Int. J. Radiat. Biol.* **2019**, *95*, 54–63. [CrossRef]
51. Berardinelli, F.; Sgura, A.; Di Masi, A.; Leone, S.; Cirrone, G.A.P.; Romano, F.; Tanzarella, C.; Antoccia, A. Radiation-Induced Telomere Length Variations in Normal and in Nijmegen Breakage Syndrome Cells. *Int. J. Radiat. Biol.* **2014**, *90*, 45–52. [CrossRef]
52. De Vitis, M.; Berardinelli, F.; Coluzzi, E.; Marinaccio, J.; O'Sullivan, R.J.; Sgura, A. X-Rays Activate Telomeric Homologous Recombination Mediated Repair in Primary Cells. *Cells* **2019**, *8*, 708. [CrossRef]
53. Alsner, J.; Rødningen, O.K.; Overgaard, J. Differential Gene Expression before and after Ionizing Radiation of Subcutaneous Fibroblasts Identifies Breast Cancer Patients Resistant to Radiation-Induced Fibrosis. *Radiother. Oncol.* **2007**, *83*, 261–266. [CrossRef]
54. Andreassen, C.N.; Overgaard, J.; Alsner, J. Independent Prospective Validation of a Predictive Test for Risk of Radiation Induced Fibrosis Based on the Gene Expression Pattern in Fibroblasts Irradiated in Vitro. *Radiother. Oncol.* **2013**, *108*, 469–472. [CrossRef]
55. Borgmann, K.; Hoeller, U.; Nowack, S.; Bernhard, M.; Röper, B.; Brackrock, S.; Petersen, C.; Szymczak, S.; Ziegler, A.; Feyer, P.; et al. Individual Radiosensitivity Measured with Lymphocytes May Predict the Risk of Acute Reaction after Radiotherapy. *Int. J. Radiat. Oncol. Biol. Phys.* **2008**, *71*, 256–264. [CrossRef]
56. Paul, S.; Barker, C.A.; Turner, H.C.; McLane, A.; Wolden, S.L.; Amundson, S.A. Prediction of In Vivo Radiation Dose Status in Radiotherapy Patients Using Ex Vivo and In Vivo Gene Expression Signatures. *Radiat. Res.* **2011**, *175*, 257–265. [CrossRef] [PubMed]
57. Huang, L.; Snyder, A.R.; Morgan, W.F. Radiation-Induced Genomic Instability and Its Implications for Radiation Carcinogenesis. *Oncogene* **2003**, *22*, 5848–5854. [CrossRef]
58. Willis, N.A.; Rass, E.; Scully, R. Deciphering the Code of the Cancer Genome: Mechanisms of Chromosome Rearrangement. *Trends Cancer* **2015**, *1*, 217–230. [CrossRef] [PubMed]
59. Ward, J.F. DNA Damage Produced by Ionizing Radiation in Mammalian Cells: Identities, Mechanisms of Formation, and Reparability. In *Progress in Nucleic Acid Research and Molecular Biology*; Cohn, W.E., Moldave, K., Eds.; Academic Press: Cambridge, MA, USA, 1988; Volume 35, pp. 95–125.
60. Behjati, S.; Gundem, G.; Wedge, D.C.; Roberts, N.D.; Tarpey, P.S.; Cooke, S.L.; Van Loo, P.; Alexandrov, L.B.; Ramakrishna, M.; Davies, H.; et al. Mutational Signatures of Ionizing Radiation in Second Malignancies. *Nat. Commun.* **2016**, *7*. [CrossRef]
61. Mosesso, P.; Cinelli, S. In Vitro Cytogenetic Assays: Chromosomal Aberrations and Micronucleus Tests. In *Genotoxicity Assessment: Methods and Protocols*; Dhawan, A., Bajpayee, M., Eds.; Methods in Molecular Biology; Springer: New York, NY, USA, 2019; pp. 79–104. ISBN 978-1-4939-9646-9.
62. Ray, F.A.; Zimmerman, E.; Robinson, B.; Cornforth, M.N.; Bedford, J.S.; Goodwin, E.H.; Bailey, S.M. Directional Genomic Hybridization for Chromosomal Inversion Discovery and Detection. *Chromosome Res.* **2013**, *21*, 165–174. [CrossRef]
63. Pella, A.; Cambria, R.; Riboldi, M.; Jereczek-Fossa, B.A.; Fodor, C.; Zerini, D.; Torshabi, A.E.; Cattani, F.; Garibaldi, C.; Pedroli, G.; et al. Use of Machine Learning Methods for Prediction of Acute Toxicity in Organs at Risk Following Prostate Radiotherapy. *Med. Phys.* **2011**, *38*, 2859–2867. [CrossRef] [PubMed]
64. Fan, J.; Wang, J.; Chen, Z.; Hu, C.; Zhang, Z.; Hu, W. Automatic Treatment Planning Based on Three-Dimensional Dose Distribution Predicted from Deep Learning Technique. *Med. Phys.* **2019**, *46*, 370–381. [CrossRef]
65. Lee, S.; Liang, X.; Woods, M.; Reiner, A.S.; Concannon, P.; Bernstein, L.; Lynch, C.F.; Boice, J.D.; Deasy, J.O.; Bernstein, J.L.; et al. Machine Learning on Genome-Wide Association Studies to Predict the Risk of Radiation-Associated Contralateral Breast Cancer in the WECARE Study. *PLoS ONE* **2020**, *15*, e0226157. [CrossRef]
66. Chen, T.; Guestrin, C. XGBoost: A Scalable Tree Boosting System. In Proceedings of the 22nd ACM SIGKDD International Conference on Knowledge Discovery and Data Mining—KDD '16, San Francisco, CA, USA, 13–17 August 2016; pp. 785–794. [CrossRef]
67. Taninaga, J.; Nishiyama, Y.; Fujibayashi, K.; Gunji, T.; Sasabe, N.; Iijima, K.; Naito, T. Prediction of Future Gastric Cancer Risk Using a Machine Learning Algorithm and Comprehensive Medical Check-up Data: A Case-Control Study. *Sci. Rep.* **2019**, *9*, 1–9. [CrossRef]
68. Yu, D.; Liu, Z.; Su, C.; Han, Y.; Duan, X.; Zhang, R.; Liu, X.; Yang, Y.; Xu, S. Copy Number Variation in Plasma as a Tool for Lung Cancer Prediction Using Extreme Gradient Boosting (XGBoost) Classifier. *Thorac. Cancer* **2020**, *11*, 95–102. [CrossRef]
69. Wang, J.; Yang, P.; Zhao, Y.; Elhalawani, H.; Liu, R.; Zhu, H.; Mohamed, A.S.; Fuller, C.D.; Zhu, H. A Predictive Model of Radiation-Related Fibrosis Based on Radiomic Features of Magnetic Resonance Imaging. *Int. J. Radiat. Oncol. Biol. Phys.* **2019**, *105*, E599. [CrossRef]
70. Poon, S.S.S.; Lansdorp, P.M. Quantitative Fluorescence In Situ Hybridization (Q-FISH). *Curr. Protoc. Cell Biol.* **2001**, *12*, 18.4.1–18.4.21. [CrossRef]
71. Howe, B.; Umrigar, A.; Tsien, F. Chromosome Preparation From Cultured Cells. *J. Vis. Exp.* **2014**. [CrossRef]
72. Williams, E.S.; Bailey, S.M. Chromosome Orientation Fluorescence in Situ Hybridization (CO-FISH). *Cold Spring Harb. Protoc.* **2009**, *2009*, pdb.prot5269. [CrossRef]
73. Schneider, C.A.; Rasband, W.S.; Eliceiri, K.W. NIH Image to ImageJ: 25 Years of Image Analysis. *Nat. Methods* **2012**, *9*, 671–675. [CrossRef]

74. Wong, H.-P.; Slijepcevic, P. Telomere Length Measurement in Mouse Chromosomes by a Modified Q-FISH Method. *CGR* **2004**, *105*, 464–470. [CrossRef]
75. Seabold, S.; Perktold, J. Statsmodels: Econometric and Statistical Modeling with Python. In Proceedings of the 9th Python in Science Conference, Austin, TX, USA, 9–15 July 2010; pp. 92–96.
76. Virtanen, P.; Gommers, R.; Oliphant, T.E.; Haberland, M.; Reddy, T.; Cournapeau, D.; Burovski, E.; Peterson, P.; Weckesser, W.; Bright, J.; et al. SciPy 1.0: Fundamental Algorithms for Scientific Computing in Python. *Nat. Methods* **2020**, *17*, 261–272. [CrossRef]
77. Pedregosa, F.; Varoquaux, G.; Gramfort, A.; Michel, V.; Thirion, B.; Grisel, O.; Blondel, M.; Müller, A.; Nothman, J.; Louppe, G.; et al. Scikit-Learn: Machine Learning in Python. *arXiv* **2018**, arXiv:1201.0490.
78. Garrett-Bakelman, F.E.; Darshi, M.; Green, S.J.; Gur, R.C.; Lin, L.; Macias, B.R.; McKenna, M.J.; Meydan, C.; Mishra, T.; Nasrini, J.; et al. The NASA Twins Study: A Multidimensional Analysis of a Year-Long Human Spaceflight. *Science* **2019**, *364*. [CrossRef]
79. Luxton, J.J.; McKenna, M.J.; Lewis, A.; Taylor, L.E.; George, K.A.; Dixit, S.M.; Moniz, M.; Benegas, W.; Mackay, M.J.; Mozsary, C.; et al. Telomere Length Dynamics and DNA Damage Responses Associated with Long-Duration Spaceflight. *Cell Rep.* **2020**, *33*, 108457. [CrossRef]
80. Bergstra, J.; Bengio, Y. Random Search for Hyper-Parameter Optimization. *J. Mach. Learn. Res.* **2012**, *13*, 281–305.
81. Stone, M. Cross-Validatory Choice and Assessment of Statistical Predictions. *J. R. Stat. Soc. Ser. B (Methodol.)* **1974**, *36*, 111–133. [CrossRef]
82. Cornforth, M.N.; Anur, P.; Wang, N.; Robinson, E.; Ray, F.A.; Bedford, J.S.; Loucas, B.D.; Williams, E.S.; Peto, M.; Spellman, P.; et al. Molecular Cytogenetics Guides Massively Parallel Sequencing of a Radiation-Induced Chromosome Translocation in Human Cells. *Radiat. Res.* **2018**, *190*, 88–97. [CrossRef]
83. Littlefield, L.G.; Colyer, S.P.; Joiner, E.E.; DuFrain, R.J. Sister Chromatid Exchanges in Human Lymphocytes Exposed to Ionizing Radiation during G0. *Radiat. Res.* **1979**, *78*, 514–521. [CrossRef]
84. Morgan, W.F.; Crossen, P.E. X Irradiation and Sister Chromatid Exchange in Cultured Human Lymphocytes. *Environ. Mutagen.* **1980**, *2*, 149–155. [CrossRef]
85. Ballarini, F.; Altieri, S.; Bortolussi, S.; Carante, M.; Giroletti, E.; Protti, N. The Role of DNA Cluster Damage and Chromosome Aberrations in Radiation-Induced Cell Killing: A Theoretical Approach. *Radiat. Prot. Dosim.* **2015**, *166*, 75–79. [CrossRef] [PubMed]
86. Carrano, A.V. Chromosome Aberrations and Radiation-Induced Cell Death: II. Predicted and Observed Cell Survival. *Mutat. Res./Fundam. Mol. Mech. Mutagen.* **1973**, *17*, 355–366. [CrossRef]

Journal of *Personalized Medicine*

MDPI

Review

Prediction of the Acute or Late Radiation Toxicity Effects in Radiotherapy Patients Using Ex Vivo Induced Biodosimetric Markers: A Review

Volodymyr Vinnikov [1,*], Manoor Prakash Hande [2], Ruth Wilkins [3], Andrzej Wojcik [4], Eduardo Zubizarreta [5] and Oleg Belyakov [5,*]

1 S.P. Grigoriev Institute for Medical Radiology and Oncology, National Academy of Medical Science of Ukraine, 61024 Kharkiv, Ukraine

2 Department of Physiology, Yong Loo Lin School of Medicine, National University of Singapore, MD9, 2 Medical Drive, Singapore 117593, Singapore; phsmph@nus.edu.sg

3 Consumer and Clinical Radiation Protection Bureau, Health Canada, 775 Brookfield Road, Ottawa, ON K1A 1C1, Canada; ruth.wilkins@canada.ca

4 Centre for Radiation Protection Research, MBW Department, Stockholm University, Svante Arrhenius väg 20C, Room 515, 10691 Stockholm, Sweden; andrzej.wojcik@su.se

5 Section of Applied Radiation Biology and Radiotherapy, Division of Human Health, Department of Nuclear Sciences and Applications, International Atomic Energy Agency, Vienna International Centre, P.O. Box 100, 1400 Vienna, Austria; E.Zubizarreta@iaea.org

* Correspondence: vlad.vinnikov@ukr.net (V.V.); O.Belyakov@iaea.org (O.B.); Tel.: +38-057-725-5013 (V.V.); +43-1-2600-21667 (O.B.)

Received: 2 November 2020; Accepted: 11 December 2020; Published: 16 December 2020

check for updates

Abstract: A search for effective methods for the assessment of patients' individual response to radiation is one of the important tasks of clinical radiobiology. This review summarizes available data on the use of ex vivo cytogenetic markers, typically used for biodosimetry, for the prediction of individual clinical radiosensitivity (normal tissue toxicity, NTT) in cells of cancer patients undergoing therapeutic irradiation. In approximately 50% of the relevant reports, selected for the analysis in peer-reviewed international journals, the average ex vivo induced yield of these biodosimetric markers was higher in patients with severe reactions than in patients with a lower grade of NTT. Also, a significant correlation was sometimes found between the biodosimetric marker yield and the severity of acute or late NTT reactions at an individual level, but this observation was not unequivocally proven. A similar controversy of published results was found regarding the attempts to apply G_2- and γH2AX foci assays for NTT prediction. A correlation between ex vivo cytogenetic biomarker yields and NTT occurred most frequently when chromosome aberrations (not micronuclei) were measured in lymphocytes (not fibroblasts) irradiated to relatively high doses (4–6 Gy, not 2 Gy) in patients with various grades of late (not early) radiotherapy (RT) morbidity. The limitations of existing approaches are discussed, and recommendations on the improvement of the ex vivo cytogenetic testing for NTT prediction are provided. However, the efficiency of these methods still needs to be validated in properly organized clinical trials involving large and verified patient cohorts.

Keywords: radiosensitivity; biodosimetry; chromosome aberrations; micronuclei; normal tissue toxicity; radiotherapy; predictive tests

1. Introduction

Radiotherapy (RT) is one of the most effective treatments for cancer. However, it is technically impossible to concentrate the impact of ionizing radiation exclusively on tumors, thus normal tissues, which are included into the treatment plan, are unavoidably exposed [1]. RT is not specific to cancer cells, and radiation-induced cytotoxic effects occur both in the tumor and in normal tissues. The "mode of action" of RT towards tumors and normal tissues, and the respective reasons for the need for well-targeted treatment that delivers the lowest dose possible to the normal tissues and organs, are fully described in special literature [1,2].

In RT there is a wide variation in the reaction of normal tissues, and in many situations, the severity of these reactions limits the dose of RT that can be administered to the tumor [3]. Well documented clinical experience shows that comprehensive normal tissue reactions occur due to differences in individual normal tissue sensitivity. If such variation in normal tissue reactions is due to differences in intrinsic cellular radiosensitivity, it should be possible to predict the former based on the measurement of the latter [4]. Ideally, results of such testing would provide a basis for personalized treatment, i.e., individualizing RT schemes [5–16]. Tactics were suggested long ago and include: (i) the identification of rare cases of extreme hyper-radiosensitivity, for which RT should be avoided and replaced by surgery and/or chemotherapy; (ii) the reduction of the total RT dose or the use of alternative fractionation scheme in 'overreacting' patients with elevated risk of severe normal tissue complication; and (iii) the escalation of the RT dose for the remaining 'radioresistant' patients to enhance the tumor control without an increase in complications [5,6,14]. The goal is strategically valuable because in many cases the individualized RT prescriptions would lead to an increased local tumor control and cure, with unchanged or improved normal tissue complication rates and higher quality life for the patient.

Many studies were carried out in order to establish whether normal cell radiosensitivity correlates with the grade of normal tissue toxicity (NTT) in RT patients [17–23]. Progress in this research, however, has been hampered by the difficulty in the translation of adverse reactions from the clinic to the laboratory. There is still no unified system for describing normal tissue reactions, and there is still no standard terminology to compare the severity of reactions in different normal tissues. Data comparisons between different radiotherapy centres are complicated by the variety of descriptions of these reactions which are difficult to quantify. It took about 20 years for the most pragmatic terminology proposed in the field of normal tissue radiosensitivity [7] to receive a comprehensive molecular and biochemical explanation [24,25], which only recently has begun to be actively explored in the theory and practice of radiation oncology [20].

In the past 30 years there were many studies that have shown some correlation between ex vivo normal cell radiosensitivity and tissue response to RT, but often these initial conclusions were challenged by the results of larger investigations. In these reports, mainly functional tests such as clonogenic, cell survival or DNA repair assays were applied to determine parameters of cellular radiosensitivity. In addition, several biochemical or molecular end-points have been tested experimentally with the hope of developing systems capable of predicting normal tissue effects to RT. It has become evident that the risk of developing side-effects is predominantly influenced by genetic factors, presumably those regulating DNA repair and relevant pathways [13–16,26–32]. Despite huge efforts and long-term research, the real progress in this area has been achieved only recently, when 'big data' became available in the framework of large-scale, international projects devoted to the validation of suggested biomarkers of the normal tissue radiotoxicity for clinical use [16,17,20,22,23,25,33–35]. Working-out and validation of molecular genetic predictors of radiosensitivity were carried out by consolidated efforts of scientific consortiums in the framework of international programs and projects: EURATOM, Multidisciplinary European Low-Dose Initiative of the European Joint Programme for the Integration of Radiation Protection Research (MELODI/CONCERT), RadGenomics,"Genetic Predictors of Adverse Radiotherapy" (Gene-PARE), "Genetic Pathways for the Prediction of the Effects of Irradiation" (GENEPI), "Assessment of Polymorphisms for Predicting the Effects of Radiotherapy" (RAPPER) or the most recent "Validating Predictive Models and Biomarkers of Radiotherapy Toxicity to Reduce Side-Effects and Improve Quality of Life in Cancer Survivors" (REQUITE) [22,23,26,33–35].

Among functional ex vivo assays there is a particular set of biomarkers, which bridges categories of radiation response and genetics. This is radiation-induced cytogenetic (chromosomal) damage, suitable for quantitative analysis and thus applicable to biological dosimetry, i.e., expressing the radiation damage yield in terms of the accumulated radiation dose, considering 'by default' the individual radiosensitivity [19]. Unlike molecular predictors based on single nucleotide polymorphisms (SNP) or constitutional gene expression, cytogenetic assays may help to evaluate the radiosensitivity according to the dose and the genetic status.

Some researchers have used cytogenetic methods in this way, but the overall outcomes of these studies appear to be quite controversial. Despite an appreciable number of relevant publications, the analysis of such reports is complicated by variations in the experimental design, end-points andthe ex vivo exposure system used, and also by the heterogeneity of patient groups and normal tissue damage evaluated in these studies. To date, none of the suggested biomarkers has been validated for clinical use as a predictor of the NTT.

The lack of robust approaches to the use of radiation biomarkers for radiation oncology is especially surprising against the background of the growing number of the specialized biodosimetry laboratories in the world in the last decade. That was recognized as a serious problem by the International Atomic Energy Agency (IAEA), and to overcome it the IAEA launched the Coordinated Research Project E35010 MEDBIODOSE, in which the improvement of the methodology of NTT prediction by the measurement of ex vivo cytogenetic damage in patients' cells comprises an important research task [36,37]. Also, the IAEA organized and coordinated the work of the group of international experts, who performed an extensive analysis of available data on the various aspects of clinical applications of biodosimetry methods. That resulted in the IAEA Human Health Series Report [38], now being prepared for publication. This current article is the supplementary part of the IAEA Human Health Series Report, being focused specifically on the application of biodosimetric markers to test cell radiosensitivity ex vivo in trying to predict NTT in RT patients, along with a discussion of limitations of these approaches. This review is addressed simultaneously to clinical radiation oncologists and radiobiologists focused on biodosimetry to stimulate their interest to collaboration.

2. A Brief Overview of Markers Used for the Cytogenetic Biodosimetry

The methodology of radiation biodosimetry has been developed in radiation protection and radiation medicine specifically to deal with scenarios of uncontrolled, accidental overexposure, for which a physical dose reconstruction is unavailable or uncertain. The main principle of the biodosimetry is the estimation of absorbed radiation dose by referring the yield of biomarkers in vivo measured in an exposed person to an appropriate dose response, generated in vitro [39].

The list of necessary characteristics of dosimetric biomarkers includes their specificity to radiation exposure, a clear dose response for a wide range of doses, a possibility to produce a calibration in vitro, and a capability to detect and quantify the heterogeneity of the dose distribution in the human body. Other important traits include responsiveness to the radiation linear energy transfer (LET) factor and an accountable dependence on the protraction or fractionation of exposure and time delay between irradiation and analysis.

Among many biochemical, biophysical, cellular and clinical end-points, tested as potential radiation dosimetric markers, only a few were found to be suitable for this purpose, and all are based on cytogenetic damage observed in metaphase spreads of cultured human cells. These include:

- dicentrics and centric rings (Dic+CR);
- stable chromosome exchanges (mainly, translocations (Tn)) and complex chromosomal rearrangements (CCR) visualized using a fluorescence in situ hybridization (FISH) technique;
- fragments and/or rings quantified among prematurely condensed chromosomes (PCC);
- micronuclei (MN) scored in cytokinesis blocked binucleated cells.

Dic+CR, PCC rings and fragments and MN are considered as 'unstable' biomarkers, because they are eliminated through cell divisions. The essential proportion of Tn are transmissible to daughter cells, but not all of them. Therefore the quantitative measurement of the radiation-induced yield of cytogenetic damage must be restricted to the 1st post-radiation mitosis. That is achieved by identifying the cell cycle number of each metaphase, if Bromodeoxiuridine (BrdU) is added to a cell culture. This technique is not applicable to the MN assay, thus scoring of micronuclei must be carried out in binucleated cells only.

Also, phosphorylated histones γH2AX, representing sites of DNA double strand break repair in interphase lymphocyte nuclei (γH2AX foci), can be used for biodosimetric purposes, but with strong limitations on time scale. The γH2AX foci appear within minutes of exposure and increase until about 1 h, after which they decline back to near background levels. This rapid change limits their ability for accurate dosimetry but still allows their use for an indication of exposure and their applicability for the radiosensitivity assessment testing in well-controlled experimental conditions.

Human peripheral blood lymphocytes (PBL) are now preferred for assays based on radiation biomarkers, particularly, as an alternative to fibroblasts, because of the ease of obtaining samples and the rapid results that can be generated. Technical aspects of the cytogenetic biodosimetry are well refined [39,40] and have reached the level of the international standard (see [37] for review). Advanced cytogenetic biodosimetry methods provide the results formalized as a mean dose of radiation of a certain quality absorbed in a certain volume fraction of lymphocytes, both values supplied with respective confidence intervals.

All existing external RT regimens, including total and partial body irradiation, most therapeutic radionuclides and diagnostic radiology procedures cause a considerable increase of the yield of bioindicators used in biodosimetry in patients' PBL (summarized data of the literature on this issue will be published as the IAEA Human Health Series Report [38]).

The use of radiation dose response biomarkers for practical purposes in radiation oncology and medical radiology has several clear advantages. These markers are recognized as measures of genotoxicity due to their relationship to DNA-damage response and, therefore, may be used for direct assessment of the risk of radiation-related pathology, including both deterministic and stochastic effects. All validated biomarkers show strong dependence on radiation dose, dose rate, irradiated volume [39] and thus theoretically can respond to the impact of radiation modifiers. Therefore, such dosimetric biomarkers can be considered as an effective tool for quantifying individualized radiation load in patients, either in vivo or ex vivo.

The theory for the application of cytogenetic damage for the prediction of normal tissue response to radiation is based on three main points. First, chromosomal aberrations (ChA) are the direct outcome of DNA repair, which is one of the core determinants of cellular radiosensitivity. Studies on DNA repair-deficient cells have demonstrated that any alterations in DNA repair genes or malfunctions of their proteins can have a significant impact on the ChA yield [41–43]. Second, some ChA (e.g., unbalanced exchanges and fragments) are the direct cause of mitotic cell death [44,45] and are, therefore, mechanistically linked to clonogenic cell survival [46,47]. Consequently, it can be expected that ChA (or their precursors—DNA breaks, or their products—MN) would also correlate with the tissue repair maintained by cell proliferation, and hence with the time of on-set and the severity of radiation-induced NTT. Third, in studies on cells of mono- and disigotic twins a significant hereditary impact on the manifestation of individual cellular radiosensitivity had been demonstrated for various end-points, including ChA or MN [29,48–55].

Combining all three reasons, the extrapolation from the cytogenetic damage induction, as a genetically controlled trait, to a radiosensitive phenotype seems to be reasonable.

3. Review of Existing Studies

Attempts to apply biodosimetric markers to the prognosis of normal tissue response to RT have been made many times. The main hypothesis tested in this research was that cancer patients with a higher yield of ex vivo radiation-induced cytogenetic damage in lymphocytes or other cells are more likely to develop RT-related morbidity. Three main biodosimetry end-points were used forex vivo testing of the patients' cells: Dic+CR, MN, and Tn or CCR visualized by FISH. Occasionally PCC methods were also applied for assessing chromosome damage, and in recent years the quantification of DNA double strand breaks (DSBs) by γH2AX foci analysis has been actively introduced into practice. In these studies, typically, cells from patients are irradiated ex vivo to X-rays or γ-rays with different radiation doses and dose rates. Some researchers have used several biodosimetric techniques in one study, e.g., dicentrics, translocations and γH2AX foci, in an attempt to determine the best end-point for predicting clinical radiosensitivity [56–58]. Among various cellular test-systems used for the assessment of chromosomal radiosensitivity, human PBL appear to be the most appropriate due the lack of a need for long cell culture periods, standardized culturing conditions and a well-developed methodology of cytogenetic marker quantification.

3.1. Cytogenetic Expertise of Individual Cases Showing Elevated Normal Tissue Toxicity (NTT)

In clinical practice of radiation oncology, the unexpected, extreme tissue reactions are still frequently attributed to the malfunction of radiotherapy devices or erroneous dosimetry. In such situations expertise is needed to clarify the reason: the accident or patient's intrinsic over-reactive status. It should be noted that, from the beginning, cytogenetic analyses were highly informative for confirming the radiosensitivity post factum in individual cases as identified by clinical symptoms. As a rule, patients with abnormal tissue radiosensitivity displayed a higher outcome of ChA per unit dose induced in lymphocytes by ex vivo irradiation [59–62]. Thus, radiation biomarkers can be used effectively for revealing a possible mechanism of radiosensitivity, particularly a malfunction of the DNA repair machinery involved in the ChA formation. Results from cytogenetic testing have led to an active exploration of tests based on quantifying DNA damage repair functionality, primarily the kinetics of DNA DSB, assessed by specific methods like γH2AX foci, which will be discussed later.

Importantly, elevated rates of ChA induced in vitro have been observed in clinically radiosensitive patients who did not have any constitutional chromosomal abnormalities [59], known genetic disorders with increased radiosensitivity [60,62], or apparent hereditary chromosome instability, cancer prone syndromes [61]. The relationship between the two latter categories is not simple. Genetic syndromes, which are linked to radiosensitivity, are generally associated with high cancer risk, while patients with syndromes linked to increased rates of tumor occurrence, are not necessarily have radiosensitive cells or tissues [18]. Nevertheless, many authors consider a high number of ex vivo induced ChA or MN as a hallmark of a genetically based radio-sensitive phenotype in patients showing enhanced tissue radiosensitivity.

3.2. Group Studies of Ex Vivo Cytogenetic Response in Cells of Patients with Various NTT Grades

In contrast to individualized studies, which focused on one or few patients, those cytogenetic predictive assays, which were performed in larger, randomly formed groups of patients and especially in a prospective, screening mode, gave rather ambiguous results.

Tables 1 and 2 summarize briefly the data obtained by different research groups in their attempts to correlate G_0 cytogenetic radiosensitivity with normal tissue reactions in RT patients. The non-exhaustive list includes 16 reports based on ChA analysis (Table 1) and 16 studies using MN test (Table 2). It can be seen that the study design varied considerably between laboratories. The most common tumor location studied was breast cancer, with head and neck, prostate and gynecological cancers being the next most popular. About half of the publications (17 out of 32) presented retrospective studies, while the prospective studies were less frequent (11 out 32), and 4 reports contained both types of studies. Furthermore, early/acute RT reactions of normal tissues and organs were considered in 9 studies, late NTT toxicity were the focus of interest in 12 reports, and 11 publications contained data on both categories of clinical effects.

Table 1. Ex vivo tests for normal tissue toxicity (NTT) prediction: chromosome aberrations in human blood lymphocytes.

Reference	Patients and Study Type	Test System and Ex Vivo Exposure Details	Normal Tissue Toxicity	Correlation
Dicentrics and fragments—conventional analysis in metaphases or prematurely condensed chromosome (PCC)spreads				
Jones et al., 1995 [63]	Retrospective; 16 breast cancer patients. Exaggerated acute or late radiation reaction of normal tissues after radiotherapy RT; no positive control (i.e., matched RT patients without acute or late reactions)	LDR [1] (0.0031 Gy min^{-1}) and HDR [2] (0.17 Gy min^{-1}) irradiation to 3 Gy γ-rays	Early reactions: erythema, moist desquamation. Late complications: fibrosis, telangiectasia.	Abnormal chromosomal radiosensitivity was found in 5 of 7 patients with excessive early skin reactions. The mean ChA [3] yield after LDR for early over-reactions was significantly higher than for healthy controls and average sparing was less. LDR-induced yields were above the control range in 2 out of 10 patients with late complications. The mean yield for late over-reactors was not significantly above that of controls. Also, one early overreactor and one late overreactor had LDR aberration yields below the control range.
Kondrashova et al., 1997 [64]	Retrospective; 12 patients with different cancers, all with late radiation skin damage, studied 0.4–31 years after RT (no positive control, i.e., matched RT patients without acute or late reactions)	Acute irradiation (0.2 Gy min^{-1}) to 2 Gy γ-rays	Late radiation skin injuries (grade not specified)	In 3 out of 12 patients the frequency of ex vivo induced chromosome type fragments significantly exceeded the control value.
Borgmann et al., 2002 [65]	Retrospective; 16 pair-wise matched head and neck cancer patients, exhibiting maximum differences (8 grade 1 vs. 8 grade 3) in late normal tissue reactions 2–7 years after RT.	Acute irradiation (2 Gy min^{-1}) to 2, 4 and 6 Gy X-rays. Conventional dicentrics and 'fusion' PCC methods.	Fibrosis, telangiectasia, mucositis and xerostomia assessed using the RTOG [4] score	At 6 Gy ex vivo irradiation the mean yield of aberrations and PCC fragments in PBL [5] of overreacting patients was significantly higher than in cells from patients with mild reactions and healthy controls. The pair-wise match of patients revealed that in all except one case the grade 1 individual had less ex vivo aberrations than the grade 3 counterpart.

Table 1. *Cont.*

Reference	Patients and Study Type	Test System and Ex Vivo Exposure Details	Normal Tissue Toxicity	Correlation
Hoeller et al., 2003 [66]	Retrospective; 86 breast cancer patients with or without late fibrosis 5–17 years after RT.	Acute irradiation (2 Gy min^{-1}) to 6 Gy X-rays	Fibrosis, LENT-SOMA [6] score, grades 0, 1, 2 or 3	Patients with high cellular radiosensitivity (ex vivo yield > mean + 1 standard deviation) showed a higher annual rate forfibrosisthan patients with low or intermediate radiosensitivity (3.6% versus 1.6% per year).
Borgmann et al., 2008 [67]	Prospective; (A) 51 patients with different tumor sites, and (B) 87 breast cancer patients.	Acute irradiation (2 Gy min^{-1}) to 3 or 6 Gy X-rays. Culturing for 72 h with noBrdU [7] control!	Acute reactions assessed using the RTOG score	The fraction of patients with Grade 2–3 reaction increased with increasing individual radiosensitivity, measured by the yield of chromosome fragments at 6 Gy.
Tang et al., 2008 [68]	Retrospective; pair-wise matched nasopharyngeal carcinoma patients with (26 persons) or without (26 persons) radiation encephalo-pathy	Acute irradiation (2 Gy min^{-1}) to 6 Gy photons (6 MeV linear accelerator)	Radiation encephalopathy assessed using the RTOG score	The mean aberration yield ex vivo in patients with Grade 3–4 reaction was higher than that in patients with Grade 1–2 reactions and controls. Patients with high cellularradiosensitivity (ex vivo yield > mean + 1 standard deviation) showed shorter latency for the encephalopathy development compared to those with a low or intermediate radiosensitivity.
Chua et al., 2011 [69]	Retrospective; 14 pair-wise matched breast cancer patients (7 cases with late radiation skin damage and 7 controls with no damage)	Acute irradiation (0.5 Gy min^{-1}) to 6 Gy X-rays. Culturing for 72 h with no BrdU control!	Scores of severe radiation-induced change (cases) or very little/no change (controls) in the breast on photos taken before RT and at 2 and 5 years post-RT	In 5 out of 7 clinically radiosensitive cases the total yield of aberrations ex vivo remarkably exceeded its top level in the matched control group. The mean yields of dicentrics and excess acentrics ex vivo were statistically higher in cases than in controls.
Padjas et al., 2012 [70]	Prospective; 35 patients with breast cancer and 34 with gynaecological cancer	Acute irradiation (2 Gy min^{-1}) to 2 Gy photons (6 MeV linear accelerator)	Early and late side effects assessed using the RTOG score	No correlation was observed between the results of the cellular radiosensitivity assay and the severity of side effects.

Table 1. *Cont.*

Reference	Patients and Study Type	Test System and Ex Vivo Exposure Details	Normal Tissue Toxicity	Correlation
Beaton et al., 2013 [56]	Retrospective; 10 prostate cancer patients with grade 3 late radiation proctitis and 20 matched patients with grade 0 proctitis.	Acute irradiation (1.7 Gy min^{-1}) to 6 Gy X-rays. Culturing for 72 h with BrdU control.	Late proctitis assessed using the RTOG score	The mean yields of dicentrics and excess acentric fragments were statistically higher in clinically radiosensitive patients than in the control group. A sufficient proportion of Grade 3 patients showed the induced acentric yield above the upper limit for this end-point observed in Grade 0 group.
FISH-detectable breaks, Tn and/or CCR in metaphases or PCC spreads				
Dunst et al., 1995 [60]	Retrospective; 16 patients (12 breast cancer and 4 other cancers), including 4 persons with increased clinical radiosensitivity and 12 with normal tolerance to RT, examined 1 to 108 months after treatment.	Acute irradiation to 0.7 or 2 Gy X-rays from 6 MeV linear accelerator. Radiation-induced breaks per mitoses assessed by FISH/CISS [8] technique	1 severe acute reaction in bladder; 1 acute skin reaction with subsequent fibrosis of breast; 1 radiation myelitis; 1 severe acute reaction after mediastinal irradiation	4 patients with increased clinical radiosensitivity showed statistically increased chromosomal radiation-induced damage as compared to the 12 patients with normal radiation tolerance at both ex vivo radiation doses.
Neubauer et al., 1997 [71]	Prospective group: 33 breast cancer patients; retrospective group: 28 breast cancer patients and 19 other tumor locations. In total 66 patients (some investigated before and after RT)	Acute irradiation (2.2 Gy min^{-1}) to 0.7 or 2 Gy X-rays from 6 MeV linear accelerator. Radiation-induced breaks and CCR per mitoses assessed by FISH/CISS technique	Acute effects assessed using the WHO [9] grading system and late side effects assessed using the RTOG score	The proportion of breaks, involved in CCR, after 0.7 Gy ex vivo, was remarkably higher in 27 samples patients with high toxic reactions, compared with 20 samples from patients with average clinical reactions and 19 healthy controls. The yield of mitoses with CCR was increased proportionally to the clinical reactivity at both ex vivo radiation doses, but the tendency was especially pronounced at 2 Gy.
Dunst et al., 1998 [72]	Prospective group: 26 patients; retrospective group 26 patients. In total 52 patients: 41 with breast cancer, 11—other sites (lung, head and neck prostate, bladder, rectal cancer and Hodgkin's disease).	Acute irradiation to 0.7 or 2 Gy X-rays (6 MeV linear accelerator). Radiation-induced breaks per mitoses assessed by FISH/CISS technique	Acute effects assessed using the WHO grading system and late side effects assessed using the RTOG score	A significantly higher number of chromosomal breaks were found after both radiation doses ex vivo in lymphocytes of 9 patients with severe or extreme radiation reaction of normal tissues as compared to 43 patients with no or mild to moderate radiation reactions.

Table 1. *Cont.*

Reference	Patients and Study Type	Test System and Ex Vivo Exposure Details	Normal Tissue Toxicity	Correlation
Keller et al., 2004 [73]	Retrospective group: 5 patients with severe radiation-induced late effects of Grade ≥3, 18–76 months after RT for cancers of different locations, versus 11 healthy individuals; no positive control, (i.e., matched RT patients without late reactions).	Acute irradiation (2.2 Gy min^{-1}) to 0.7 or 2 Gy X-rays from 6 MeV linear accelerator. Radiation- induced FISH-detectable breaks and CCR, dicentrics, translocations, excess acentrics per mitoses assessed by FISH/CISS technique	Late effects assessed using the RTOG score	The ratio of the mean yields in radiosensitive patients to that of in healthy donors after 2 Gy ex vivo varied from 1.2 to 1.8 for breaks, translocations, dicentrics and excess acentrics, and increased to 3.2 for CCRs. The "frequency of breaks per metaphase", "CCR per metaphase" and "translocations per metaphase" appeared to be the most suitable parameters to detect a difference in chromosomal sensitivity between healthy and clinically radiosensitive individuals.
Huber et al., 2011 [74]	Prospective group: 47 breast cancer patients. Acute skin reactions: 4 patients showed grade 0, 30 patients grade 1, 12 patients grade 2, and 1 patient grade 3.	Acute irradiation (0.5 Gy min^{-1}) to 3 Gy X-rays. Radiation-induced FISH-detectable dicentrics, Tn and colour junctions assessed by FISH technique (Dic were counted only in painted chromosomes)	Acute effects scored according to the NCI-CTC [10] scale. Also according to the time of the skin reaction occurrence, patients were divided into "early", "in between reaction" and "late reaction".	Three out of 4 patients with increased chromosomal radiosensitivity showed either more severe side effects (1 patient) or early onset of the skin reactions (2 patients). A significant overall correlation was found between the ex vivo frequencies of Tn and the latency of side effects of the skin. With a definite cut-off for Tn yield, 22 of the 30 short latency patients were correctly detected (73.3% sensitivity) and 11 of the 17 longer latency patients (were correctly assigned (64.7% specificity).
Beaton et al., 2013 [57]	Retrospective group: 10 prostate cancer patients with Grade 3 late proctitis versus matched 10 prostate cancer patients with no proctitis.	Acute irradiation (1.7 Gy min^{-1}) to 4 Gy X-rays. Radiation-induced, FISH-detectable ChA and colour junctions	Late proctitis assessed using RTOG/EORTC Late Toxicity Scale	After 4 Gy ex vivo irradiation, the clinically radiosensitive group had significantly higher rates of chromosome damage in the number of colour junctions per cell, the number of deletions per cell and the number of dicentrics per cell, compared to proctitis-free control.

Table 1. *Cont.*

Reference	Patients and Study Type	Test System and Ex Vivo Exposure Details	Normal Tissue Toxicity	Correlation
Schmitz et al., 2013 [75]	Retrospective group: 10 prostate cancer patients with acute (0 or 2 months after RT) or late side effect (16 months after RT) versus 10 patients without severe side effects versus 11 healthy controls	Acute irradiation (0.74 Gy min^{-1}) to 0.5, 1.0 and 2.0 Gy ^{137}Cs γ-rays. Culturing for 72 h with no BrdU control! Radiation-induced FISH-detectable dicentrics, Tn, centric rings, excess acentrics per mitoses assessed by FISH technique	Early and late severe side effects assessed with the validated Expanded Prostate Cancer Index Composite questionnaire (EPIC)	Prostate cancer patients with and without side effects cannot be distinguished from healthy donors based on the mean aberration yield after ex vivo irradiation. The distribution pattern of the aberrations per donor did not differ in each donor group after exposure to any dose ex vivo.

[1] LDR—Low dose-rate. [2] HDR—High dose-rate. [3] ChA—chromosome aberrations. [4] RTOG (also RTOG/EORTC)—The Radiation Therapy Oncology Group and the European Organization for Research and Treatment of Cancer criteria. [5] PBL—peripheral blood lymphocytes. [6] LENT-SOMA—The Late Effects in Normal Tissue—Subjective, Objective, Management, Analytic criteria. [7] BrdU—Bromodeoxiuridine, a reagent typically used in radiation cytogenetics for the control of the number of cell cycles passed by a particular cell in culture [39].[8] CISS—Chromosomal in Situ Suppression Hybridization technique. [9] WHO—World Health Organization. [10] NCI-CTC—Common Toxicity Criteria of the United States National Cancer Institute.

Table 2. Ex vivo testsfor NTT prognoses: micronuclei in human blood lymphocytes as the end-point.

Reference	Patients and Study Type	Test System and Ex Vivo Exposure Details	Normal Tissue Toxicity	Correlation
Rached et al., 1998 [76]	Retrospective group: 15 patients with various cancers experiencing severe acute reaction of normal tissue, 15 non-matched cancer patients without reactions and 15 healthy donors.	Acute irradiation (1.08 Gy min^{-1}) to 4 Gy X-rays.	Mucositis, diarrhea, epitheliolysis, proctitis	There was no difference between cancer patients with or without acute reactions in normal tissues in their MN scores after ex vivo irradiation.
Barber et al., 2000 [77]	Breast cancer patients. Prospective group: 123 patients studied before RT, 116 tested with the HDR assay, 73 with the LDR assay. Retrospective group: 8–14 years after RT, 47 tested with the HDR assay, 26 with the LDR assay.	HDR assay: Acute irradiation (3.0 Gy min^{-1}) to 3.5 Gy ^{137}Cs γ-rays. LDR assay: protracted irradiation (dose rate 0.15 cGy min^{-1}, total exposure time 38.8 h) to 3.5 Gy ^{137}Cs γ-rays. Throughout the LDR irradiation period the samples were maintained at 37 °C in 5% CO_2 atmosphere. Culturing for 90 h!	Acute skin reactions scored as minimum erythema, moderate erythema or severe erythema/moist desquamation/edema. Late effects assessed according to the LENT-SOMA	In the prospective group with and without acute reactions there was no significant difference between clinically hyper-sensitive (HR) and non-HR patients for the MN yield induced ex vivo either at HDR or LDR. Regarding late effects: mean HDR and LDR MN scores were higher in 4 patients with severe telangiectasia than in those with normal reactions and 8 patients with severe fibrosis had higher HDR MN scores than the normal reactors. However, the HDR assay's sensitivity for detecting HR cases was 0/6 for acute reactions, 4/8 for late fibrosis, 2/9 for breast retraction and 2/4 for telangiectasia. For LDR assay's sensitivity that was 0/2, 0/5, 0/3 and 2/4, respectively.

Table 2. *Cont.*

Reference	Patients and Study Type	Test System and Ex Vivo Exposure Details	Normal Tissue Toxicity	Correlation
Słonina et al., 2000 [78]	Prospective group: 12 cervical cancer patients and 11 head and neck cancer patients. Retrospective group: 9 cervical cancer patients and 1 head and neck cancer patient, all late reactors (4–14 years after RT).	Acute irradiation (0.73 Gy min^{-1}) to 0, 2.0 and 4.0 Gy ^{60}Co γ-rays.	Acute and late reactions were assessed according to RTOG/EORTC grading system for 8–50 months in prospective group.	There was no correlation between the radiosensitivity, assessed as induced ex vivo MN yield, and acute or late clinically observed side effects in RT patients.
Lee et al., 2000 [79]	Prospective group: 8 prostate cancer patients. Blood taken before RT and during RT.	Before RT: Acute irradiation (0.8 Gy min^{-1}) to 0, 1.0, 2.0, 3.0 and 4.0 Gy ^{137}Cs γ-rays. During RT: Acute irradiation (0.8 Gy min^{-1}) to 0 and 2.0 ^{137}Cs γ-rays.	Acute side effects: cystitis, diarrhea	In 2 of 3 patients with Grade I RT-induced early side effects the MN yield in PBL induced by ex vivo irradiation before RT was significantly higher than in the other patients without RT-induced side effects. For the second blood samples obtained during the second half of RT course the MN yields in PBL induced by 2 Gy ex vivo irradiation had no predictive value.
Lee et al., 2003 [80]	Prospective group: 38 prostate cancer patients: over-reactors (OR, 13 patients with Grade ≥2 RT-related morbidity) and average reactors (AR, 25 patients with Grade 0–1 RT-related morbidity). Strict patient selection criteria.	Acute irradiation (0.9 Gy min^{-1}) to 0, 1.0, 2.0, 3.0 and 4.0 Gy ^{137}Cs γ-rays.	Gastrointestinal (GI) and genitourinary (GU) morbidity assessed according to the RTOG criteria.	The averaged dose response for ex vivo induced MN was remarkably more intensive in OR than in AR; the differences in MN yield were highly significant at doses ≥2 Gy. Also, for both AR and OR groupss, the inter-individual variation of the ex vivo dose response of MN yields was greater than that of the intra-individual variation.
Widel et al., 2003 [81]	Prospective group: 55 cervical carcinoma patients. Verified group due to strict patient selection criteria. Control group—25 healthy female donors.	Acute irradiation (0.8–1.0 Gy min^{-1}) to 0, 2.0 and 4.0 Gy ^{60}Co γ-rays.	Acute reactions during RT and up to 3 months after RT assessed by the Common Toxicity Criteria of the National Cancer Institute and RTOG. The late effects were classified according to the RTOG/ EORTC grading system	In lymphocytes irradiated ex vivo to 4 Gy the mean yield of MN was significantly higher in samples from patients, who suffered from acute and/or late normal tissue reactions, than in those from patients with no reactions, but in healthy donors the value fit in between two patients groups. A significant correlation was found between individual MN yield at 4 Gy and the severity of acute reactions and late reactions. However, the essential overlap between the distributions of individual MN frequencies in patients with high-grade and low-grade reactions does not clearly allow identification of persons at risk by MN test.

Table 2. *Cont.*

Reference	Patients and Study Type	Test System and Ex Vivo Exposure Details	Normal Tissue Toxicity	Correlation
Bustos et al., 2002 [82]; Di Giorgio et al., 2004 [83]	Retrospective group: 19 head andneck cancer patients 6–18 months after RT	Acute irradiation to 0 and 2.0 Gy ^{60}Co γ-rays.	"Late" reactions to RT: osteonecrosis, fibrosis and trismus	In 3 out of 4 patients, who had developed late reactions, the ex vivo induced MN yield was significantly higher than in lymphocytes from the rest of the patients. The individual cytogenetic response ex vivo showed a correlation with the maximum grade of late reactions.
Taghavi-Dehaghani et al., 2005 [84]	Retrospective group: 26 breast cancer patients, including 15 with acute reactions and 11 with late reactions (no positive control, i.e., matched RT patients without acute or late reactions). Time after RT not specified.	Acute irradiation to 0 and 4.0 Gy ^{60}Co γ-rays.	Early tissue damage: erythema, dry desquamation, moist desquamation. Late tissue damage: fibrosis, skin telangiectasia, pigmentation.	The mean yield of MN after 4 Gy ex vivo was significantly (1.6 times) higher in lymphocytes of patients with early reactions, than that of patients with late reactions.
Rzeszowska-Wolny et al., 2008 [85]	Prospective group: 34 head andneck cancer patients.	Acute irradiation (1.14 Gy min^{-1}) to 0, 2.0 and 4.0 Gy ^{60}Co γ-rays.	Acute reactions measured using the Dische scale	In a subgroup of 14 patients with a high level of induced residual DNA damage, measured using a 'comet' assay ex vivo, a statistical correlation occurred between the MN yield after 4 Gy ex vivoandacutetoxicity score.
Encheva et al., 2011 [86]	Prospective group: 23 cervical cancer and 17 endometrial cancer patients.	Acute irradiation (1.0 Gy min^{-1}) to 0 and 1.5 Gy ^{60}Co γ-rays.	Acute normal tissue reactions were graded according to the NCI-CTC for Adverse Events v.3.0.	Great variations in MN yield ex vivo were found, but no correlation occurred between cytogenetic effect and clinical radiosensitivity. The resultant conclusion is against a recommendation of ex vivo MN test for clinical use.
Finnon et al., 2012 [87]	Retrospective group: breast cancer patients with marked (31 cases) or mild (28 controls) late adverse reaction to adjuvant breast RT	Acute irradiation to 3.5 Gy X-rays. Cell culturing for 90 h!	Scores of severe radiation-induced change (cases) or very little/no change (controls) in the breast on photos taken before and after RT.	Significant inter-individual variations in radiation-induced MN were observed, but there was no evidence of a differential response in cases and controls in matched or unmatched analyses, e.g., variations in cytogenetic ex vivo radiosensitivity did not correlate with normal tissue response to RT.

Table 2. *Cont.*

Reference	Patients and Study Type	Test System and Ex Vivo Exposure Details	Normal Tissue Toxicity	Correlation
Vandevoorde et al., 2016 [88]	Retrospective group: 12 breast cancer patients expressing severe radiation toxicity matched to 12 controls with no or minimal reactions, with a follow-up for at least 3 years	Acute irradiation (0.14 Gy min^{-1}) to 5 doses from 0.2 to 3.0 Gy ^{60}Co γ-rays.	Late adverse reactions assessed by LENT-SOMA scale and by comparing standardized photographs pre- and post-RT resulting in an overall cosmetic score.	The average dose response curve of the ex vivo induced MN yield for cases lies significantly above the average dose response curve of the controls, and the coefficients of the LQ dose response do not overlap between cases and controls. However the shift in the dose response from case to control on an individual basis was not systematic, indicating no direct correlation of the MN induction with the clinical radiotoxic effects.
Batar et al., 2016 [89] Batar et al., 2018 [90]	Prospective group: 40 [89] and later on 100 [90] breast cancer patients, including 20 [89] or 50 [90] 'cases' with acute reactions (grades 2, 3 or 4) and 20 [89] or 50 [90] 'controls' with no or mild adverse.	Acute irradiation (1.0 Gy min^{-1}) to 0 and 2.0 Gy ^{60}Co γ-rays.	Acute normal tissue reactions were followed during 6 weeks after RT and graded using CTC: Grade: 0 (no adverse effect), 1 (mild adverse effect), 2 (moderate adverse effect), 3 (severe side effect) and 4 (life-threatening adverse effect).	The MN yield was higher in the group with acute reactions (2.10 ± 0.27) than in control patients (1.67 ± 0.20), but the difference was not statistically significant. There was no difference in the mean MN frequency between the group with acute reactions (6.8 ± 4.2) and controls (6.9 ± 2.6).
Guogytė et al., 2017 [91]	Prospective group: 4 prostate cancer patients and 1 uterine cancer patient.	Acute irradiation to 0 and 2.0 Gy X-rays.	Acute normal tissue reactions, including GI and GU were graded according to the RTOG/EORTC.	The ex vivo MN yield in 2 patients with Grade 1 side effects increases by 8% compared with that in 2 patients without side effects. The patient with Grade 2 side effects had the ex vivo MN yield 9% higher than that in Grade 0 case and 1% higher than in patients with Grade 1 side effects.
da Silva et al., 2020 [92]	Prospective group: 10 cervical cancer patients, including 3 patients treated with teletherapy alone and 7 receiving teletherapy and brachytherapy.	Acute irradiation (2 Gy min^{-1}) to 2.0 Gy X-rays on a linear accelerator.	Acute normal tissue reactions, that were developed in patients 5–10 days after starting the radiation treatment, were graded according to the RTOG.	The ex vivo MN yield showed a significant correlation with the RTOG score ($r = 0.96$). However, the baseline MN yield in non-irradiated cultures also had a significant correlation with the severity of adverse effects ($r = 0.86$). The re-analysis of the original data showed a strong association between MN yields in ex vivo irradiated and sham irradiated samples ($r = 0.90$) and very moderate correlation of the truly induced MN yield (the difference between irradiated and non-irradiated samples) with the toxicity score ($r = 0.44$). Actually, only 1 out of 3 patients with severe NTT can be identified confidently by the ex vivo induced MN yield.

Table 2. *Cont.*

Reference	Patients and Study Type	Test System and Ex Vivo Exposure Details	Normal Tissue Toxicity	Correlation
Chaouni et al., 2020 [93]	Retrospective group: 18 patients with Merkel Cell Carcinomas, including 9 patients with Grade ≤2 and 9 patients with Grade ≥3 NTT in skin. Exact time after RT not specified.	Acute irradiation (2 Gy min^{-1}) to 2.0 Gy and 10.0 Gy photons on 6 MeV linear accelerator.	Late skin reactions assessed according to RTOG/EORTC grading system.	Inverse correlation between the ex vivo induced MN yield and NTT. The difference between 0 Gy and 2.0 Gy points were 333 MN per 1000 BN in Grade ≤2 group and 218 MN per 1000 BN in Grade ≥3 group; between 0 Gy and 10.0 Gy that, respectively, were 2663 MN per 1000 BN and 854 MN per 1000 BN. The 3.1-fold difference between groups with Grades ≤2 and ≥3 NTT for the MN yield after 10 Gy was statistically significant.

In 6 studies, positive controls (i.e., matched patients with no normal tissue damage) were not specifically included, so that the ex vivo induced cytogenetic damage yield in overreacting patients was compared with that of healthy donor cells [63,64,73], or between overreactors with different NTT types [84], or with the yield in a single patient with no toxic reactions at the time of study [91,92]. Although such results have some academic interest, they cannot be fully used for analysis.

3.2.1. Efficacy of Different End-Points

Considering acute and late NTT effects separately, and excluding study [84] from the score, the distribution of the results in 41 analyzed datasets (22 with on ChA and 19 with MN data) is as follows. A positive correlation between cytogenetic damage induced in PBL ex vivo and clinical radiation toxicity grade was observed in 11 reports with acute reactions (6 using ChA and 5 using MN assay) and 14 reports involving late effects (10 using ChA and 4 using MN assay). In one of these studies, the correlation occurred in a subgroup of patients, initially selected for a high level of induced residual DNA damage measured using a 'comet' assay ex vivo. In this case, the MN test was a secondary discriminative tool within a multiparametric approach [85]. A significant correlation between the ex vivo frequencies of Tn and the latency of skin side effects but not with the grade of the effect was observed in another study [74]. Nevertheless, these results demonstrated a rather high sensitivity and specificity. In two reports claiming a positive correlation between the ex vivo MN yield and the severity of adverse NTT effects [91,92] both research groups did not subtract the background MN frequency from the yield observed in irradiated samples prior to correlation analysis, therefore the authors' conclusions are rendered suspect. Also, in one of the most recent studies the inverse (!) correlation was found between the NTT grades and MN yields induced by ex vivo radiation doses 2.0 and 10.0 Gy; no explanation for this phenomenon was provided [93].

The absence of a link between cytogenetic and clinical radiosensitivity was shown in 15 datasets. That included 6 studies based on ChA analysis: 2 reports contained respective data on acute effects, and 4 on late NTT. Among 9 observations based on MN assay, 6 were focused on acute and 3 on late NTT effects. Interestingly, one of the research groups, which found no correlation between the induced MN yields and acute NTT grades in breast cancer patients, reported quite different MN yields in their two consequent publications [89,90], and the reasons for such a discrepancy are unclear.

Thus, in general, the analysis of ChAs in conventionally stained or FISH-painted metaphases or PCC spreads appeared to be more suitable for clinical ex vivo irradiation tests compared to the MN assay. Among various types of chromosomal damage registered during the analysis, chromosome fragments (excess acentrics or PCC fragments) and color junctions or CCR detectable by FISH were the most sensitive ex vivo markers for acute NTT effects or late lesions.

No clear mechanistic explanation for the predictive ability of chromosome fragment-type breakage has been suggested yet. Meanwhile, the elevated numbers of CCR observed in metaphases of clinical over-reactors may be linked to defects in one or several of the cell-cycle checkpoints, which when functioning normally, prevent heavily damaged cells from entering mitosis [71].

Besides a compromised cell cycle regulation, cytogenetic radiation biomarkers, which are in the focus of current review, have strong mechanistic linkage to the complex interplay of several DNA DSB repair pathways, including their cell cycle-specific impairment, which causes a shift from the canonical non-homologous end-joining (NHEJ) or homologous recombination (HR) towards alternative, more error-prone mechanisms [94–96]. In line with this, it was shown that genes of both HR and NHEJ pathways in PBL of severe reacting patients were less induced by ex vivo irradiation in compare with that in patients without late reactions [97]. Obviously, acell cycle-dependent analysis of DSB repair may be valuable for the expression of clinical hypersensitivity to ionizing radiation, e.g., as shown by Zahnreich et al. [98]. However, the overall problem of the correlation between radiosensitivity and DSB repair is very broad, and its discussion is beyond the scope of our review.

3.2.2. The Role of Dose and Dose Rate of Ex Vivo Exposures

It should be noted, that in two studies using the MN test [77,87] and in one using the ChA test [75], which did not detect a predictive value of cytogenetics, the irradiated lymphocytes were cultured longer than is normally done according to biodosimetry standards [39] and without an indicator for cell cycle (such as BrdU for ChAs), even though the doses used for ex vivo irradiation (2–3.5 Gy) were not high enough to cause a significant mitotic delay. The absence of correlation between cytogenetic and clinical radiosensitivity in these reports can, therefore, be partially attributed to aberration-free cells surviving into 2nd divisions while damaged cells would more likely be eliminated in the 1st division. There are other studies in the list, which also involved similar longer-term cell culturing, but in which a correlation was found. In these reports the radiation dose (6 Gy) was high enough to produce both a mitotic delay and aberrant status in 100% of irradiated lymphocytes [67,69]. However, due to the absence of BrdU in cultures it cannot be excluded that some chromosome damage actually occurred in the 2nd mitoses (M2 cells), so perhaps the more damaged cells were being lost and the less damaged cells passed through to M2. This methodological defect may essentially contribute to the overall heterogeneity of the estimates of individual chromosomal radiosensitivity.

One important question is: which radiation doses and dose rates should be used for ex vivo irradiations? In all reports, in which biodosimetric markers showed a notable predictive value, the authors used relatively high ex vivo radiation doses (6 Gy for Dic+CR method and 2–4 Gy for FISH and MN assays). It seems that the approach 'The Dose must be As High As Possible' (DAHAP) is applicable here. From the point of classical biodosimetry, such doses are the highest normally used for constructing calibration curves in vitro [39]. After 6 Gy of γ- or X-rays, all metaphase cells carry unstable aberrations, but accurate quantification of chromosome rearrangements is still possible ([99] and references therein). By using caffeine or other chemicals that overcome the G_2/M block, or by applying a PCC method, higher doses might be attainable. However, this will also artificially increase the yield of chromosome rearrangements being visible in cells, which normally would have been arrested and dead. If the correlation between ex vivo ChA yields and NTT is somehow relevant to the inter-individual differences in the G_2/M block, then its intentional abrogation may lead to the lesser heterogeneity of this radiobiological index in the patients group, and thus reduce the separation power of the assay, worsening the overall prediction of the risk of NTT.

Also, with FISH painting, the total detectable yield of ChAs per unit dose is much higher than with conventional solid stain analysis due to inclusion of Tn and CCR, thus aberration scoring becomes difficult at doses above 4 Gy. Similarly, the MN yield in binucleated cells reaches a plateau and shows a faulty dose response at doses higher than 5 Gy [100,101]. It should be noted that 10 Gy, used in the study with an unusual result [93], essentially exceeds the upper dose threshold of the practical application of the MN assay in human PBLs. However, the lower doses, particularly <2 Gy, did not provide enough discrimination of an ex vivo effect among patients.

The role of the radiation dose can be illustrated by the data presented by Borgman et al. [67]: the number of chromosomal deletions induced ex vivo was plotted as a function of dose and, although there was already some inter-patient variation at 3 Gy, it became clearer at 6 Gy. Importantly, there was a poor correlation between the aberration yields at the two doses, and as a consequence, the classifications between resistant, normal, and sensitive patients obtained at 3 and 6 Gy were not identical. This discrepancy can be partially explained by the lack of a cell cycle control using BrdU that would cause some unknown proportion of the 2nd division metaphases to be included in the analysis at 3 Gy, contributing to intra-individual heterogeneity, while at 6 Gy this effect would be much lower. The overall problem of reproducibility of ex vivo data will be discussed in more detail below, but regardless of the mechanism, these results showed that the association between individual cytogenetic radiosensitivity and NTT risk can be different for different dose levels. The authors [67] concluded that in order to obtain a robust discrimination between the radiation responses of patients a sufficiently high dose is required. This is a prerequisite for detecting a clear association with the risk of clinical effects.

Previously, a similar conclusion was made in the study [80], in which the authors compared complete dose responses (0–4 Gy) generated for MN yield ex vivo in prostate cancer patients: "We believe that an assessment of individual intrinsic radiosensitivity at only one radiation dose level can be misleading, and that the accurate discrimination of individual radiation sensitivity differences necessitates the determination of the dose–response from baseline (0 Gy) to 4 Gyex vivo irradiation". This theory was supported by the comparison of the entire area under the curve (AUC) of the dose response generated for MN in the dose range 0.2–3 Gy in a case-control study [88]. Using this parameter, 10 out of 12 NTT cases scored higher than their matched controls, however, 6 of the 12 pairs showed overlap in their standard deviations.

Regarding the dose rate, the majority of studies involved an acute irradiation performed at high dose rates (HDR). Based on the experience of non-cytogenetic, cellular testing, as well as from cytogenetic research unrelated to NTT on cells of healthy individuals, carriers of DNA-repair-deficiency syndromes and cancer patients, it is known that the low dose rate (LDR) approach allows better discrimination (stratifying) of patients according to their intrinsic cellular radiosensitivity [63,102]. Nevertheless, only one NTT-related report was found that used a LDR for the ChA assay [63] and one for the MN assay [77]. In the former study, the LDR approach revealed a difference between over-reacting patients and healthy donors, however, the fact that no normal RT patients were included casts doubts on these conclusions. Furthermore, in the latter study, the LDR approach was not conclusive. It should be kept in mind that the main advantage of using a LDR is the dose rate sparing effect, which can be estimated only in comparison with HDR exposure results. Ideally, both ex vivo dose rates would be used for each patient, doubling the resources needed. The necessity of keeping cells at physiological conditions (temperature of 37 °C and 5% CO_2 atmosphere) during a prolonged irradiation time also makes the LDR method more technically demanding. These considerations highlight the unsuitability of the LDR approach for NTT predictive testing in clinical practice. The HDR approach provides meaningful results with much higher success, especially when the correct methodology of the NTT data analysis is used.

3.2.3. Clinical, Methodological and Statistical Confounders

There are three parameters to be considered in view of RT induced normal tissue damage: the severity (grade), the frequency and the onset time or latency period for its occurrence. The NTT grade is the basic factor by which patient groups are stratified in retrospective studies, and for which the correlation with ex vivo cytogenetic radiosensitivity is usually evaluated. Only a few reports showed a linkage between ChA or MN yields and the frequency of NTT cases [67], or the actuarial rate of NTT occurrence [66], or the latency period of NTT development [68,74]. It has become apparent that the validity of cytogenetic predictive tests should be defined by stratifying patients according to their chromosomal radiosensitivity, followed by the comparison of the predicted versus observed clinical radiation sequelae. This might also explain why several studies, which stratified according to the observed NTT effect instead of to the cytogenetic test result, failed to demonstrate an association between individual cellular radiosensitivity and NTT. By contrast, in the listed studies that stratified groups according to predicted radiosensitivity, the conclusions about the predictive value of ex vivo tests were the most accurate.

Individual radiosensitivity, assessed by induced cytogenetic damage yield ex vivo, was usually described by normal distribution of individual levels of ChA or MN, exactly as expected from the stochastic nature of chromosomal rearrangements [66,67,75,81,103,104]. However, not all the studies of the possible NTT predictors included statistical analysis of that distribution. Sometimes it was shown that cancer patients, especially those who showed elevated NTT grades, had a much broader spectrum of aberration yields per donor when compared to healthy individuals (e.g., [75]).

Also, in contrast to standard biodosimetry methodology, the ChA or MN per cell distribution was rarely tested for consistency with expected Poisson statistics in ex vivo NTT-related radiosensitivity studies. Moreover, if it was done, any significant over dispersion was not explained [75]. Meanwhile, retrospective studies involve taking blood from patients, who were irradiated in the past and thus carry a certain elevated 'baseline' yield of radiation-induced ChA or MN, as compared to normal spontaneous level in healthy control donors. In most such reports the ChA or MN frequencies observed in ex vivo irradiated cells were corrected for the frequencies in unirradiated cells. Usually, the total number of ChA in the control samples was subtracted from the total number of ChA in the irradiated ones without controlling for the specific type of aberration (e.g., in [75]). This ignores the fact that different types of chromosomal rearrangement make different quantitative contributions to spontaneous levels, RT-induced 'baseline' yields or ex vivo induced aberrations. Moreover, in particular for FISH-based testing, subtracting the baseline yield brings a lot of uncertainty due to the presence of metaphases with multiple aberrations in RT patients. While it is well known from the biodosimetry practice that the inclusion or rejection of just one or two such cells during the analysis may substantially change the overall aberration yield [105].

The FISH-based end-point, CCR, appears to be especially vulnerable to confounding factors: Lymphocytes of patients having just undergone RT exhibit high baseline frequencies of CCR, which are also dependent on the time since the previous RT and influenced by previous cytostatic therapy. The most important factor, however, is that cells taken from patients during or after RT may respond to ex vivo irradiation with a more drastic increase of CCR than lymphocytes of non-exposed patients [71]. Even the most successful parameter identified to datė for predicting NTT, i.e., the proportion of breaks involved in CCRs, which according to [71] are not affected by previous cytostatic treatment and the magnitude of ex vivo dose, should be treated with caution, because their quantification may be affected by the scoring system applied in the study: Protocol for Aberration Identification and Nomenclature Terminology (PAINT) or Savage and Simpson (S&S) nomenclature. Thus, when planning the research and interpretation of results in terms of the linkage between cytogenetic radiosensitivity and clinical NTT, such factors have to be considered carefully.

It should be noted that the general methodology of ex vivo testing is far from complete and cohesive. There have been specific studies addressing the question of which cytogenetic parameters are the most suitable for discriminating patients with increased chromosomal radiosensitivity from healthy individuals [73], and how many metaphases need to be analyzed [106]. However, there has been no such study focused specifically on patients with different grades of clinical radiosensitivity. Furthermore, in NTT studies, the numbers of cells scored at different ex vivo radiation doses were chosen arbitrarily, e.g., 200 metaphase spreads were scored for chromosomal aberrations at 2 Gy, 400 metaphases at 0.7 Gy and 1000 metaphases at 0 Gy [71,72]. These studies did not take into account the recommendations for biodosimetry [39] for either the optimal number of metaphases scored (500 for conventional and 1500 for FISH analysis), or for determining the required accuracy of the estimate (the ratio of the error to the yield) based on the Poisson statistics for the aberration mean yield and per-cell distribution.

The main issues are the intra-individual heterogeneity and overall reproducibility of ex vivo testing results, particularly because the biodosimetric markers measured in these NTT prediction studies are stochastic radiation effects, which show a certain natural variability. Unfortunately, examples of systematic repeated testing of RT patients' cells, which are needed to examine this natural variability, are rare. In one study, samples from seven patients were analyzed two or three times after RT and showed a stable general pattern of cytogenetic reaction, including CCR induction [71]. In a second study, repeat samples were tested in 13 patients with the time between sampling ranging from 3 to 9 months. Good reproducibility of the HDR MN assay results was demonstrated by a strong correlation between the repeat samples [77].

Among other RT patient-related publications, the reproducibility of the ex vivo assay has been mentioned twice, but both times with respect to blood samples taken from healthy donors [81,103]. Thus, a quality assurance and quality control (QA/QC) system still needs to be developed for the area of clinical use of ex vivo radiation biomarkers for NTT prediction in RT patients, starting with basic validation steps: sensitivity, specificity, reproducibility, confounders.

3.3. Studies Using Non-Lymphocyte Cell Systems

In trying to use a cytogenetic test-system closely linked to cell survival assays, some researchers have measured the yield of radiation-induced biomarkers in cultured skin fibroblasts, keratinocytes or lymphoblastoid cell lines.

An extensive analysis of ex vivo MN was performed in cultured skin fibroblasts of 17 patients with increased acute and/or late side effects along with 10 patients with no excessive reactions [107]. Dose response curves were generated individually for each patient in the range of 1–7 Gy, however a saturation or decrease in MN yield at doses ≥4 Gy occurred nearly in all cases. The cells of the majority of the sensitive patients showed a higher MN induction than the average of the donors with a normal response. Only two of the patients with acute reactions and four with late effects had a dose response clearly below or similar to the average of the normal patients.

In a study performed on fibroblasts of 8 retrospectively examined patients with cervical or head andneck cancers, no significant correlation was found between the rate of ex vivo MN induction in fibroblasts (2–5 Gy) and acute and late normal tissue reaction scores [78]. In addition, no relationship was observed between the ex vivo cytogenetic radiosensitivity of lymphocytes and fibroblasts derived from the same individuals in this work (6 cancer patients plus 5 healthy donors).

Dermal fibroblast lines were established from skin biopsies of 26 patients with soft tissue sarcoma and subjected to 2.4 Gy of low dose-rate (0.0194 Gy min^{-1})^{60}Co γ-rays [108]. The MN frequency in irradiated fibroblasts did not correspond to differences in normal tissue responses, which were wound-healing complications and subcutaneous fibrosis.

Later a more sophisticated study was performed in order to compare the dose responses for MN in cultured primary fibroblasts (2–4 Gy γ-rays in vitro) and long-term lymphocyte cell lines (1–2 Gy γ-rays in vitro) derived from 36 patients who had severe acute or late reactions from RT [109]. Heterogeneity of MN frequency in irradiated fibroblasts and lymphocyte cell lines (LCLs) was apparent. Across the different doses, the average MN frequency consistently trended towards being higher in cells obtained from clinically radiosensitive individuals versus those of normal responders (controls). Also, in separately examined subgroups of LCLs derived from patients who had breast cancer, the severe acute reactors showed a significant difference of the average number of cells with multiple MN compared with controls. Among 7 paired fibroblast lines and LCLs derived from the same clinically radiosensitive patients, only one individual with late reactions showed a significant correlation between the two cell lineages for their radiosensitivity, presenting as very high MN frequency.

Also, in a perspective study of 32 cervical cancer patients, an ex vivo MN assay dose response (0.05–4 Gy ^{60}Co γ-rays) in fibroblasts and keratinocytes was compared to the normal tissue reactions [110]. Despite the presence of 6 patients with a hyper-radiosensitivity (HRS)-like ex vivo response, the radiation-induced MN did not correlate, either in fibroblasts or keratinocytes, with the grade of acute or late reactions in patients. Five of the 6 patients with HRS cells did not suffer from any mild or severe side effects after RT. Thus, the MN assay showed no predictive value.

The most recent and the largest study to date aimed at establishing possible quantitative links between RT-related overreaction grades and MN yield induced ex vivo (2 Gy γ-rays) in fibroblasts. The study involved more than 100 patient skin biopsy specimens [25]. The MN yield remaining 24 h post-irradiation discriminated three patient subpopulations: radioresistant, overreacting and hyper-radiosensitive patients as classified using the Common Terminology Criteria for Adverse Events (CTCAE). These sub-populations corresponded to three groups of DNA-repair based radiosensitivity defined initially in that study which, by surprise, appeared to be in line with the pragmatic clinical classification [7]. However, within the overreacting cohort the MN test could not discriminate between patients with different clinical radiosensitivity, whether classified using the CTCAE or RTOG scales. These results suggest that ex vivo radiation-induced MN can only distinguish large differences in radiosensitivity.

Based on these studies, MN analysis in fibroblasts, keratinocytes and LCLs does not seem to provide a strong predictive value for radiosensitivity. In addition, these assays take a long time to conduct, requiring cells to be grown from biopsies or transformed from lymphocytes. Therefore, these assays are not effective or practical for the clinical setting. As shown above, PBL have higher potential to be a more appropriate test-system for cytogenetic research aimed at the assessment of chromosomal radiosensitivity for NTT prediction.

3.4. *Prediction of NTT Using Ex Vivo Tests Based on Other DNA or Chromosome Damage Biomarkers*

There are three radiation-induced cellular effects which are promising ex vivo irradiation assays for predicting patient clinical radiosensitivity: γ-H2AX foci, which appear in response to DNA DSBs, chromatid aberrations induced in the G_2 phase of the cell cycle and alterations of the length of telomeres. These radiation biomarkers are not adapted in classic biodosimetry, thus are subjected only to very brief analysis in the current review.

3.4.1. γ-H2AX Foci

A brief overview of the state of the art of using γ-H2AX in clinical settings has been presented by Redon et al. [111]. The induction of γ-H2AX foci is directly related to DNA DSB recognition and repair, thus a possible relation of their initially-induced or residual yield to clinical radiosensitivity should be considered along with other DNA repair-based assays (e.g., Comet assay). The number of publications highlighting the possibilities and limitations of surrogate end points based on DNA damage repair as predictors of NTT far exceeds the limits of this review. Nevertheless, γ-H2AX foci is claimed as a useful tool in triage biodosimetry and recommended for inclusion into the toolbox of radiation cytogenetic laboratories [112–116], thus it is appropriate to present a brief analysis of the predictive value of this particular end-point.

In our non-exhaustive list of publications about ex vivo induced γ-H2AX foci yield in isolated PBL in patients with various NTT effects there are 13 reports showing that quantification of γ-H2AX foci by microscopy or flow cytometry is not predictive of acute or late radiation toxicity [58,87,88,117–126]. On the other hand, there are a number of reports showing the opposite result. Earlier, there was a report about a patient who had previously shown severe side effects after RT, and whose lymphocytes in vivo displayed levels of γ-H2AX foci at various sampling times after Computed Tomography (CT) that were several times higher than those of normal individuals. Furthermore, fibroblasts from the same patient also showed significant ex vivo radiosensitivity by γ-H2AX foci analysis [127]. More recently, ex vivo testing of lymphocytes by this technique has shown remarkable differences between groups of patients with high and low NTT grades, and/or enabled identification of patients at risk for higher grade toxicities in at least 13 publications [69,128–138]. The main conclusion made in these studies was that the γ-H2AX assay may have a high potential for screening individual radiosensitivity among RT patients. Various methodological aspects of these reports, including radiation doses used, time points investigated, the role of mutations in DNA repair genes, as well as reproducibility and intra-patient variability, are awaiting a specific meta-analysis.

In addition to γ-H2AX, other surrogate markers of DNA DSB repair (e.g., Rad51, BRCA1, 53BP1, pATM, etc.) are specific indicators of different DSB repair pathways that may play a role in the development of NTT [123]. However, none of them have been yet implemented in radiation biodosimetry.

3.4.2. G_2 Assay

Historically, cytogenetic radiosensitivity tests with irradiation of unstimulated PBL (or other quiescent cells) is called the G_0 assay, in contrast to the G_2 assay in which radiation exposure is performed on proliferating cells. The latter method is based on quantification of chromatid-type fragments and is not used for biodosimetry. The reports analysing chromosomal radiosensitivity detected by the G_2 assay are rather numerous. A rough search in the literature identified 14 papers on the use of G_2 damage as a marker of genetic predisposition to clinical NTT effects. Seven of these reports contain the conclusion that no direct correlation exists between G_2 damage and NTT grade [70,75,87,122,126,139,140]. In equal number of studies the opposite result was observed, i.e., cells from patients with severe acute or late NTT effects had a mean G_2 sensitivity significantly higher than that of the patients without RT-induced normal tissue damage [77,88,91,141–144]. It should be noted that two positive findings were made using a modification of the G_2 assay, in which MN were scored instead of chromatid breaks [88,144], and in two studies caffeine was added to the irradiated lymphocyte culture for G_2-checkpoint abrogation [88,91]. Other known hybrids of the G_2 approach and DNA damage end-points, like G_2+γ-H2AX foci (e.g., [145]) or G_2+PCC (e.g., [146]) have not been reported yet in studies aimed at ex vivo sensitivity related to NTT effects in RT patients.

The G_2 assay was often used along with the G_0 test in the same study. In all such reports the authors found that there was no individual correlation between G_2 and G_0 damage yields, and each assay identified different patients as radiosensitive [70,75,77,141]. These results suggest that, since different molecular machinery is involved in chromosomal breakage and repair at different stages of the cell cycle, different mechanisms of chromosomal radiosensitivity are likely to operate in G_2 and G_0 cells. In general, chromosomally radiosensitive patients may be defective in only one such mechanism, possibly through mutation (or polymorphism) of a single gene. Such mutations may lead to cancer predisposition, of low penetrance, in a large proportion of patients [141]. This hypothesis was supported by a study demonstrating the Mendelian heritability of chromosomal radiosensitivity in family members of breast cancer cases [147,148]. Later, strong evidence for heritability of the G_2 radiosensitive phenotype was confirmed in another cohort [149].

More information about the possibilities and limitations of the G_2 assay, covering various aspects of the technique performance, can be found in numerous reports on the use of the G_2 score as a marker of cancer predisposition. A compilation of data from such studies is beyond the scope of current review. However, one important issue is the intra-individual variations of G_2 which were investigated in a special study [149]. The heterogeneity was so significant that the authors concluded that too much reliance should not be placed on the result from a single sample when assessing individual radiosensitivity status by the G_2 assay.

3.4.3. Telomere Length

One more cytogenetic end-point is telomere length. There is some evidence suggesting a link between this parameter and cellular or clinical radiosensitivity. However, the data on the nature of correlation between telomere length and cancer susceptibility (i.e., is the dependence positive or negative?) is rather inconclusive [150]. Moreover, a comparison of telomere length, determined by a flow cytometric FISH assay in PBL of breast cancer patients, failed to reveal differences in cellular radiosensitivity in groups with normal and severe skin reactions to RT [151].

3.5. Combination of Biodosimetric Markers with Other Biomarkers of Radiation Response. Multiparametric Approach

The prevalence of a mitotic death pathway for most irradiated normal tissues makes the quantification of ex vivo induced ChA and MN a reliable approach to link the intrinsic radiosensitivity to the NTT in RT patients. However, it should be kept in mind that cytogenetic damage may cover a only a certain range of intrinsic radiosensitivity occurring within a certain range of radiation doses, and may predict not all the types of NTT, but might be best working if the analysis is restricted to specific radiotherapy side effects in patients with one tumor location [152].

On the other hand, it is increasingly accepted that clinical radiosensitivity is likely to be a complex genetic phenotype controlled by genes involved in many cellular processes, including DNA damage recognition and repair, cell proliferation and inter- and intra-tissue signaling. This combination of contributors underlies the inter-individual heterogeneity in radiation effects (damage and repair) in tissues and organs. The genetic determinants of individual radiation susceptibility can be revealed by genomic technologies like mutation detection, SNP analysis or genome-wide association studies. Among prognostic factors, apart from cytogenetic damage (G_0 ChAs and MN, G_2 chromatid breaks, γ-H2AX foci), there are a large number of biological end-points, which can serve as a measure of radiation response: DNA breakage and repair, apoptosis, G_2/M checkpoint arrest, cell survival, colony-forming ability, expression of certain genes, intra- and inter-cell signaling and various biochemical and metabolic changes.

However, for various reasons, the discriminatory power of all known radiation response assays is too low to be used alone in clinical settings, particularly for ex vivo tests. This is not surprising, if one considers that the adverse reactions in patients' normal tissues may arise from more than one type of underlying defect at cellular level, e.g., the enhanced ChA production may be coupled to the altered apoptosis. Therefore, in clinical practice these biomarkers should not be taken alone, but instead should be included in a compendium of end-points. This is fully applicable to cytogenetic biomarkers. There are many papers presenting the results of ex vivo radiosensitivity assessment using several methods in one study, however, in most such reports, only a simple comparison of prognostic accuracy of different end-points was made. A truly multiparametric approach, where measured effects are combined into an entire prognostic profile, might provide better discrimination.

In the area of interest of this review, there are some examples of such an approach. De Ruyck et al. [143] determined that the G_2 radiosensitivity assay results, coupled to the risk allele model based on a combination of diverse polymorphisms in DNA repair genes, allowed identification of 23% of the patients with late normal tissue reactions, without false-positive results. In the study of Rzeszowska-Wolny et al. [85], radiosensitive patients were initially selected by a DNA repair test, and then a correlation with NTT in this subgroup was established with the MN assay. Beaton et al. [56] detected a significant increase in the unstable aberration yield in 1st post-radiation mitoses and simultaneously a reduced proportion of cells in 2nd metaphase in ex vivo irradiated lymphocytes of prostate patients, who showed adverse late radiation effects as compared to matched patients exhibiting no adverse effects. In a recent multi-assay study on patients' fibroblasts, Granzotto et al. [25] showed that the best discrimination among clinically over-reacting patients was provided by the maximal number of pATM foci, and a significant correlation with the NTT severity grade was reached when γ-H2AX foci analysis was added to the results of pATM foci assay, independent of tumor localization and of the early or late nature of the reactions. Further research may help to establish the best combinations of such assays and the "confidence zone" of their application [95].

Among the PBL-based biodosimetry methods currently under development, the most promising are transcriptomics or single gene expression analysis. These technologies have proven to be quite an effective tool for detecting radiation exposure to humans [153,154], including such a complex scenarios as fractionated RT [153,155,156]. There have been several studies that attempted to link ex vivo radiation-induced changes in the expression level of certain genes in patients' PBLs with their NTT; success in establishing the desired correlation has been regularly reported [87,97,121,157–162]. Corresponding changes in gene expression have also been found in RT patients with different grades of NTT in vivo [32,163]. It seems possible that both dose-response markers and NTT predictors can be measured simultaneously within the same transcriptomic platform, providing an 'all-in-one' approach with the advantage of full automation and high throughput.

Clearly, more research is needed, in which two or more radiation response biomarkers measured under ex vivo conditions and showing a moderate rate of correlation between them, could be combined using multiple linear regression in order to improve the sensitivity/specificity of prediction of RT-induced NTT.

3.6. General Concerns Regarding the Ex Vivo Chromosomal Radiosensitivity as a Predictor of NTT Effects

The intra-individual variability and reproducibility of the cytogenetic assays based on ex vivo irradiation is a very important issue for the radiosensitivity testing and, therefore, requires more comments. In several studies a significant intra-donor variation of radiation-induced cytogenetic damage incidence was found. It was shown that, for the ex vivo assay, the contribution of intra-individual variance to the overall heterogeneity of radiation-induced MN frequencies may be as high as 75% [164]. After both HDR and LDR irradiation regimens, a significant inter-experiment variability was observed in MN yields as well as the dose-rate sparing effect (i.e., reduction in MN yield at LDR compared with HDR) in control donors' lymphocytes [102]. However, in another study the same researchers noted good reproducibility of the MN assay performed on lymphocytes of 5 normal control donors, whose blood was repeatedly tested 6 times [165]. The conclusions about the ratio of inter-individual to intra-individual variability of cytogenetic radiation response in healthy donors' cells are contradictory. Some authors showed that the inter-individual variation was significantly higher than intra-individual [166], but other researchers pointed out that there was a high variability between experiments, such that it was not possible to demonstrate inter-individual differences in chromosomal sensitivity. This was true in spite of the use of a control sample from the same normal donor in each experiment [167]. A remarkable, 2-fold increase in variations in radiation-induced cytogenetic damage yields in the same donors' cells was observed with longer time intervals between repeated samples ranging from 1–3 months to 1 year [81]. The inclusion of the reproducibility test on lymphocytes from healthy control donors has become standard in intrinsic radiosensitivity studies [103,165], but has not changed the overall concern about the results, as the RT patients were only tested once.

Inter- and intra-individual variations of the G_0 ex vivo MN assay were investigated thoroughly by A. Vral and colleagues [168–170]. Repeated experiments on blood cells taken from the same donors over a 1-year period demonstrated that there was no significant difference between intra- and inter-individual variability. Since reproducibility of the assay is determined by the intra-individual variability, these results highlighted the limitations of cytogenetic end points in detecting real, reproducible differences in radiation sensitivity between individuals within a normal population. For example, some healthy donors in the population were identified as being radiosensitive (based on the 90th percentile criterion) but turned out to be normal (non-sensitive) when the assay was repeated at later time points [168,169]. Prolongation of the follow up period up to 3 years did not change the results of testing the repeat samples [170]. The authors stated that the determination of individual radiosensitivity using cytogenetic assays is unreliable when based only on one blood sample, as it may lead to erroneous conclusions. Multiple blood sampling may be necessary to draw reliable conclusions.

There are no reports in the literature presenting a tactics, which can be an alternative to that of suggested by A. Vral et al. [168–170] for overcoming the problem of intra-individual variations and low reproducibility of ex vivo radiation cytogenetic assays. As mentioned above, even two radiation doses used in one testing round can produce different classifications for the same individuals [67].

Possibly, building up an entire dose response and further comparison of the curve coefficients or AUCs is a solution for this limitation [80,88].

There are two additional scientific questions, which are somewhat relevant to the problem of the intrinsic chromosomal radiosensitivity. These are (i) the natural general variability of the cytogenetic radiation response in human of lymphocytes, and (ii) the specific traits of chromosomal radiosensitivity in cancer patients versus healthy donors. A large number of reports can be found in the literature on each of these questions, but these studies did not register clinical NTT effects, therefore their results have limited value for radiation oncology. Their detailed analysis is beyond the scope of the current work; however, these issues will be highlighted in the forthcoming IAEA Health Series Report [38] in relevance to other clinical applications of cytogenetic biodosimetry. Actually, in the correctly executed NTT studies a possible impact of the aforementioned factors can be minimized by (i) the presence of a sufficient number of cases in the study, and (ii) the inclusion of positive controls, i.e., patients without radiation lesions, and negative controls, i.e., unirradiated healthy donors.

As was mentioned at the beginning of this review, the key idea of the prediction of the NTT by ex vivo tests is that elevated chromosomal radiosensitivity and a predisposition to the abnormal NTT response to RT are both attributable to patients' genetics. Therefore, it is very tempting to assume the presence of a mechanistic link between these two traits. Data obtained by Widel et al. [81] best supports this assumption: In lymphocytes irradiated ex vivo, the mean yield of MN was significantly higher in samples from patients demonstrating acute and/or late normal tissue reactions, than in those from patients showing no reactions; however, healthy donors fell between the two patient groups. This may suggest that the control healthy donors group may contain both radiosensitive and radioresistant individuals, and that some of them may be potential clinical over-reactors. Therefore, it should be recommended that a matched (or at least, large enough) group of healthy donors always be included in the ex vivo radiosensitivity testing in order to guarantee the quality control of the studied population.

Also the aspect of the patient's age might play a very important, dual role. First, aging tissues might intrinsically harbor more DNA damage that could sensitize (or not) to RT, thus modulating the NTT occurrence. Second, there are serious concerns about the equality of the cytogenetic dose response (i.e., chromosomal radiosensitivity) in cells of young vs. old donors [171,172]. To the best of our knowledge, no one research group specifically considered the age factor in their studies on ex vivo cytogenetic tests for the NTT prediction. This might be a task for future research.

Also, it is important to determine the best method for the initial stratification of patient cohorts for data analysis: either according to the chromosomal radiosensitivity or clinical response. If the former is chosen as a discriminator, then the shape of the ChA or MN frequency distribution within a cohort should be thoroughly analysed, and the cut-off criteria must be clearly defined. The most frequent approach is to check the observed distribution for consistency with Gaussian statistics and to carry out a classification based on the arbitrarily chosen definitions ≤MV–SD as resistant, MV ± SD as normal and ≥MV + SD as sensitive, where MV is mean value and SD is standard deviation of the mean. It is apparent, that such a classification does not consider the normal probability for any individual in the group to be located in any of three categories after a single sampling. Therefore, "two doses, two times" can be recommended as a minimum experimental design for unbiased assigning of a patient to a certain category of cytogenetic radiosensitivity. However, it is not yet clear whether the definition based on MV and SD is applicable and how it should be modified, if the test is performed two or more times, or is based on two or more radiation dose points.

If it is possible to create a full ex vivo dose response curve for each patient in the study, then the efficacy of the AUC versus curve coefficients ± error as a discriminator have to be evaluated.

Irrespective of study design, it should be kept in mind that the difference in radiation-induced aberration yield per unit radiation dose between individuals can be rather small. Therefore, in order to validate the suggested assays, QA/QC actions aimed at strengthening the reproducibility should be supplemented with normalization of the individual data using internal standards, as was suggested earlier for clonogenic end-points of cellular radiosensitivity, which also suffer from intra-individual variation [173,174].

Another aspect of the problem is the evaluation of NTT per se. Focusing the study on one type/location of normal tissue damage (e.g., skin) reduces uncertainties compared to the inclusion of various NTT effects graded by a certain scoring system. Also it is plausible that different cytogenetic assays could identify different response phenotypes associated with acute or late reactions [77].

A prospective study design seems to be the best for the development of prognostic test, as it avoids the uncertainty caused by RT induced ChA or MN yields. For the analysis of late NTT effects, patients should be surveyed long enough after RT to cover the latency period for clinical effects.

If in the radiosensitivity study the cytogenetic data are used as the primary factor for patient group stratification, and the NTT effect is a dependent parameter, then the latter should be assessed for the grade, the frequency and the on-set time. Thus, the most comprehensive approach for clinical practice includes the stratification of patients according to the results of the comparison of AUCs of their individual ex vivo dose responses, followed by generating the predictive risk-analysis actuarial curves for complication-free survival for a given grade of the certain NTT effect.

Recently a method was suggested, by which the patients were identified on the basis of moderate/marked or minimal/no NTT adverse effect despite the absence or presence of variables predisposing the patient to this particular effect [137]. Risk factors for adverse RT effects can then be established by multivariate analysis of the NTT outcomes. For example, in that report the favourable factors (lower NTT risk) in breast cancer patients were the lower whole breast RT dose, 3D dosimetry, no boost dose to the tumor bed, small breast size, minimal surgical cavity and no axillary RT. Patients with striking adverse effects despite favourable parameters were classified as 'RT-Sensitive', and unmatched patients with no changes even with unfavourable parameters were considered as 'RT-Resistant'. This approach allows maximum separation in terms of intrinsic factors predisposing the patient to the presence or absence of adverse NTT effects. In this report a significant association between the NTT effects and ex vivo γ-H2AX foci yields was established particularly in lymphocytes, whereas no such correlations was observed in cultured skin cells (fibroblasts, endothelium, keratinocytes and epidermis [137]. However, to the best of our knowledge, such a classifier based on the 'despite-predisposing-variables' principle, has not yet been applied in NTT-radiosensitivity studies using biodosimetric markers. Surely, more validation studies on the reliability of such an approach are required.

Other aspects of radiation biomarker research in relation to clinical radiosensitivity, including the underlying rationale, the necessity formeticulous recruitment of patients, study design that accounts for clinical factors, which modify normal tissue responses, as well as some limitations and confounding factors that affect tests of association between predictive markers and clinical radiosensitivity, have been highlighted in reviews [16–23,31,32,95].

4. Conclusions and Recommendations

In RT, normal tissue reactions are often the regulating factor for treatment. As such, there is no robust screening method to predict normal tissue reactions to RT, particularly in comparison to tumor tissue. Such a screening method would allow radiation dose to be tailored to each patient. On the basis of numerous studies, it is reasonable to conclude that the severity of RT-related complications is essentially determined by genetic predisposition, which can be revealed and quantified in normal cells. Human PBL are the preferred tissue for assays of NTT response (particularly, as an alternative to fibroblasts) due to the ease of obtaining samples and the rapid generation of the results. In cancer patients, evidence suggests that enhanced PBL radiosensitivity, assessed by various end-points, associates with the development of RT-related morbidity. Therefore, the attempts to develop clinically applicable tests based on radiation cyto- or genotoxicity in lymphocytes as a rapid predictive biomarker of normal tissue radiosensitivity are convincing and logical.

ChA frequency is considered a good indicator, because cytogenetic damage is usually related to an altered DNA repair function, which is in turn linked to cellular radiosensitivity, for which a dysfunction of many elements of DNA damage sensing and repair have been demonstrated. This has been strongly supported by the clear success of cytogenetic analysis of cases with inherited DNA repair defects, identified by molecular or clinical signs, which are always confirmed by abnormal results of post-ex vivo irradiation cytogenetic analysis.

However, for the rest of the over-reacting patients, the results appear to be rather controversial. In approximately 50% of the reports, the average yield of biodosimetric markers was higher in over-reacting patients than in patients with lower grade NTT. Also, a significant correlation was sometimes found between the biomarker yield and the severity of acute or late NTT reactions at an individual level, but this observation was not unequivocally proven. Both the presence and the absence of correlations between cytogenetic damage frequency and acute or late normal tissue effects after RT were reported by the same and by different research teams. Thus, it is possible that, for different cytogenetic radiosensitivity phenotypes, their associations with NTT effect might be irradiation site- and damaged organ/tissue-specific.

The inter-individual variations of ex vivo ChA or MN yields in over-reacting patients is similar to or wider than that of patients without adverse NTT effects. In the majority of studies the overlap between the distributions of individual frequencies of cytogenetic damage in cells taken from patients with high-grade and low-grade NTT reactions did not allow clear identification of persons at risk by an ex vivo test. That is one of the main reasons for the limited application of biodosimetric markers for identifying radiosensitive individuals among RT patients. The second reason is the intra-individual heterogeneity, which determines the reproducibility of the assay, and which has not been studied thoroughly enough in RT cohorts. Instead, there is a serious concern, coming from cancer risk studies, that the determination of individual radiosensitivity with cytogenetic assays is unreliable when based on a single measurement, and multiple blood sampling is necessary to get reliable patient classification.

Thus, a general conclusion is that the assays based on ex vivo biodosimetric markers in PBL in their present form are unlikely to result in the development of a reliable 'stand-alone' assay of radiosensitivity, which can be of assistance for the prediction of NTT effects in the clinic and lead to individualized patient RT schedules. The following are some suggestions how these issues can be addressed:

- Patient groups, selected for prospective studies, should be large enough to provide a sufficient number of cases of adverse NTT. In retrospective studies, a case-control design is preferable with well-matched control patients. A healthy donors group should also be included in the study.
- The formation of "teaching" datasets for the primary search for a correlation between ex vivo induced biomarker yield and the NTT should be undertaken through stratifying the patients according to their clinical effects. A "despite-predisposing-variables" approach [137] should be used, where possible, to guarantee the maximum separation of clinically radiosensitive and radioresistant patients in terms of intrinsic factors predisposing to the presence or absence of adverse NTT effects.
- It is highly desirable to maintain the second means of patient stratification according to molecular classification of human radiosensitivity [25]. Respective predictive assays should be performed to separate the radioresistance group; the group of moderate radiosensitivity caused by delay of nucleoshuttling of ATM (includes majority over-reacting patients), and the group of hyper-radiosensitivity caused by a gross DSB repair defect. The biodosimetric markers may be applied for further partition of the over-responding patient group.
- A set of criteria of excellence for these types of study should be maintained:
    - minimum confounders, i.e., one tumor site, one irradiation scheme and irradiated sites locations;
    - one type of NTT (one organ or tissue) per study; NTT grade, frequency and latency assessed;

- ChAs are more preferable than MN;
- at least 2 radiation doses ex vivo (the higher of two doses has to be AHAP), at least 2 repeats of the assay for each individual in the studied cohort;
- alternatively, a full dose response should be built for each individual according to classical biodosimetric methodology (minimum 6 dose response points to estimate 3 coefficients of the classic linear quadratic model); the result is the set of coefficients with their errors or the entire AUC.

- The "teaching" phase should be finalized by generating prognostic risk-analysis actuarial curves for complication-free survival (frequency and latency time) for various grades of the studied NTT effect.
- In the validation phase of the ex vivo biomarker study, its predictive efficacy should be assessed by a common test for general accuracy (sensitivity/specificity), and re-evaluated by stratifying patients according to their intrinsic cytogenetic radiosensitivity and calculating the annual risk for a given grade of the NTT effect using the actuarial curves.
- The use of internal standards for the determination of the intrinsic radiosensitivity in patients' lymphocytes at each stage of the research should aid the development and evaluation of the prognostic tests.

To make cytogenetic ex vivo irradiation-based assays more attractive for clinical applications, they can be combined with automated scoring of cytogenetic damage using flow cytometry or computerized image analysis systems [175,176].

These recommendations may help to develop the ex vivo tests, which would be feasible in clinical practice and could be used as supplementary markers in radiobiological control for radiation oncology. To accomplish this, more retrospective, case-control studies are needed, along with larger prospective studies to confirm existing findings. This will help validate the use of ex vivo cytogenetic assays in the future to predict normal tissue radiosensitivity and discriminate individuals with marked early and late normal tissue reactions after RT. A coordinated approach among different laboratories would be useful to set the relevant standards and increase sample numbers to allow for robust analysis and strong conclusions that will help convince the radiation oncology community to adopt these predictive assays.

Author Contributions: Conceptualization, O.B. and E.Z.; Methodology, V.V. and O.B.; Investigation and Analysis, V.V., R.W., M.P.H., A.W.; Writing—Original Draft Preparation, V.V.; Writing—Review andEditing, R.W., M.P.H., A.W., O.B.; Supervision, E.Z.; Project Administration, O.B. All authors have read and agreed to the published version of the manuscript.

Funding: This research was supported by the International Atomic Energy Agency (IAEA), Coordinated Research Project E3.50.10 "MEDBIODOSE", that provided funds to cover the APC.

Acknowledgments: The authors are very grateful to the IAEA for provision administrative support for this work.

Conflicts of Interest: The authors declare no conflict of interest. The IAEA made a choice of the research topic, but had no role in the design, execution, interpretation, or writing of this review.

References

1. Joiner, M.C.; van der Kogel, A.J.; Steel, G.G. (Eds.) Introduction: The significance of radiobiology and radiotherapy for cancer treatment. In *Basic Clinical Radiobiology*, 5th ed.; CRC Press/Taylor & Francis Group: Boca Raton, FL, USA, 2018; pp. 1–8. [CrossRef]
2. Wenz, F. (Ed.) *Radiation Oncology*; Springer Nature: Cham, Switzerland, 2020. [CrossRef]
3. Baumann, M.; Krause, M.; Overgaard, J.; Debus, J.; Bentzen, S.M.; Daartz, J.; Richter, C.; Zips, D.; Bortfeld, T. Radiation oncology in the era of precision medicine. *Nat. Rev. Cancer.* **2016**, *16*, 234–249. [CrossRef] [PubMed]
4. Burnet, N.G.; Nyman, J.; Turesson, I.; Wurm, R.; Yarnold, J.R.; Peacock, J.H. The relationship between cellular radiation sensitivity and tissue response may provide the basis for individualising radiotherapy schedules. *Radiother. Oncol.* **1994**, *33*, 228–238. [CrossRef]

5. Tucker, S.L.; Geara, F.B.; Peters, L.J.; Brock, W.A. How much could the radiotherapy dose be altered for individual patients based on a predictive assay of normal-tissue radiosensitivity? *Radiother. Oncol.* **1996**, *38*, 103–113. [CrossRef]
6. Bentzen, S.M. Potential clinical impact of normal-tissue intrinsic radiosensitivity testing. *Radiother. Oncol.* **1997**, *43*, 121–131. [CrossRef]
7. Burnet, N.G.; Johansen, J.; Turesson, I.; Nyman, J.; Peacock, J.H. Describing patients' normal tissue reactions: Concerning the possibility of individualising radiotherapy dose prescriptions based on potential predictive assays of normal tissue radiosensitivity. Steering Committee of the BioMed2 European Union Concerted Action Programme on the Development of Predictive Tests of Normal Tissue Response to Radiation Therapy. *Int. J. Cancer.* **1998**, *79*, 606–613.
8. Mackay, R.I.; Hendry, J.H. The modelled benefits of individualizing radiotherapy patients' dose using cellular radiosensitivity assays with inherent variability. *Radiother. Oncol.* **1999**, *50*, 67–75. [CrossRef]
9. Sanchez-Nieto, B.; Nahum, A.E.; Dearnaley, D.P. Individualization of dose prescription based on normal-tissue dose-volume and radiosensitivity data. *Int. J. Radiat. Oncol. Biol. Phys.* **2001**, *49*, 487–499. [CrossRef]
10. Russell, N.S.; Begg, A.C. Predictive assays for normal tissue damage. *Radiother. Oncol.* **2002**, *64*, 125–129. [CrossRef]
11. Torres-Roca, J.F.; Stevens, C.W. Predicting response to clinical radiotherapy: Past, present, and future directions. *Cancer Control* **2008**, *15*, 151–156. [CrossRef]
12. Lacombe, J.; Riou, O.; Solassol, J.; Mangé, A.; Bourgier, C.; Fenoglietto, P.; Pèlegrin, A.; Ozsahin, M.; Azria, D. Intrinsic radiosensitivity: Predictive assays that will change daily practice. *Cancer Radiother.* **2013**, *17*, 337–343. [CrossRef]
13. Barnett, G.C.; West, C.M.; Dunning, A.M.; Elliott, R.M.; Coles, C.E.; Pharoah, P.D.; Burnet, N.G. Normal tissue reactions to radiotherapy: Towards tailoring treatment dose by genotype. *Nat. Rev. Cancer* **2009**, *9*, 134–142. [CrossRef] [PubMed]
14. Scaife, J.E.; Barnett, G.C.; Noble, D.J.; Jena, R.; Thomas, S.J.; West, C.M.L.; Burnet, N.G. Exploiting biological and physical determinants of radiotherapy toxicity to individualize treatment. *Br. J. Radiol.* **2015**, *88*, 20150172. [CrossRef] [PubMed]
15. Bergom, C.; West, C.M.; Higginson, D.S.; Abazeed, M.E.; Arun, B.; Bentzen, S.M.; Bernstein, J.L.; Evans, J.D.; Gerber, N.K.; Kerns, S.L.; et al. The Implications of genetic testing on radiation therapy decisions: A guide for radiation oncologists. *Int. J. Radiat. Oncol. Biol. Phys.* **2019**, *105*, 698–712. [CrossRef] [PubMed]
16. Sørensen, B.S.; Andreassen, C.N.; Alsner, J. Molecular biomarkers in radiation oncology. In *Radiation Oncology*; Wenz, F., Ed.; Springer Nature: Cham, Switzerland, 2019; 18p. [CrossRef]
17. Granzotto, A.; Joubert, A.; Viau, M.; Devic, C.; Maalouf, M.; Thomas, C.; Vogin, G.; Malek, K.; Colin, C.; Balosso, J.; et al. Individual response to ionising radiation: What predictive assay(s) to choose? *C. R. Biol.* **2011**, *334*, 140–157. [CrossRef] [PubMed]
18. Foray, N.; Colin, C.; Bourguignon, M. 100 Years of individual radiosensitivity: How we have forgotten the evidence. *Radiology* **2012**, *264*, 627–631. [CrossRef] [PubMed]
19. Chua, M.L.; Rothkamm, K. Biomarkers of radiation exposure: Can they predict normal tissue radiosensitivity? *Clin. Oncol. R. Coll. Radiol.* **2013**, *25*, 610–616. [CrossRef] [PubMed]
20. Foray, N.; Bourguignon, M.; Hamada, N. Individual response to ionizing radiation. *Mutat. Res.* **2016**, *770 Pt B*, 369–386. [CrossRef]
21. Habash, M.; Bohorquez, L.C.; Kyriakou, E.; Kron, T.; Martin, O.A.; Blyth, B.J. Clinical and functional assays of radiosensitivity and radiation-induced second cancer. *Cancers* **2017**, *9*, 147. [CrossRef] [PubMed]
22. Gomolka, M.; Blyth, B.; Bourguignon, M.; Badie, C.; Schmitz, A.; Talbot, C.; Hoeschen, C.; Salomaa, S. Potential screening assays for individual radiation sensitivity and susceptibility and their current validation state. *Int. J. Radiat. Biol.* **2020**, *96*, 280–296. [CrossRef] [PubMed]
23. Seibold, P.; Auvinen, A.; Averbeck, D.; Bourguignon, M.; Hartikainen, J.M.; Hoeschen, C.; Laurent, O.; Noël, G.; Sabatier, L.; Salomaa, S.; et al. Clinical and epidemiological observations on individual radiation sensitivity and susceptibility. *Int. J. Radiat. Biol.* **2020**, *96*, 324–339. [CrossRef] [PubMed]
24. Bodgi, L.; Foray, N. The nucleo-shuttling of the ATM protein as a basis for a novel theory of radiation response: Resolution of the linear-quadratic model. *Int. J. Radiat. Biol.* **2016**, *92*, 117–131. [CrossRef] [PubMed]

25. Granzotto, A.; Benadjaoud, M.A.; Vogin, G.; Devic, C.; Ferlazzo, M.L.; Bodgi, L.; Pereira, S.; Sonzogni, L.; Forcheron, F.; Viau, M.; et al. Influence of nucleoshuttling of the ATM protein in the healthy tissues response to radiation therapy: Toward a molecular classification of human radiosensitivity. *Int. J. Radiat. Oncol. Biol. Phys.* **2016**, *94*, 450–460. [CrossRef] [PubMed]
26. West, C.M.; Elliott, R.M.; Burnet, N.G. The genomics revolution and radiotherapy. *Clin. Oncol. R. Coll. Radiol.* **2007**, *19*, 470–480. [CrossRef] [PubMed]
27. Gatti, R. The inherited basis for human radiosensitivity. *Radiat. Res.* **2008**, *170*, 669–670. [CrossRef] [PubMed]
28. Andreassen, C.N. Searching for genetic determinants of normal tissue radiosensitivity—Are we on the right track? *Radiother. Oncol.* **2010**, *97*, 1–8. [CrossRef]
29. West, C.M.; Barnett, G.C. Genetics and genomics of radiotherapy toxicity: Towards prediction. *Genome Med.* **2011**, *3*, 52. [CrossRef]
30. Barnett, G.C.; Kerns, S.L.; Noble, D.J.; Dunning, A.M.; West, C.M.; Burnet, N.G. Incorporating genetic biomarkers into predictive models of normal tissue toxicity. *Clin. Oncol. R. Coll. Radiol.* **2015**, *27*, 579–587. [CrossRef]
31. Andreassen, C.N.; Schack, L.M.H.; Laursen, L.V.; Alsner, J. Radiogenomics–current status, challenges and future directions. *Cancer Lett.* **2016**, *382*, 127–136. [CrossRef]
32. Palumbo, E.; Piotto, C.; Calura, E.; Fasanaro, E.; Groff, E.; Busato, F.; El Khouzai, B.; Rigo, M.; Baggio, L.; Romualdi, C.; et al. Individual radiosensitivity in oncological patients: Linking adverse normal tissue reactions and genetic features. *Front. Oncol.* **2019**, *9*, 987. [CrossRef]
33. Baumann, M.; Hölscher, T.; Begg, A.C. Towards genetic prediction of radiation responses: ESTRO's GENEPI project. *Radiother. Oncol.* **2003**, *69*, 121–125. [CrossRef]
34. Burnet, N.G.; Barnett, G.C.; Summersgill, H.R.; Dunning, A.M.; West, C.M.L. RAPPER—A success story for collaborative translational radiotherapy research. *Clin. Oncol.* **2019**, *31*, 416–419. [CrossRef] [PubMed]
35. Seibold, P.; Webb, A.; Aguado-Barrera, M.E.; Azria, D.; Bourgier, C.; Brengues, M.; Briers, E.; Bultijnck, R.; Calvo-Crespo, P.; Carballo, A.; et al. REQUITE: A prospective multicentre cohort study of patients undergoing radiotherapy for breast, lung or prostate cancer. *Radiother. Oncol.* **2019**, *138*, 59–67. [CrossRef] [PubMed]
36. Vinnikov, V.; Belyakov, O. Clinical applications of biomarker of radiation exposure: Limitations and possible solutions through coordinated research. *Radiat. Prot. Dosim.* **2019**, *186*, 3–8. [CrossRef] [PubMed]
37. Vinnikov, V.; Belyakov, O. Radiation exposure biomarkers in the practice of medical radiology: Cooperative research and the role of the International Atomic Energy Agency (IAEA) Biodosimetry/Radiobiology Laboratory. *Health Phys.* **2020**, *119*, 83–94. [CrossRef] [PubMed]
38. International Atomic Energy Agency (IAEA). *Clinical Application of Biomarkers of Radiation Exposure in Radiation Oncology*; IAEA Human Health Series; IAEA: Vienna, Austria, 2021; in press.
39. International Atomic Energy Agency (IAEA). *Cytogenetic Dosimetry: Application in Preparedness for and Response to Radiation Emergencies*; IAEA Emergency Preparedness and Response Series EPR-Biodosimetry; IAEA: Vienna, Austria, 2011.
40. Kato, T.A.; Wilson, P.F. (Eds.) *Radiation Cytogenetics. Methods and Protocols*; Methods in Molecular Biology; Springer Science + Business Media, LLC: Cham, Switzerland, 2019. [CrossRef]
41. Rosen, E.M.; Fan, S.; Goldberg, I.D.; Rockwell, S. Biological basis of radiation sensitivity. Part 2: Cellular and molecular determinants of radiosensitivity. *Oncol. Williston Park* **2000**, *14*, 741–757, discussion 757–758, 761–766.
42. Bourguignon, M.H.; Gisone, P.A.; Perez, M.R.; Michelin, S.; Dubner, D.; Giorgio, M.D.; Carosella, E.D. Genetic and epigenetic features in radiation sensitivity. Part II: Implications for clinical practice and radiation protection. *Eur. J. Nucl. Med. Mol. Imaging.* **2005**, *32*, 351–368. [CrossRef]
43. Jeggo, P.; Lavin, M.F. Cellular radiosensitivity: How much better do we understand it? *Int. J. Radiat. Biol.* **2009**, *85*, 1061–1081. [CrossRef]
44. Carrano, A.V.; Heddle, J.A. The fate of chromosome aberrations. *J. Theor. Biol.* **1973**, *38*, 289–304. [CrossRef]
45. Bauchinger, M.; Schmid, E.; Braselmann, H. Cell survival and radiation induced chromosome aberrations. II. Experimental findings in human lymphocytes analysed in first and second post-irradiation metaphases. *Radiat. Environ. Biophys.* **1986**, *25*, 253–260. [CrossRef]
46. Prosser, J.S.; Edwards, A.A.; Lloyd, D.C. The relationship between colony-forming ability and chromosomal aberrations induced in human T-lymphocytes after gamma-irradiation. *Int. J. Radiat. Biol.* **1990**, *58*, 293–301. [CrossRef]

47. Rave-Fränk, M.; Virsik-Köpp, P.; Pradier, O.; Nitsche, M.; Grünefeld, S.; Schmidberger, H. In vitro response of human dermal fibroblasts to X-irradiation: Relationship between radiation-induced clonogenic cell death, chromosome aberrations and markers of proliferative senescence or differentiation. *Int. J. Radiat. Biol.* **2001**, *77*, 1163–1174. [CrossRef] [PubMed]
48. Wu, X.; Spitz, M.R.; Amos, C.I.; Lin, J.; Shao, L.; Gu, J.; de Andrade, M.; Benowitz, N.L.; Shields, P.G.; Swan, G.E. Mutagen sensitivity has high heritability: Evidence from a twin study. *Cancer Res.* **2006**, *66*, 5993–5996. [CrossRef] [PubMed]
49. Camplejohn, R.S.; Hodgson, S.; Carter, N.; Kato, B.S.; Spector, T.D. Heritability of DNA-damage-induced apoptosis and its relationship with age in lymphocytes from female twins. *Br. J. Cancer.* **2006**, *95*, 520–524. [CrossRef] [PubMed]
50. Borgmann, K.; Haeberle, D.; Doerk, T.; Busjahn, A.; Stephan, G.; Dikomey, E. Genetic determination of chromosomal radiosensitivities in G_0- and G_2-phase human lymphocytes. *Radiother. Oncol.* **2007**, *83*, 196–202. [CrossRef]
51. Schmitz, A.; Bayer, J.; Dechamps, N.; Goldin, L.; Thomas, G. Heritability of susceptibility to ionizing radiation-induced apoptosis of human lymphocyte subpopulations. *Int. J. Radiat. Oncol. Biol. Phys.* **2007**, *68*, 1169–1177. [CrossRef]
52. Finnon, P.; Robertson, N.; Dziwura, S.; Raffy, C.; Zhang, W.; Ainsbury, L.; Kaprio, J.; Badie, C.; Bouffler, S. Evidence for significant heritability of apoptotic and cell cycle responses to ionising radiation. *Hum. Genet.* **2008**, *123*, 485–493. [CrossRef]
53. Curwen, G.B.; Cadwell, K.K.; Winther, J.F.; Tawn, E.J.; Rees, G.S.; Olsen, J.H.; Rechnitzer, C.; Schroeder, H.; Guldberg, P.; Cordell, H.J.; et al. The heritability of G_2 chromosomal radiosensitivity and its association with cancer in Danish cancer survivors and their offspring. *Int. J. Radiat. Biol.* **2010**, *86*, 986–995. [CrossRef]
54. Surowy, H.; Rinckleb, A.; Luedeke, M.; Stuber, M.; Wecker, A.; Varga, D.; Maier, C.; Hoegel, J.; Vogel, W. Heritability of baseline and induced micronucleus frequencies. *Mutagenesis* **2011**, *26*, 111–117. [CrossRef]
55. Zyla, J.; Kabacik, S.; O'Brien, G.; Wakil, S.; Al-Harbi, N.; Kaprio, J.; Badie, C.; Polanska, J.; Alsbeih, G. Combining CDKN1A gene expression and genome-wide SNPs in a twin cohort to gain insight into the heritability of individual radiosensitivity. *Funct. Integr. Genomics* **2019**, *19*, 575–585. [CrossRef]
56. Beaton, L.A.; Ferrarotto, C.; Marro, L.; Samiee, S.; Malone, S.; Grimes, S.; Malone, K.; Wilkins, R.C. Chromosome damage and cell proliferation rates in in vitro irradiated whole blood as markers of late radiation toxicity after radiation therapy to the prostate. *Int. J. Radiat. Oncol. Biol. Phys.* **2013**, *85*, 1346–1352. [CrossRef]
57. Beaton, L.A.; Marro, L.; Samiee, S.; Malone, S.; Grimes, S.; Malone, K.; Wilkins, R.C. Investigating chromosome damage using fluorescent in situ hybridization to identify biomarkers of radiosensitivity in prostate cancer patients. *Int. J. Radiat. Biol.* **2013**, *89*, 1087–1093. [CrossRef] [PubMed]
58. Beaton, L.A.; Marro, L.; Malone, S.; Samiee, S.; Grimes, S.; Malone, K.; Wilkins, R.C. Investigating γ H2AX as a biomarker of radiosensitivity using flow cytometry methods. *ISRN Radiol.* **2013**, *2013*, 704659. [CrossRef] [PubMed]
59. Matsubara, S.; Saito, F.; Suda, T.; Fijibayashi, H.; Shibuya, H.; Horiuchi, J.; Suzuki, S. Radiation injury in a patient with unusually high sensitivity to radiation. *Acta Oncol.* **1988**, *27*, 67–71. [CrossRef] [PubMed]
60. Dunst, J.; Gebhart, E.; Neubauer, S. Can an extremely elevated radiosensitivity in patients be recognized by the in-vitro testing of lymphocytes? *Strahlenther. Onkol.* **1995**, *171*, 581–586. [PubMed]
61. Greulich-Bode, K.M.; Zimmermann, F.; Muller, W.-U.; Pakisch, B.; Molls, M.; Wurschmidt, F. Clinical, molecular and cytogenetic analysis of a case of severe radio-sensitivity. *Curr. Genomics* **2012**, *13*, 426–432. [CrossRef] [PubMed]
62. Fahrig, A.; Koch, T.; Lenhart, M.; Rieckmann, P.; Fietkau, R.; Distel, L.; Schuster, B. Lethal outcome after pelvic salvage radiotherapy in a patient with prostate cancer due to increased radiosensitivity: Case report and literature review. *Strahlenther. Onkol.* **2018**, *194*, 60–66. [CrossRef]
63. Jones, L.A.; Scott, D.; Cowan, R.; Roberts, S.A. Abnormal radiosensitivity of lymphocytes from breast cancer patients with excessive normal tissue damage after radiotherapy: Chromosome aberrations after low dose-rate irradiation. *Int. J. Radiat. Biol.* **1995**, *67*, 519–528. [CrossRef]
64. Kondrashova, T.V.; Ivanova, T.I.; Katsalap, S.N. Chromosome aberrations in cultured peripheral lymphocytes from persons with elevated skin radiosensitivity. *Environ. Health Perspect.* **1997**, *105* (Suppl. 6), 1437–1439.

65. Borgmann, K.; Roper, B.; El-Awady, R.; Brackrock, S.; Bigalke, M.; Dork, T.; Alberti, W.; Dikomey, E.; Dahm-Daphi, J. Indicators of late normal tissue response after radiotherapy for head and neck cancer: Fibroblasts, lymphocytes, genetics, DNA repair, and chromosome aberrations. *Radiother. Oncol.* **2002**, *64*, 141–152. [CrossRef]
66. Hoeller, U.; Borgmann, K.; Bonacker, M.; Kuhlmey, A.; Bajrovic, A.; Jung, H.; Alberti, W.; Dikomey, E. Individual radiosensitivity measured with lymphocytes may be used to predict the risk of fibrosis after radiotherapy for breast cancer. *Radiother. Oncol.* **2003**, *69*, 137–144. [CrossRef]
67. Borgmann, K.; Hoeller, U.; Nowack, S.; Bernhard, M.; Röper, B.; Brackrock, S.; Petersen, C.; Szymczak, S.; Ziegler, A.; Feyer, P.; et al. Individual radiosensitivity measured with lymphocytes may predict the risk of acute reaction after radiotherapy. *Int. J. Radiat. Oncol. Biol. Phys.* **2008**, *71*, 256–264. [CrossRef] [PubMed]
68. Tang, Y.; Zhang, Y.; Guo, L.; Peng, Y.; Luo, Q.; Xing, Y. Relationship between individual radiosensitivity and radiation encephalopathy of nasopharyngeal carcinoma after radiotherapy. *Strahlenther. Onkol.* **2008**, *184*, 510–514. [CrossRef] [PubMed]
69. Chua, M.L.; Somaiah, N.; A'Hern, R.; Davies, S.; Gothard, L.; Yarnold, J.; Rothkamm, K. Residual DNA and chromosomal damage in ex vivo irradiated blood lymphocytes correlated with late normal tissue response to breast radiotherapy. *Radiother. Oncol.* **2011**, *99*, 362–366. [CrossRef] [PubMed]
70. Padjas, A.; Kedzierawski, P.; Florek, A.; Kukolowicz, P.; Kuszewski, T.; Góźdz, S.; Lankoff, A.; Wojcik, A.; Lisowska, H. Comparative analysis of three functional predictive assays in lymphocytes of patients with breast and gynaecological cancer treated by radiotherapy. *J. Contemp. Brachyther.* **2012**, *4*, 219–226. [CrossRef]
71. Neubauer, S.; Dunst, J.; Gebhart, E. The impact of complex chromosomal rearrangements on the detection of radiosensitivity in cancer patients. *Radiother. Oncol.* **1997**, *43*, 189–195. [CrossRef]
72. Dunst, J.; Neubauer, S.; Becker, A.; Gebhart, E. Chromosomal in-vitro radiosensitivity of lymphocytes in radiotherapy patients and AT-homozygotes. *Strahlenther. Onkol.* **1998**, *174*, 510–516. [CrossRef] [PubMed]
73. Keller, U.; Kuechler, A.; Liehr, T.; Müller, E.; Grabenbauer, G.; Sauer, R.; Distel, L. Impact of various parameters in detecting chromosomal aberrations by FISH to describe radiosensitivity. *Strahlenther. Onkol.* **2004**, *180*, 289–296. [CrossRef]
74. Huber, R.; Braselmann, H.; Geinitz, H.; Jaehnert, I.; Baumgartner, A.; Thamm, R.; Figel, M.; Molls, M.; Zitzelsberger, H. Chromosomal radiosensitivity and acute radiation side effects after radiotherapy in tumour patients—A follow-up study. *Radiat. Oncol.* **2011**, *6*, 32. [CrossRef]
75. Schmitz, S.; Brzozowska, K.; Pinkawa, M.; Eble, M.; Kriehuber, R. Chromosomal radiosensitivity analyzed by FISH in lymphocytes of prostate cancer patients and healthy donors. *Radiat. Res.* **2013**, *180*, 465–473. [CrossRef]
76. Rached, E.; Schindler, R.; Beer, K.T.; Vetterli, D.; Greiner, R.H. No predictive value of the micronucleus assay for patients with severe acute reaction of normal tissue after radiotherapy. *Eur. J. Cancer* **1998**, *34*, 378–383. [CrossRef]
77. Barber, J.B.; Burrill, W.; Spreadborough, A.R.; Levine, E.; Warren, C.; Kiltie, A.E.; Roberts, S.A.; Scott, D. Relationship between in vitro chromosomal radiosensitivity of peripheral blood lymphocytes and the expression of normal tissue damage following radiotherapy for breast cancer. *Radiother. Oncol.* **2000**, *55*, 179–186. [CrossRef]
78. Słonina, D.; Klimek, M.; Szpytma, T.; Gasinska, A. Comparison of the radiosensitivity of normal-tissue cells with normal-tissue reactions after radiotherapy. *Int. J. Radiat. Biol.* **2000**, *76*, 1255–1264. [CrossRef] [PubMed]
79. Lee, T.K.; O'Brien, K.F.; Naves, J.L.; Christie, K.I.; Arastu, H.H.; Eaves, G.S.; Wiley, A.L., Jr.; Karlsson, U.L.; Salehpour, M.R. Micronuclei in lymphocytes of prostate cancer patients undergoing radiation therapy. *Mutat. Res.* **2000**, *469*, 63–70. [CrossRef]
80. Lee, T.K.; Allison, R.R.; O'Brien, K.F.; Johnke, R.M.; Christie, K.I.; Naves, J.L.; Kovacs, C.J.; Arastu, H.; Karlsson, U.L. Lymphocyte radiosensitivity correlated with pelvic radiotherapy morbidity. *Int. J. Radiat. Oncol. Biol. Phys.* **2003**, *57*, 222–229. [CrossRef]
81. Widel, M.; Jedrus, S.; Lukaszczyk, B.; Raczek-Zwierzycka, K.; Swierniak, A. Radiation-induced micronucleus frequency in peripheral blood lymphocytes is correlated with normal tissue damage in patients with cervical carcinoma undergoing radiotherapy. *Radiat. Res.* **2003**, *159*, 713–721. [CrossRef]

82. Bustos, E.; Di Giorgio, M.; Sardi, M.; Aguilar Paredes, J.; Taja, M.R. Micronucleus assay as radiosensitivity indicator in head and neck tumor patients. Retrospective and prospective study. In Proceedings of the Annual Meeting of the American Academy of Otolaryngology-Head and Neck Surgery, San Diego, CA, USA, 21–25 September 2002; pp. 305–309.
83. Di Giorgio, M.; Sardi, M.; Bustos, E.; Vallerga, M.B.; Taja, M.R.; Mairal, L. Assessment of individual radiosensitivity in human lymphocytes using micronucleus and microgel electrophoresis "Comet" assays. In Proceedings of the 11th International Congress on the International Radiation Protection Association, Madrid, Spain, 23–28 May 2004; pp. 53–60.
84. Taghavi-Dehaghani, M.; Mohammadi, S.; Ziafazeli, T.; Sardari-Kermani, M. A study on differences between radiation-induced micronuclei and apoptosis of lymphocytes in breast cancer patients after radiotherapy. *Z. Naturforsch. C* **2005**, *60*, 938–942. [CrossRef]
85. Rzeszowska-Wolny, J.; Palyvoda, O.; Polanska, J.; Wygoda, A.; Hancock, R. Relationships between acute reactions to radiotherapy in head and neck cancer patients and parameters of radiation-induced DNA damage and repair in their lymphocytes. *Int. J. Radiat. Biol.* **2008**, *84*, 635–642. [CrossRef]
86. Encheva, E.; Deleva, S.; Hristova, R.; Hadjidekova, V.; Hadjieva, T. Investigating micronucleus assay applicability for prediction of normal tissue intrinsic radiosensitivity in gynecological cancer patients. *Rep. Pract. Oncol. Radiother.* **2011**, *17*, 24–31. [CrossRef]
87. Finnon, P.; Kabacik, S.; MacKay, A.; Raffy, C.; A'Hern, R.; Owen, R.; Badie, C.; Yarnold, J.; Bouffler, S. Correlation of in vitro lymphocyte radiosensitivity and gene expression with late normal tissue reactions following curative radiotherapy for breast cancer. *Radiother. Oncol.* **2012**, *105*, 329–336. [CrossRef]
88. Vandevoorde, C.; Depuydt, J.; Veldeman, L.; De Neve, W.; Sebastià, N.; Wieme, G.; Baert, A.; De Langhe, S.; Philippé, J.; Thierens, H.; et al. In vitro cellular radiosensitivity in relationship to late normal tissue reactions in breast cancer patients: A multi-endpoint case-control study. *Int. J. Radiat. Biol.* **2016**, *92*, 823–836. [CrossRef]
89. Batar, B.; Guven, G.; Eroz, S.; Bese, N.S.; Guven, M. Decreased DNA repair gene XRCC1 expression is associated with radiotherapy-induced acute side effects in breast cancer patients. *Gene* **2016**, *582*, 33–37. [CrossRef] [PubMed]
90. Batar, B.; Mutlu, T.; Bostanci, M.; Akin, M.; Tuncdemir, M.; Bese, N.; Guven, M. DNA repair and apoptosis: Roles in radiotherapy-related acute reactions in breast cancer patients. *Cell. Mol. Biol.* **2018**, *64*, 64–70. [CrossRef]
91. Guogytė, K.; Plieskienė, A.; Ladygienė, R.; Vaisiūnas, Ž.; Sevriukova, O.; Janušonis, V.; Žiliukas, J. Assessment of correlation between chromosomal radiosensitivity of peripheral blood lymphocytes after in vitro irradiation and normal tissue side effects for cancer patients undergoing radiotherapy. *Genome Integr.* **2017**, *8*, 1. [CrossRef] [PubMed]
92. Da Silva, E.B.; Cavalcanti, B.M.; Ferreira Da Silva, C.S.; de Salazar E Fernandes, T.; Melo, J.A.; Lucena, L.; Netto, A.M.; Amaral, A. Micronucleus assay for predicting side effects of radiotherapy for cervical cancer. *Biotech. Histochem.* **2020**, 1–7. [CrossRef] [PubMed]
93. Chaouni, S.; Lecomte, D.D.; Stefan, D.; Leduc, A.; Barraux, V.; Leconte, A.; Grellard, J.M.; Habrand, J.L.; Guillamin, M.; Sichel, F.; et al. The possibility of using genotoxicity, oxidative stress and inflammation blood biomarkers to predict the occurrence of late cutaneous side effects after radiotherapy. *Antioxidants* **2020**, *9*, 220. [CrossRef] [PubMed]
94. Joubert, A.; Zimmerman, K.M.; Bencokova, Z.; Gastaldo, J.; Chavaudra, N.; Favaudon, V.; Arlett, C.F.; Foray, N. DNA double-strand break repair defects in syndromes associated with acute radiation response: At least two different assays to predict intrinsic radiosensitivity? *Int. J. Radiat. Biol.* **2008**, *84*, 107–125. [CrossRef] [PubMed]
95. Massart, C.; Joubert, A.; Granzotto, A.; Viau, M.; Seghier, F.; Balosso, J.; Foray, N. Prediction of the human radiosensitivity: What is the most relevant endpoint? Gene expressions, mutations or functions? Chapter XI. In *Genotoxicity: Evaluation, Testing and Prediction*; Kocsis, A., Molna, H., Eds.; Nova Science Publishers Inc.: Hauppauge, NY, USA, 2009; pp. 275–291, ISBN 978-1-60741-714-9.
96. Iliakis, G.; Murmann, T.; Soni, A. Alternative end-joining repair pathways are the ultimate backup for abrogated classical non-homologous end-joining and homologous recombination repair: Implications for the formation of chromosome translocations. *Mutat. Res. Genet. Toxicol. Environ. Mutagen.* **2015**, *793*, 166–175. [CrossRef] [PubMed]

97. Van Oorschot, B.; Hovingh, S.E.; Moerland, P.D.; Medema, J.P.; Stalpers, L.J.; Vrieling, H.; Franken, N.A. Reduced activity of double-strand break repair genes in prostate cancer patients with late normal tissue radiation toxicity. *Int. J. Radiat. Oncol. Biol. Phys.* **2014**, *88*, 664–670. [CrossRef]
98. Zahnreich, S.; Weber, B.; Rösch, G.; Schindler, D.; Schmidberger, H. Compromised repair of radiation-induced DNA double-strand breaks in Fanconi anemia fibroblasts in G2. *DNA Repair Amst.* **2020**, *96*, 102992. [CrossRef]
99. Vinnikov, V.A.; Maznyk, N.A. Cytogenetic dose-response in vitro for biological dosimetry after exposure to high doses of gamma-rays. *Radiat. Prot. Dosim.* **2013**, *154*, 186–197. [CrossRef]
100. Müller, W.U.; Rode, A. The micronucleus assay in human lymphocytes after high radiation doses (5–15 Gy). *Mutat. Res.* **2002**, *502*, 47–51. [CrossRef]
101. Kacprzak, J.; Kuszewski, T.; Lankoff, A.; Müller, W.U.; Wojcik, A.; Lisowska, H. Individual variations in the micronucleus assay for biological dosimetry after high dose exposure. *Mutat. Res.* **2013**, *756*, 196–200. [CrossRef] [PubMed]
102. Scott, D.; Hu, Q.; Roberts, S.A. Dose-rate sparing for micronucleus induction in lymphocytes of controls and ataxia-telangiectasia heterozygotes exposed to ^{60}Co gamma-irradiation in vitro. *Int. J. Radiat. Biol.* **1996**, *70*, 521–527. [CrossRef] [PubMed]
103. Distel, L.V.; Neubauer, S.; Keller, U.; Sprung, C.N.; Sauer, R.; Grabenbauer, G. Individual differences in chromosomal aberrations after in vitro irradiation of cells from healthy individuals, cancer and cancer susceptibility syndrome patients. *Radiother. Oncol.* **2006**, *81*, 257–263. [CrossRef] [PubMed]
104. Moquet, J.; Rothkamm, K.; Barnard, S.; Ainsbury, E. Radiation biomarkers in large scale human health effects studies. *J. Pers. Med.* **2020**, *10*, 155. [CrossRef]
105. Ainsbury, E.A.; Livingston, G.K.; Abbott, M.G.; Moquet, J.E.; Hone, P.A.; Jenkins, M.S.; Christensen, D.M.; Lloyd, D.C.; Rothkamm, K. Interlaboratory variation in scoring dicentric chromosomes in a case of partial-body x-ray exposure: Implications for biodosimetry networking and cytogenetic "triage mode" scoring. *Radiat. Res.* **2009**, *172*, 746–752. [CrossRef]
106. Keller, U.; Grabenbauer, G.; Kuechler, A.; Sauer, R.; Distel, L. Technical report. Radiation sensitivity testing by fluorescence in-situ hybridization: How many metaphases have to be analysed? *Int. J. Radiat. Biol.* **2004**, *80*, 615–620. [CrossRef]
107. Nachtrab, U.; Oppitz, U.; Flentje, M.; Stopper, H. Radiation-induced micronucleus formation in human skin fibroblasts of patients showing severe and normal tissue damage after radiotherapy. *Int. J. Radiat. Biol.* **1998**, *73*, 279–287. [CrossRef]
108. Akudugu, J.M.; Bell, R.S.; Catton, C.; Davis, A.M.; O'Sullivan, B.; Waldron, J.; Wunder, J.S.; Hill, R.P. Clonogenic survival and cytokinesis-blocked binucleation of skin fibroblasts and normal tissue complications in soft tissue sarcoma patients treated with preoperative radiotherapy. *Radiother. Oncol.* **2004**, *72*, 103–112. [CrossRef]
109. Sprung, C.N.; Chao, M.; Leong, T.; McKay, J. Chromosomal radiosensitivity in two cell lineages derived from clinically radiosensitive cancer patients. *Clin. Cancer Res.* **2005**, *11*, 6352–6358. [CrossRef]
110. Słonina, D.; Biesaga, B.; Urbanski, K.; Kojs, Z. Comparison of chromosomal radiosensitivity of normal cells with and without HRS-like response and normal tissue reactions in patients with cervix cancer. *Int. J. Radiat. Biol.* **2008**, *84*, 421–428. [CrossRef] [PubMed]
111. Redon, C.E.; Weyemi, U.; Parekh, P.R.; Huang, D.; Burrell, A.S.; Bonner, W.M. γ-H2AX and other histone post-translational modifications in the clinic. *Biochim. Biophys. Acta* **2012**, *1819*, 743–756. [CrossRef] [PubMed]
112. Roch-Lefèvre, S.; Mandina, T.; Voisin, P.; Gaëtan, G.; Mesa, J.E.; Valente, M.; Bonnesoeur, P.; García, O.; Voisin, P.; Roy, L. Quantification of gamma-H2AX foci in human lymphocytes: A method for biological dosimetry after ionizing radiation exposure. *Radiat. Res.* **2010**, *174*, 185–194. [CrossRef] [PubMed]
113. Roch-Lefèvre, S.; Valente, M.; Voisin, P.h.; Barquinero, J.-F. Suitability of the γH2AX Assay for Human Radiation Biodosimetry. In *Current Topics in Ionizing Radiation Research*; Nenoi, M., Ed.; IntechOpen: London, UK, 2012. Available online: https://www.intechopen.com/books/current-topics-in-ionizing-radiation-research/suitability-of-the-gamma-h2ax-assay-for-human-radiation-biodosimetry (accessed on 2 December 2020). [CrossRef]
114. Moquet, J.; Barnard, S.; Rothkamm, K. Gamma-H2AX biodosimetry for use in large scale radiation incidents: Comparison of a rapid '96 well lyse/fix' protocol with a routine method. *Peer J.* **2014**, *2*, e282. [CrossRef] [PubMed]

115. Viau, M.; Testard, I.; Shim, G.; Morat, L.; Normil, M.D.; Hempel, W.M.; Sabatier, L. Global quantification of γH2AX as a triage tool for the rapid estimation of received dose in the event of accidental radiation exposure. *Mutat. Res.* **2015**, *793*, 123–131. [CrossRef]
116. Raavi, V.; Perumal, V.; Paul, S.F.D. Potential application of γ-H2AX as a biodosimetry tool for radiation triage. *Mutat. Res.* **2020**, 108350. [CrossRef]
117. Olive, P.L.; Banáth, J.P.; Keyes, M. Residual gamma H2AX after irradiation of human lymphocytes and monocytes in vitro and its relation to late effects after prostate brachytherapy. *Radiother. Oncol.* **2008**, *86*, 336–346. [CrossRef]
118. Werbrouck, J.; De Ruyck, K.; Beels, L.; Vral, A.; Van Eijkeren, M.; De Neve, W.; Thierens, H. Prediction of late normal tissue complications in RT treated gynaecological cancer patients: Potential of the gamma-H2AX foci assay and association with chromosomal radiosensitivity. *Oncol. Rep.* **2010**, *23*, 571–578. [CrossRef]
119. Werbrouck, J.; Duprez, F.; De Neve, W.; Thierens, H. Lack of a correlation between γH2AX foci kinetics in lymphocytes and the severity of acute normal tissue reactions during IMRT treatment for head and neck cancer. *Int. J. Radiat. Biol.* **2011**, *87*, 46–56. [CrossRef]
120. Fleckenstein, J.; Kühne, M.; Seegmüller, K.; Derschang, S.; Melchior, P.; Gräber, S.; Fricke, A.; Rübe, C.E.; Rübe, C. The impact of individual in vivo repair of DNA double-strand breaks on oral mucositis in adjuvant radiotherapy of head-and-neck cancer. *Int. J. Radiat. Oncol. Biol. Phys.* **2011**, *81*, 1465–1472. [CrossRef]
121. Greve, B.; Bölling, T.; Amler, S.; Rössler, U.; Gomolka, M.; Mayer, C.; Popanda, O.; Dreffke, K.; Rickinger, A.; Fritz, E.; et al. Evaluation of different biomarkers to predict individual radiosensitivity in an inter-laboratory comparison–lessons for future studies. *PLoS ONE* **2012**, *7*, e47185. [CrossRef] [PubMed]
122. Brzozowska, K.; Pinkawa, M.; Eble, M.J.; Müller, W.U.; Wojcik, A.; Kriehuber, R.; Schmitz, S. In vivo versus in vitro individual radiosensitivity analysed in healthy donors and in prostate cancer patients with and without severe side effects after radiotherapy. *Int. J. Radiat. Biol.* **2012**, *88*, 405–413. [CrossRef] [PubMed]
123. Schuler, N.; Palm, J.; Kaiser, M.; Betten, D.; Furtwängler, R.; Rübe, C.; Graf, N.; Rübe, C.E. DNA-damage foci to detect and characterize DNA repair alterations in children treated for pediatric malignancies. *PLoS ONE* **2014**, *9*, e91319. [CrossRef] [PubMed]
124. Djuzenova, C.S.; Zimmermann, M.; Katzer, A.; Fiedler, V.; Distel, L.V.; Gasser, M.; Waaga-Gasser, A.M.; Flentje, M.; Polat, B. A prospective study on histone γ-H2AX and 53BP1 foci expression in rectal carcinoma patients: Correlation with radiation therapy-induced outcome. *BMC Cancer* **2015**, *15*, 856. [CrossRef]
125. Marková, E.; Somsedíková, A.; Vasilyev, S.; Pobijaková, M.; Lacková, A.; Lukačko, P.; Belyaev, I. DNA repair foci and late apoptosis/necrosis in peripheral blood lymphocytes of breast cancer patients undergoing radiotherapy. *Int. J. Radiat. Biol.* **2015**, *91*, 934–945. [CrossRef]
126. Pinkawa, M.; Brzozowska, K.; Kriehuber, R.; Eble, M.J.; Schmitz, S. Prediction of radiation-induced toxicity by in vitro radiosensitivity of lymphocytes in prostate cancer patients. *Future Oncol.* **2016**, *12*, 617–624. [CrossRef]
127. Löbrich, M.; Rief, N.; Kuhne, M.; Heckmann, M.; Fleckenstein, J.; Rube, C.; Uder, M. In vivo formation and repair of DNA double-strand breaks after computed tomography examinations. *Proc. Natl. Acad. Sci. USA* **2005**, *102*, 8984–8989. [CrossRef]
128. Rübe, C.E.; Fricke, A.; Schneider, R.; Simon, K.; Kühne, M.; Fleckenstein, J.; Gräber, S.; Graf, N.; Rübe, C. DNA repair alterations in children with pediatric malignancies: Novel opportunities to identify patients at risk for high-grade toxicities. *Int. J. Radiat. Oncol. Biol. Phys.* **2010**, *78*, 359–369. [CrossRef]
129. Bourton, E.C.; Plowman, P.N.; Smith, D.; Arlett, C.F.; Parris, C.N. Prolonged expression of the gamma-H2AX DNA repair biomarker correlates with excess acute and chronic toxicity from radiotherapy treatment. *Int. J. Cancer* **2011**, *129*, 2928–2934. [CrossRef]
130. Goutham, H.V.; Mumbrekar, K.D.; Vadhiraja, B.M.; Fernandes, D.J.; Sharan, K.; Parashiva, G.K.; Kapaettu, S.; Sadashiva, S.R.B. DNA double-strand break analysis by γ-H2AX foci: A useful method for determining the overreactors to radiation-induced acute reactions among head-and-neck cancer patients. *Int. J. Radiat. Oncol. Biol. Phys.* **2012**, *84*, e607–e612. [CrossRef]
131. Li, P.; Du, C.R.; Xu, W.C.; Shi, Z.L.; Zhang, Q.; Li, Z.B.; Fu, S. Correlation of dynamic changes in γ-H2AX expression in peripheral blood lymphocytes from head and neck cancer patients with radiation-induced oral mucositis. *Radiat. Oncol.* **2013**, *8*, 155. [CrossRef] [PubMed]

132. Djuzenova, C.S.; Elsner, I.; Katzer, A.; Worschech, E.; Distel, L.V.; Flentje, M.; Polat, B. Radiosensitivity in breast cancer assessed by the histone γ-H2AX and 53BP1 foci. *Radiat. Oncol.* **2013**, *8*, 98. [CrossRef] [PubMed]
133. Mumbrekar, K.D.; Fernandes, D.J.; Goutham, H.V.; Sharan, K.; Vadhiraja, B.M.; Satyamoorthy, K.; Sadashiva, S.R.B. Influence of double-strand break repair on radiation therapy-induced acute skin reactions in breast cancer patients. *Int. J. Radiat. Oncol. Biol. Phys.* **2014**, *88*, 671–676. [CrossRef] [PubMed]
134. Chua, M.L.; Horn, S.; Somaiah, N.; Davies, S.; Gothard, L.; A'Hern, R.; Yarnold, J.; Rothkamm, K. DNA double-strand break repair and induction of apoptosis in ex vivo irradiated blood lymphocytes in relation to late normal tissue reactions following breast radiotherapy. *Radiat. Environ. Biophys.* **2014**, *53*, 355–364. [CrossRef]
135. Pouliliou, S.E.; Lialiaris, T.S.; Dimitriou, T.; Giatromanolaki, A.; Papazoglou, D.; Pappa, A.; Pistevou, K.; Kalamida, D.; Koukourakis, M.I. Survival fraction at 2 Gy and γH2AX expression kinetics in peripheral blood lymphocytes from cancer patients: Relationship with acute radiation-induced toxicities. *Int. J. Radiat. Oncol. Biol. Phys.* **2015**, *92*, 667–674. [CrossRef]
136. Van Oorschot, B.; Hovingh, S.; Dekker, A.; Stalpers, L.J.; Franken, N.A. Predicting radiosensitivity with gamma-H2AX foci assay afters single High-Dose-Rate and Pulsed Dose-Rate ionizing irradiation. *Radiat. Res.* **2016**, *185*, 190–198. [CrossRef]
137. Somaiah, N.; Chua, M.L.; Bourne, S.; Daley, F.; A'Hern, R.; Nuta, O.; Gothard, L.; Boyle, S.; Herskind, C.; Pearson, A.; et al. Correlation between DNA damage responses of skin to a test dose of radiation and late adverse effects of earlier breast radiotherapy. *Radiother. Oncol.* **2016**, *119*, 244–249. [CrossRef]
138. Lobachevsky, P.; Leong, T.; Daly, P.; Smith, J.; Best, N.; Tomaszewski, J.; Thompson, E.R.; Li, N.; Campbell, I.G.; Martin, R.F.; et al. Compromized DNA repair as a basis for identification of cancer radiotherapy patients with extreme radiosensitivity. *Cancer Lett.* **2016**, *383*, 212–219. [CrossRef]
139. Papworth, R.; Slevin, N.; Roberts, S.A.; Scott, D. Sensitivity to radiation-induced chromosome damage may be a marker of genetic predisposition in young head and neck cancer patients. *Br. J. Cancer.* **2001**, *84*, 776–782. [CrossRef]
140. Lisowska, H.; Lankoff, A.; Wieczorek, A.; Florek, A.; Kuszewski, T.; Góźdź, S.; Wojcik, A. Enhanced chromosomal radiosensitivity in peripheral blood lymphocytes of larynx cancer patients. *Int. J. Radiat. Oncol. Biol. Phys.* **2006**, *66*, 1245–1252. [CrossRef]
141. Scott, D.; Barber, J.B.; Spreadborough, A.R.; Burrill, W.; Roberts, S.A. Increased chromosomal radiosensitivity in breast cancer patients: A comparison of two assays. *Int. J. Radiat. Biol.* **1999**, *75*, 1–10. [CrossRef] [PubMed]
142. Scott, D. Chromosomal radiosensitivity, cancer predisposition and response to radiotherapy. *Strahlenther. Onkol.* **2000**, *176*, 229–234. [CrossRef] [PubMed]
143. De Ruyck, K.; Van Eijkeren, M.; Claes, K.; Morthier, R.; De Paepe, A.; Vral, A.; De Ridder, L.; Thierens, H. Radiation-induced damage to normal tissues after radiotherapy in patients treated for gynecologic tumors: Association with single nucleotide polymorphisms in XRCC1, XRCC3, and OGG1 genes and in vitro chromosomal radiosensitivity in lymphocytes. *Int. J. Radiat. Oncol. Biol. Phys.* **2005**, *62*, 1140–1149. [CrossRef] [PubMed]
144. Djuzenova, C.S.; Mühl, B.; Fehn, M.; Oppitz, U.; Müller, B.; Flentje, M. Radiosensitivity in breast cancer assessed by the Comet and micronucleus assays. *Br. J. Cancer.* **2006**, *94*, 1194–1203. [CrossRef] [PubMed]
145. Kato, T.A.; Wilson, P.F.; Nagasaw, H.; Peng, Y.; Weil, M.M.; Little, J.B.; Bedford, J.S. Variations in radiosensitivity among individuals: A potential impact on risk assessment? *Health Phys.* **2009**, *97*, 470–480. [CrossRef] [PubMed]
146. Cadwell, K.K.; Curwen, G.B.; Tawn, E.J.; Winther, J.F.; Boice, J.D., Jr. G2 checkpoint control and G2 chromosomal radiosensitivity in cancer survivors and their families. *Mutagenesis* **2011**, *26*, 291–294. [CrossRef]
147. Roberts, S.A.; Spreadborough, A.R.; Bulman, B.; Barber, J.B.; Evans, D.G.; Scott, D. Heritability of cellular radiosensitivity: A marker of low-penetrance predisposition genes in breast cancer? *Am. J. Hum. Genet.* **1999**, *65*, 784–794. [CrossRef]
148. Scott, D. Chromosomal radiosensitivity and low penetrance predisposition to cancer. *Cytogenet. Genome Res.* **2004**, *104*, 365–370. [CrossRef]
149. Curwen, G.B.; Cadwell, K.K.; Tawn, E.J.; Winther, J.F.; Boice, J.D., Jr. Intra-individual variation in G2 chromosomal radiosensitivity. *Mutagenesis* **2012**, *27*, 471–475. [CrossRef]

150. Sprung, C.N.; Davey, D.S.; Withana, N.P.; Distel, L.V.; McKay, M.J. Telomere length in lymphoblast cell lines derived from clinically radiosensitive cancer patients. *Cancer Biol. Ther.* **2008**, *7*, 638–644. [CrossRef]
151. Iwasaki, T.; Robertson, N.; Tsigani, T.; Finnon, P.; Scott, D.; Levine, E.; Badie, C.; Bouffler, S. Lymphocyte telomere length correlates with in vitro radiosensitivity in breast cancer cases but is not predictive of acute normal tissue reactions to radiotherapy. *Int. J. Radiat. Biol.* **2008**, *84*, 277–284. [CrossRef]
152. Twardella, D.; Chang-Claude, J. Studies on radiosensitivity from an epidemiological point of view-overview of methods and results. *Radiother. Oncol.* **2002**, *62*, 249–260. [CrossRef]
153. Abend, M.; Badie, C.; Quintens, R.; Kriehuber, R.; Manning, G.; Macaeva, E.; Njima, M.; Oskamp, D.; Strunz, S.; Moertl, S.; et al. Examining radiation-induced in vivo and in vitro gene expression changes of the peripheral blood in different laboratories for biodosimetry purposes: First RENEB gene expression study. *Radiat. Res.* **2016**, *185*, 109–123. [CrossRef] [PubMed]
154. Macaeva, E.; Mysara, M.; De Vos, W.H.; Baatout, S.; Quintens, R. Gene expression-based biodosimetry for radiological incidents: Assessment of dose and time after radiation exposure. *Int. J. Radiat. Biol.* **2019**, *95*, 64–75. [CrossRef]
155. O'Brien, G.; Cruz-Garcia, L.; Majewski, M.; Grepl, J.; Abend, M.; Port, M.; Tichý, A.; Sirak, I.; Malkova, A.; Donovan, E.; et al. FDXR is a biomarker of radiation exposure in vivo. *Sci. Rep.* **2018**, *8*, 684. [CrossRef]
156. Tichý, A.; Kabacik, S.; O'Brien, G.; Pejchal, J.; Sinkorova, Z.; Kmochova, A.; Sirak, I.; Malkova, A.; Beltran, C.G.; Gonzalez, J.R.; et al. The first in vivo multiparametric comparison of different radiation exposure biomarkers in human blood. *PLoS ONE* **2018**, *13*, e0193412. [CrossRef]
157. Rieger, K.E.; Hong, W.J.; Tusher, V.G.; Tang, J.; Tibshirani, R.; Chu, G. Toxicity from radiation therapy associated with abnormal transcriptional responses to DNA damage. *Proc. Natl. Acad. Sci. USA* **2004**, *101*, 6635–6640. [CrossRef]
158. Svensson, J.P.; Stalpers, L.J.; Esveldt-vanLange, R.E.; Franken, N.A.; Haveman, J.; Klein, B.; Turesson, I.; Vrieling, H.; Giphart-Gassler, M. Analysis of gene expression using gene sets discriminates cancer patients with and without late radiation toxicity. *PLoS Med.* **2006**, *3*, e422. [CrossRef] [PubMed]
159. Wiebalk, K.; Schmezer, P.; Kropp, S.; Chang-Claude, J.; Celebi, O.; Debus, J.; Bartsch, H.; Popanda, O. In vitro radiation-induced expression of XPC mRNA as a possible biomarker for developing adverse reactions during radiotherapy. *Int. J. Cancer* **2007**, *121*, 2340–2345. [CrossRef] [PubMed]
160. Badie, C.; Dziwura, S.; Raffy, C.; Tsigani, T.; Alsbeih, G.; Moody, J.; Finnon, P.; Levine, E.; Scott, D.; Bouffler, S. Aberrant CDKN1A transcriptional response associates with abnormal sensitivity to radiation treatment. *Br. J. Cancer* **2008**, *98*, 1845–1851. [CrossRef]
161. Henríquez-Hernández, L.A.; Lara, P.C.; Pinar, B.; Bordón, E.; Gallego, C.R.; Bilbao, C.; Pérez, L.F.; Morales, A.F. Constitutive gene expression profile segregates toxicity in locally advanced breast cancer patients treated with high-dose hyperfractionated radical radiotherapy. *Radiat. Oncol.* **2009**, *4*, 17. [CrossRef] [PubMed]
162. Mayer, C.; Popanda, O.; Greve, B.; Fritz, E.; Illig, T.; Eckardt-Schupp, F.; Gomolka, M.; Benner, A.; Schmezer, P. A radiation-induced gene expression signature as a tool to predict acute radiotherapy-induced adverse side effects. *Cancer Lett.* **2011**, *302*, 20–28. [CrossRef] [PubMed]
163. Manning, G.; Tichý, A.; Sirák, I.; Badie, C. Radiotherapy-associated long-term modification of expression of the inflammatory biomarker genes *ARG1*, *BCL2L1*, and *MYC*. *Front. Immunol.* **2017**, *8*, 412. [CrossRef] [PubMed]
164. Huber, R.; Braselmann, H.; Bauchinger, M. Intra- and inter-individual variation of background and radiation-induced micronucleus frequencies in human lymphocytes. *Int. J. Radiat. Biol.* **1992**, *61*, 655–661. [CrossRef]
165. Scott, D.; Barber, J.B.; Levine, E.L.; Burrill, W.; Roberts, S.A. Radiation-induced micronucleus induction in lymphocytes identifies a high frequency of radiosensitive cases among breast cancer patients: A test for predisposition? *Br. J. Cancer* **1998**, *77*, 614–620. [CrossRef]
166. Słonina, D.; Gasińska, A. Intrinsic radiosensitivity of healthy donors and cancer patients as determined by the lymphocyte micronucleus assay. *Int. J. Radiat. Biol.* **1997**, *72*, 693–701. [CrossRef]
167. Burrill, W.; Levine, E.L.; Hindocha, P.; Roberts, S.A.; Scott, D. The use of cryopreserved lymphocytes in assessing inter-individual radiosensitivity with the micronucleus assay. *Int. J. Radiat. Biol.* **2000**, *76*, 375–382. [CrossRef]

168. Vral, A.; Thierens, H.; Baeyens, A.; De Ridder, L. The micronucleus and G_2-phase assays for human blood lymphocytes as biomarkers of individual sensitivity to ionizing radiation: Limitations imposed by intraindividual variability. *Radiat. Res.* **2002**, *157*, 472–477. [CrossRef]
169. Vral, A.; Thierens, H.; Baeyens, A.; De Ridder, L. What is the reliability of chromosomal aberration assays as biomarkers of individual sensitivity towards ionising radiation? *Int. J. Low Radiat.* **2004**, *1*, 256–265. [CrossRef]
170. Vral, A.; Thierens, H.; Baeyens, A.; De Ridder, L. Chromosomal aberrations and in vitro radiosensitivity: Intra-individual versus inter-individual variability. *Toxicol. Lett.* **2004**, *149*, 345–352. [CrossRef]
171. Stephan, G.; Schneider, K.; Panzer, W.; Walsh, L.; Oestreicher, U. Enhanced yield of chromosome aberrations after CT examinations in paediatric patients. *Int. J. Radiat. Biol.* **2007**, *83*, 281–287. [CrossRef] [PubMed]
172. Vandevoorde, C.; Franck, C.; Bacher, K.; Breysem, L.; Smet, M.H.; Ernst, C.; De Backer, A.; Van DeMoortele, K.; Smeets, P.; Thierens, H. γ-H2AX foci as in vivo effect biomarker in children emphasize the importance to minimize x-ray doses in paediatric CT imaging. *Eur. Radiol.* **2015**, *25*, 800–811. [CrossRef] [PubMed]
173. Nakamura, N.; Sposto, R.; Kushiro, J.; Akiyama, M. Is interindividual variation of cellular radiosensitivity real or artifactual? *Radiat. Res.* **1991**, *125*, 326–330. [CrossRef] [PubMed]
174. Elyan, S.A.; West, C.M.; Roberts, S.A.; Hunter, R.D. Use of an internal standard in comparative measurements of the intrinsic radiosensitivities of human T-lymphocytes. *Int. J. Radiat. Biol.* **1993**, *64*, 385–391. [CrossRef]
175. Wilkins, R.C.; Rodrigues, M.A.; Beaton-Green, L.A. The application of imaging flow cytometry to high-throughput biodosimetry. *Genome Integr.* **2017**, *8*, 7. [CrossRef]
176. Li, Y.; Shirley, B.C.; Wilkins, R.C.; Norton, F.; Knoll, J.H.M.; Rogan, P.K. Radiation dose estimation by completely automated interpretation of the dicentric chromosome assay. *Radiat. Prot. Dosim.* **2019**, *186*, 42–47. [CrossRef]

Publisher's Note: MDPI stays neutral with regard to jurisdictional claims in published maps and institutional affiliations.

Journal of *Personalized Medicine*

MDPI

Article

Radiation Biomarkers in Large Scale Human Health Effects Studies

Jayne Moquet [1,*], Kai Rothkamm [1,2], Stephen Barnard [1] and Elizabeth Ainsbury [1]

1 Public Health England, Centre for Radiation, Chemical and Environmental Hazards, Chilton, Didcot, Oxfordshire OX11 0RQ, UK; k.rothkamm@uke.de (K.R.); stephen.barnard@phe.gov.uk (S.B.); liz.ainsbury@phe.gov.uk (E.A.)

2 Department of Radiotherapy & Radio-Oncology, University Medical Centre Hamburg-Eppendorf, 20251 Hamburg, Germany

* Correspondence: jayne.moquet@phe.gov.uk; Tel.: +44-(0)1235-825104

Received: 3 September 2020; Accepted: 1 October 2020; Published: 3 October 2020

check for updates

Abstract: Following recent developments, the RENEB network (Running the European Network of biological dosimetry and physical retrospective dosimetry) is in an excellent position to carry out large scale molecular epidemiological studies of ionizing radiation effects, with validated expertise in the dicentric, fluorescent in situ hybridization (FISH)-translocation, micronucleus, premature chromosome condensation, gamma-H2AX foci and gene expression assays. Large scale human health effects studies present complex challenges such as the practical aspects of sample logistics, assay costs, effort, effect modifiers and quality control/assurance measures. At Public Health England, the dicentric, automated micronucleus and gamma-H2AX radiation-induced foci assays have been tested for use in a large health effects study. The results of the study and the experience gained in carrying out such a large scale investigation provide valuable information that could help minimise random and systematic errors in biomarker data sets for health surveillance analyses going forward.

Keywords: ionizing radiation; biomarkers; dicentric assay; micronucleus assay; gamma H2AX foci assay; health surveillance analyses

1. Introduction

One of the hallmarks of ionizing radiation is its ability to induce DNA double-strand breaks, lesions that are difficult to repair and prone to mis-repair, resulting in mutations and chromosomal aberrations such as dicentrics or acentric fragments [1]. In addition, the modification or accumulation of DNA damage response proteins at the site of DNA double-strand breaks can be visualised as gamma-H2AX and 53BP1 foci [2]. These biomarkers of radiation exposure and effect are key tools to (i) support the clinical management of critically exposed individuals and reassure the 'worried well' following a radiation accident or incident, e.g., [3]; (ii) support counselling on the likelihood of long-term health radiation-induced effects such as cancer, e.g., [4]; (iii) provide dose estimates in epidemiological studies of health risks associated with radiation exposure, e.g., [5]; and (iv) predict the response of a tumour and the patient's normal tissues to radiotherapy in order to personalise treatment and thus maximise the probability of complication-free tumour control, e.g., [6].

To date, DNA and chromosome damage-associated markers have been most widely used for biological dose estimation [7]. Considerable progress has been made recently in the development, standardisation and validation of exposure biomarkers, e.g., through the European Union (EU) projects MULTIBIODOSE (Multi-disciplinary biodosimetric tools to manage high scale radiological casualties; https://cordis.europa.eu/project/id/241536) and RENEB (Realizing the European Network of Biodosimetry; http://cordis.europa.eu/project/id/295513). Progress in the area of predictive markers of individual response to radiation exposure has been much more limited, although a number of small scale studies (7–10 patients plus matched controls) and recently larger studies (42–>1000 patients) have also suggested an association of DNA double-strand break-related markers or apoptosis with clinical radiosensitivity in non-syndromic patients [8–13].

The EU RENEB project has resulted in a number of key outputs and these include harmonisation activities to strengthen radiation exposure assessment, with a training program to include periodic inter-comparisons [14], a strategic research agenda [15] and a common quality manual outlining the framework of quality assurance/quality management (QA/QM), with QA/QM criteria for all assays that make up the operational basis of the network [16]. These assays include (i) the dicentric assay; (ii) the FISH-translocation assay; (iii) the micronucleus assay; (iv) the premature chromosome condensation assay; (v) the gamma-H2AX assay; and (vi) electron paramagnetic resonance/optically stimulated luminescence. In addition, candidate techniques, such as gene or micro-RNA expression, and new partner laboratories are being evaluated for inclusion in the network [17]. The network now has a legal structure with a minor adaptation in the name, RENEB—Running the European Network of biological dosimetry and physical retrospective dosimetry (https://www.reneb.net/). As of January 2016, RENEB has 26 member organisations and is now in a position not only to respond to radiation emergencies, but also to contribute to large scale studies relevant for patient health and radiation protection that require dose assessment [14].

Recent work at Public Health England (PHE) involved a large scale study of more than 400 historically exposed breast and prostate radiotherapy patients in which a panel of DNA damage-associated markers were used for biological dose reconstruction and as indicators of individual radiosensitivity following the ex vivo radiation exposure of blood samples. Based on this experience, discussed here are the complex challenges that need to be addressed when using such assays in large scale human health effects studies. These include practical aspects such as assay costs, effort, automation, sample logistics and failure rates, effect modifiers such as inter-scorer variation and assay 'drift' over time, but also quality control/assurance measures that could help minimise random and systematic errors in biomarker data sets.

2. Materials and Methods

2.1. Patient Selection and Blood Sampling

Volunteers participating in two randomised controlled radiotherapy trials, testing of 5.7 Gy and 6.0 Gy fractions of whole breast radiotherapy FAST or Conventional Hypofractionated High Dose Intensity Modulated Radiotherapy for Prostate Cancer (CHHIP), were recruited for the present study. FAST is a prospective randomised clinical trial testing 5.7 Gy and 6.0 Gy fractions of whole breast radiotherapy in terms of late normal tissue responses and tumour control (ISRCTN62488883) [18]. CHHIP (Conventional Hypofractionated High Dose Intensity Modulated Radiotherapy for Prostate Cancer (ICRCTN97182923)) is a randomised trial to see whether hypofractionated radiotherapy schedules for localised prostate cancer could improve the therapeutic ratio by either improving tumour control or reducing normal tissue side effects [19]. Both trials test the hypothesis that fewer, larger radiotherapy doses than those delivered by standard regimens improve local control and/or reduce late adverse effects in patients treated for early stage breast cancer (FAST) or localised prostate cancer (CHHIP). The trials collected prospective clinician and patient self-assessed scores of late adverse effects and quality of life for a minimum of 5 years post-treatment. The present study was carried out in accordance with the Declaration of Helsinki (1964) and the Research Governance Framework Second edition (2005). Ethics approval was obtained from all the participating cancer centres and written informed consent was given by all the study volunteers. Patient confidentiality was maintained at all times. Heparinized venous blood was collected from a total of 406 volunteers when they came in for one of their periodic post-treatment clinical assessments, over a period of 18 months, at selected UK centres participating in the FAST and CHHIP trials. Samples were packaged according to the UN

3373 Biological Substance Category B specifications [20] and dispatched by express courier, at ambient temperature, to PHE (10 mL per patient).

2.2. Ex Vivo Irradiation of Separated Lymphocytes and Whole Blood

Upon arrival at the laboratory the next day, blood was immediately aliquoted for use in the gamma-H2AX foci assay (FCA), the dicentric (DCA) and micronucleus (MNA) assays. Prior to irradiation, the whole blood for the gamma-H2AX assay was separated on histopaque 1077 (Sigma-Aldrich, Dorset, UK) and isolated lymphocytes suspended in minimal essential medium (MEM) with 10% heat-inactivated foetal bovine serum (FBS), 100 units/mL penicillin plus 100 µg/mL streptomycin and 2 mM L-glutamine (all from Invitrogen, Paisley, UK). Separated lymphocytes and whole blood samples were irradiated with X-rays using an A.G.O. X-ray System, model CP160/1 (AGO X-ray Ltd., Martock, UK), at 250 kVp with a half value layer of 2 mm of copper and 1.5 aluminium and a dose rate of 0.5 Gy/min. Irradiation of the samples was performed at 37 °C in 15 mL centrifuge tubes, held inside a 22 mm polystyrene block on top of an 8 mm Perspex plate. Dosimetry was carried out in the same geometry as the specimens using a calibrated reference ionisation chamber. All the exposures were monitored using a calibrated UNIDOSE electrometer, traceable to a national standard, and an 'in beam' ionisation chamber (all from PTW, Freiburg, Germany). In addition, the spatial dose uniformity was checked using Gafchromic EBT2 films (Vertec Scientific Ltd., Reading, UK). Separated lymphocytes for the FCA were irradiated to 0.5 and 4 Gy and the whole blood to 6 and 2 Gy for the DCA and MNA, respectively. Small scale studies, with a highly select group of patients, have suggested that the doses used here can predict normal tissue radiosensitivity using DCA [8], MNA [21] and FCA [9]. Sham-irradiated controls were also included for the FCA and DCA, but not for the MNA, due to the limited amount of blood available. The controls were transported to the irradiation facility with the experimental samples and held inside a polystyrene block to simulate exposure. Staff carrying out the irradiations also processed and scored the samples and were not blind to the radiation doses used.

2.3. Gamma H2AX Assay for Initial and Residual Radiation-Induced Foci

Following irradiation, the separated lymphocyte samples were incubated at 37 °C in a 5% CO_2 humidified atmosphere to simulate in vivo repair. The 0.5 Gy samples were held for 0.5 h and the 4 Gy specimens for 24 h, to assess the initial and residual radiation-induced foci, respectively. Samples were then processed for the assessment of gamma-H2AX foci using a standard technique [22]. In brief, the lymphocytes were spotted onto adhesive slides, fixed with formaldehyde (Polysciences Inc., Warrington, PA, USA), permeabilised with Triton X (Sigma-Aldrich, Dorset, UK), blocked with bovine serum albumin (Fisher Scientific, Loughborough, UK) and immunostained for gamma-H2AX and 53BP1 using fluorophore-conjugated secondary antibodies (AlexaFluor 488 goat anti-mouse/AlexaFluor 555 goat anti-rabbit, Invitrogen, Paisley, UK). Fifty cells per sample were scored manually by one person, (with the exception of 8 donors), for gamma-H2AX and 53BP1 foci, using a Nikon Optiphot 2 fluorescence microscope equipped with separate filters to visualise 4′,6-diamidino-2-phenylindole (DAPI), fluorescein isothio-cyanate (FITC) and Texas Red. Only gamma-H2AX foci co-localised with 53BP1 were scored, as this reduces the possibility of erroneously scoring fluorescent antibody aggregates as foci [23].

2.4. Dicentric and Micronucleus Assays

For consistency with the standard protocol for the construction of calibration curves for biological dosimetry, whole blood samples were held for 2 h following irradiation at 37 °C, to allow for repair [3]. Whole blood was mixed with MEM for the DCA and RPMI medium (Sigma-Aldrich, Dorset, UK) for the MNA. MEM was used for the DCA for consistency with the protocol used to construct the X-ray dose–response curve used in this study [24], while RPMI has been the medium of choice in a previous study using an automated micronucleus analysis system [25]. The medium was supplemented with

10% FBS, 1% phytohaemagglutinin (Invitrogen, Paisley, UK), 100 units/mL penicillin plus 100 μg/mL streptomycin and 2 mM L-glutamine. In addition, 5-bromo-2-deoxyuridine and Colcemid (both from Sigma-Aldrich, Dorset, UK) were added to the DCA cultures at final concentrations of 10 and 0.04 μg/mL, respectively. All samples were cultured at 37 °C in a 5% CO_2 humidified atmosphere. At 70 h, metaphases were harvested for the DCA by a standard hypotonic treatment in 0.075 M potassium chloride for 7 min at 37 °C followed by three changes of 3:1 methanol:acetic acid fixative. For the MN assay, the cell cultures had cytochalasin B (Sigma) added at 24 h, giving a final concentration of 6 μg/mL to block cytokinesis. The cells were harvested after a total of 72 h in culture by treatment with 0.075 M potassium chloride pre-cooled to 4 °C followed by fixation in methanol:acetic acid (3:1) with 1% formaldehyde. There followed two further changes of 3:1 methanol:acetic acid fixative. Fixed cells were dropped onto clean microscope slides, air dried and stained with 5% Giemsa (DCA) or 200 ng/mL DAPI in antifade mounting media (MNA). DAPI was used for the MNA instead of Giemsa as the automated detection software requires fluorescent images. The culture, fixation and staining procedures followed standard protocols recommended by the International Atomic Energy Agency [3]; although some MNA preparations were washed in phosphate buffered saline solution prior to staining to try and improve the quality of the stained preparations. Fifty metaphases per donor were scored manually for chromosome aberrations for the DCA, by 3 scorers. Dose estimates, based on the number of dicentrics per cell, were calculated using Dose Estimate_v5.1 [26] and dose–response curve coefficients $C = 0.0005 \pm 0.0005$, $\alpha = 0.046 \pm 0.005$, $\beta = 0.065 \pm 0.003$ [24]. A minimum of 500 binucleated cells (BN) per patient were scored automatically for the MNA on the Metafer slide scanning platform (Metasystems, Altlussheim, Germany), using the MSearch/MNScore software [27]. The data were recorded as fully automated scoring and with a cut-off for cells containing >4 micronuclei (MN). An estimate of the nuclear division index (NDI) was also calculated [3] for each sample.

2.5. DCA Calibration Curve Construction

The construction of the DCA calibration curve has been fully described by Lloyd et al. [24]. In brief, whole blood from a healthy male donor was exposed at 37 °C to 250 kV X-rays at a dose rate of 1.0 Gy/min. Eleven doses were used in total, ranging from 0.05 to 8.0 Gy. Following irradiation, the samples were held for 2 h at 37 °C and the cultures set up as described above, but without the addition of Colcemid at the start of the culture process. Samples were cultured at 37 °C for 48 h, with Colcemid added at 45 h to give a final concentration of 0.2 μg/mL. After 48 h, the cultures were fixed as described in Section 2.4 above for the DCA. The chromosome preparations were stained with orcein and scored for unstable aberrations. A later study [28] found similar yield coefficients, demonstrating that the data were not confounded by the presence of large numbers of second division cells despite using orcein stain.

2.6. Statistical Methods

Kolmogorov–Smirnov normality testing was carried out to assess the relevance of normal statistical analysis techniques. General linear model analysis of variance (GLM ANOVA) was then carried out, with post-hoc testing using Tukey's pairwise comparisons between factors, using Minitab® 17. For DCA, the factors tested were the scorer (3 individuals, pairwise comparisons); blood collection date (random variable); blood collection time (random variable); sample origin (4 hospitals) on dicentrics/cell, excess acentrics/cell and total aberrations/cell. Regression models were also applied for the aberration endpoints over time, to investigate an apparent variation in response. For the MNA, the model considered the influence of blood collection date, blood collection time and staining technique (washed or not washed prior to DAPI staining) on MN/cell (no cut off); MN/cell (cut off > 4 MN) and NDI. Data from a subset of 239 samples were used to investigate if the length of time-fixed samples had been stored in the freezer had an effect on the MNA endpoints. To ensure consistency between the time of making slides and scoring, this subset was used as the samples were all scored within 3 days of making slides regardless of storage time in the freezer. For the FCA, the scorer, stainer (2 individuals), blood collection date and time were assessed for the number of foci per cell at 24 h following 4 Gy or 0.5 h following 0.5 Gy. In addition, correlations between the endpoints were assessed using pairwise correlation analysis, to assess whether any single assay can be used as a homologue for the other endpoints. Finally, the Anderson–Darling test was used to investigate the distribution of the dose estimates from the DCA and then chi-squared testing, with Yates correction, was applied to compare each of the measured doses with the true dose.

3. Results

Normality testing was carried out on the control and irradiated data and there was no evidence for significant deviation from normality for the majority of the DCA and foci endpoints. For the DCA, in Figure 1, the dose estimate and standard errors have been plotted for each patient in chronological order.

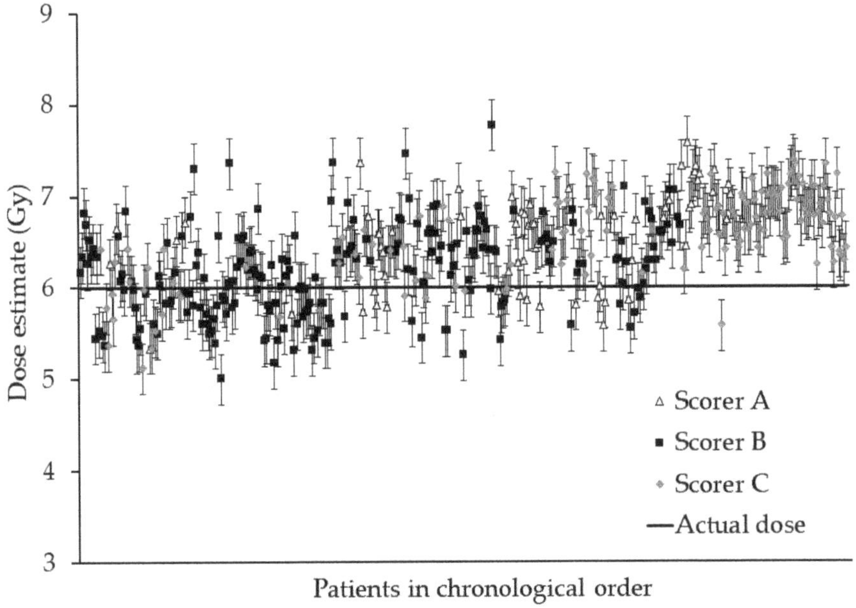

Figure 1. Graph showing the dose estimate and standard errors for each person. The data are presented in chronological order, (samples received over a continuous 18 month period) and for each scorer who analysed the sample. Every sample was given an ex vivo X-ray dose of 6 Gy.

The Anderson–Darling test revealed a slight departure from normality in the distribution of the measured doses, chiefly due to a few outliers at each end of the scale, thus the chi-squared testing with Yates correction was applied to compare each of the measured doses with the true dose of 6 Gy. However, the results revealed that no one data point was significantly different from 6 Gy (all $p > 0.6$) and as a whole, the summed Yates's chi-squared test suggests that the data are not significantly different from the true dose ($p > 0.999$).

Figure 2A shows the yield of total aberrations (dicentrics + centric rings + excess acentrics) and dicentrics + centric rings found in each patient and grouped by scorer A, B or C. Within each group, the patients are arranged in chronological order. Figure 2B shows the average yield of dicentrics + centric rings and excess acentrics analysed by scorers A, B and C. The GLM ANOVA indicated that the scorer was a significant factor for total aberrations/cell ($p = 0.008$), but not for excess acentrics/cell ($p = 0.163$) or dicentrics/cell ($p = 0.146$). The sampling time of day and the location from which it was sent had no significant influence on the aberration yields ($p \geq 0.656$). However, the date of the blood sampling was significant for all the endpoints ($p \leq 0.005$) but was independent of scorer interaction.

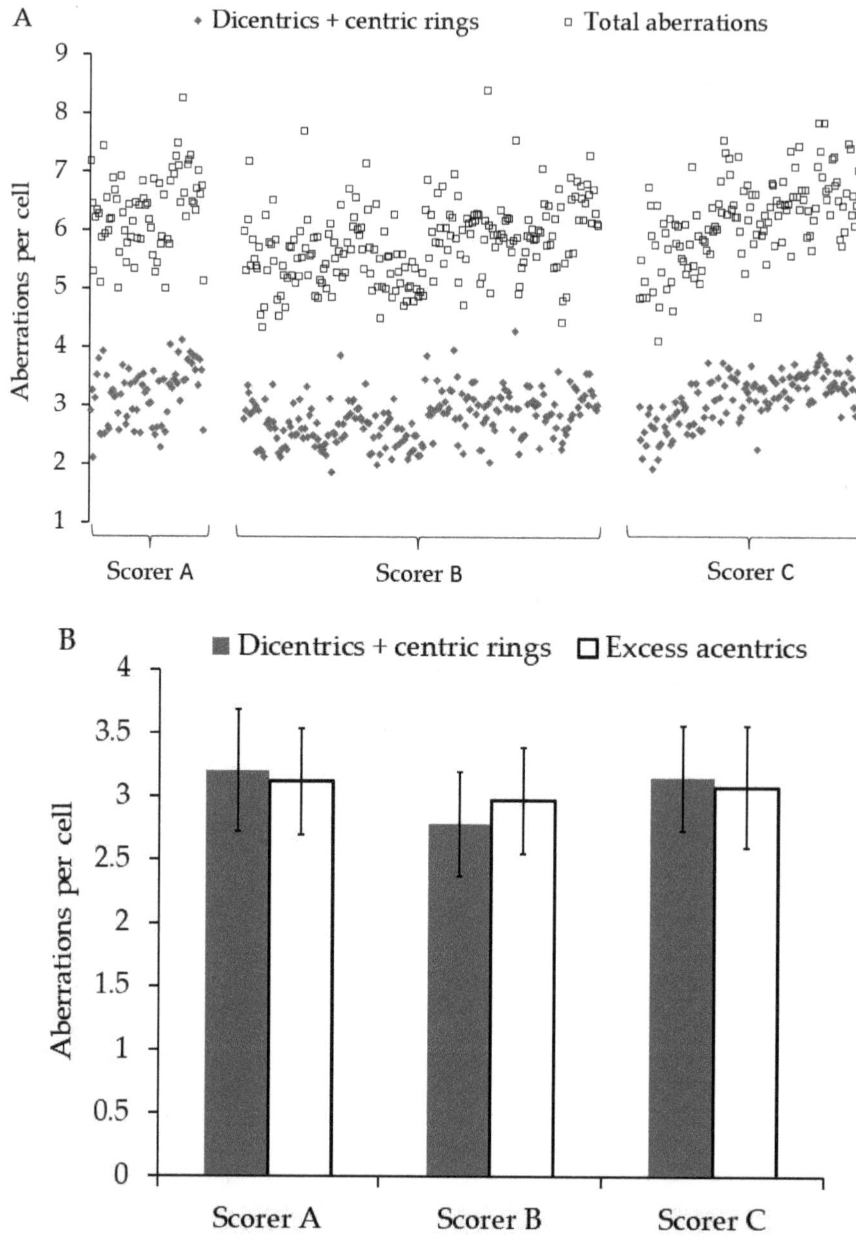

Figure 2. (**A**) Shows the yield of total aberrations (dicentrics + centric rings + excess acentrics) and dicentrics + centric rings found in each patient and grouped by scorer A, B or C. Within each group, the patients are arranged in chronological order. (**B**) shows the average yield of dicentrics + centric rings and excess acentrics analysed by scorers A, B and C. The errors bars represent the standard deviation.

Shown in Figure 3 are the results of the MNA for MN/cell (no cut off), MN/cell (cut of > 4 MN) and NDI for each patient, in chronological order. In common with the DCA, the date of the blood sampling was significant for all three MN endpoints (all $p < 0.001$). The sampling time of day was not significant for MN (cut off > 4 MN) and NDI, ($p = 0.247$ and 0.867 respectively) and only showed a borderline significance for MN (no cut off), $p = 0.049$. The staining technique did not have a significant influence on the MN/cell when no cut off was used ($p = 0.273$), but for a MN/cell with a cut off > 4 MN and for NDI, the techniques produced different results ($p = 0.049$ and 0.019, respectively). The length of time for which the fixed sample was stored in the freezer (0 to 58 weeks) had a significant effect on the MN/cell (no cut off) ($p = 0.06$), MN/cell (cut off > 4 MN) ($p = 0.033$) and NDI ($p = 0.010$).

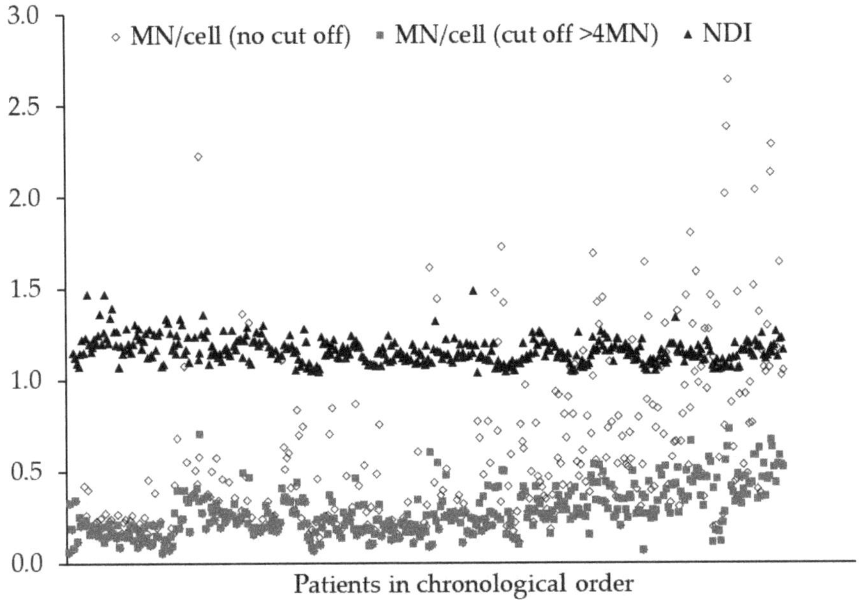

Figure 3. Graph showing the frequency of micronuclei (MN) observed and the nuclear division index (NDI) for each person after an ex vivo X-ray dose of 2 Gy. The data are presented in chronological order (samples received over a continuous 18 month period). Objects in bi-nucleated cells containing >4 MN tend to be artefacts or debris and can be eliminated using a cut off.

Figure 4 shows the foci yields for each patient in chronological order for the 0 Gy, 0.5 Gy + 0.5 h and the 4 Gy + 24 h samples. ANOVA revealed that the effect of the scorer was not significant for the actual number of foci/cell (4 Gy + 24 h), $p = 0.789$, but only one batch of eight samples was scored by another person. In addition, the sampling time of day was not significant for 0.5 Gy + 0.5 h ($p = 0.455$) or 4 Gy + 24 h ($p = 0.241$). The effect of the person staining the samples was shown to be significant ($p < 0.001$), although all samples were stained by one person except for one batch of eight 0.5 Gy + 0.5 h samples. As with the DCA and MNA, the date of the blood sampling was significant ($p = 0.001$) for the FCA.

Cross endpoint correlations were carried out on dicentrics/cell, total aberrations/cell, MN/cell (no cut off), MN/cell (cut of >4 MN), foci/cell (0.5 Gy + 0.5 h) and foci/cell (4 Gy + 24 h). Most of the endpoints showed significant cross correlation, ($p \leq 0.050$). No significant correlation occurred between foci/cell (4 Gy + 24 h) and dicentrics/cell ($p = 0.531$), total aberrations/cell ($p = 0.179$) or excess acentrics/cell ($p = 0.153$). In addition, the foci/cell (0.5 Gy + 0.5 h) were not significantly correlated with excess acentrics/cell ($p = 0.660$). MN/cell (cut of > 4 MN) showed no significant correlation with excess acentrics/cell ($p = 0.090$). However, MN (no cut off) was significantly inversely correlated with NDI $p < 0.001$, but there was no significant correlation with MN (cut off > 4 MN) and NDI $p = 0.29$.

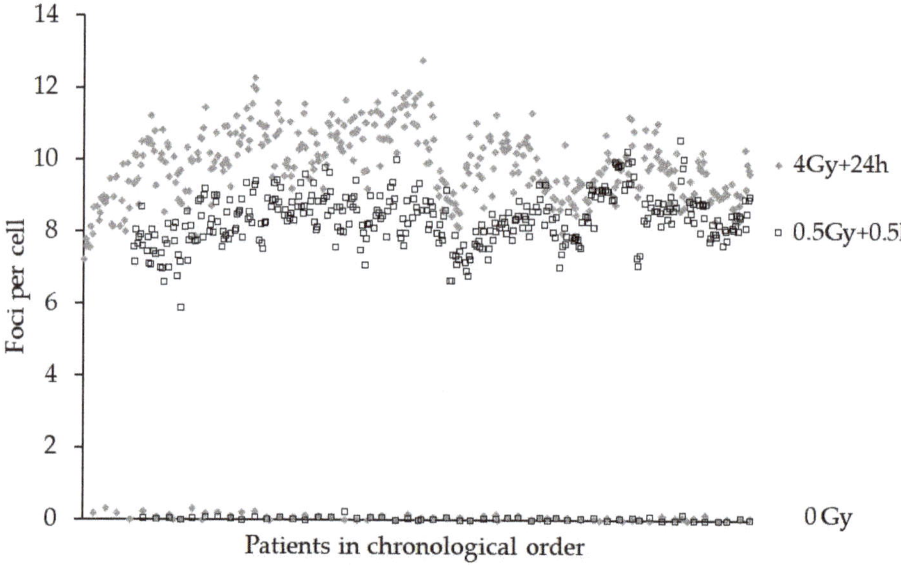

Figure 4. Graph showing the foci assay (FCA) results as gamma-H2AX foci per cell for 0 Gy, 0.5 Gy + 0.5 h and 4 Gy + 24 h ex vivo incubation at 37 °C samples. The data are presented in chronological order, (samples received over a continuous 18 month period).

4. Discussion

This paper looks at the logistics of carrying out the laboratory work and sample analysis for a large health effects study. A comparison of the cytogenetic and DNA damage data with the clinical scores of radiosensitivity will be the subject of a separate paper.

In this study, it was necessary for samples to be sent in batches, with a maximum of eight samples per batch. A total of 57 batches of samples were sent over an 18 month period. Only one batch of samples failed to arrive the next day and had to be repeated. In the present study, samples were only sent and received within the same country. Previous experience has shown that sending samples within the EU has been straight forward and that most samples arrive within 24 h [29,30]. Standard sample shipment outside of the EU, however, has been shown to be problematic, with delays as a result of country-specific import regulations that had to be overcome by using a specialised and expensive courier service [30].

The DCA was the most reliable assay with >99% of samples successfully completed, followed by the FCA (96%) and MNA (93%). Failures were caused by low cell numbers (all assays) or poor lymphocyte separation and bad staining (FCA). As a percentage of the total cost of the study, which includes reagents and staff costs (GBP 180,000), the MNA was the least expensive assay at 9% (GBP 16,000), followed by the FCA at 11% (GBP 20,000 for two time points), while the DCA was the most costly at nearly 25% (GBP 44,000). In part, this was due to the amount of effort required per sample. This was calculated to be 30, 50 and 120 min for the FCA, MNA and DCA, respectively. The use of automated scoring helped to keep the cost of the MNA low. If reagent costs alone are considered, the FCA is the most expensive and the DCA the least costly. Remarkably, the cost for the DCA, MNA and FCA together (45%) was lower than that for patient selection, recruitment, sampling and shipment in this study (55%).

All the patients had been historically exposed to ionizing radiation as treatment for either breast or prostate cancer [18,19]. The DCA and MNA assays used in this study measure unstable aberrations, for example, lymphocyte precursors carrying dicentrics or acentrics impose a hinderance to successful cell division and are eliminated over time. Dicentric yield therefore reduces with a half time of about 3 years [3], which is consistent with dicentric yields in the range of 0.005–0.070 per cell observed in patient baseline samples. In healthy non-exposed volunteers, background dicentric yields range from 0 to 0.002 per cell [31] and the excess aberrations in the patients' baseline samples were considered to be very low compared to those induced by the 6 and 2 Gy ex vivo irradiation. The situation is even less critical for the FCA, which as a surrogate marker for radiation-induced DNA double-strand breaks shows a bi-exponential loss (fast and slow) of foci with time due to repair. Half times for the fast and slow repair have been shown to be 1.6 and 38 h, respectively [23].

As Figure 1 shows, there was a tendency for individual dose estimates to be above the 6 Gy actual dose (73%), although statistical testing suggested no single data point was significantly different from the true dose. One possible reason may be the slight variation in techniques between the application of the assay and the construction of the calibration curve, where blood was cultured for 48 h and Colcemid added at 45 h in the standard manner [24]. In the present study, a culture time of 70 h was used with Colcemid added at the start, albeit at a lower concentration. It is known that more heavily damaged cells reach metaphase later than cells containing fewer aberrations [32,33]. Despite using a lower concentration of Colcemid, the cells reaching metaphase sooner may have become more condensed and less easy to score and so have been more likely to be rejected by the scorer.

As described in the materials and methods, the scorers were not blinded to the radiation doses in this experiment. The main reason for this was the fact that doses were chosen on the basis of the indications in the literature that they could be useful for the prediction of normal tissue radiosensitivity, and in order to further investigate and compare the specific responses of the assays in this large scale scenario, rather than solely to test the ability of the assays to estimate the doses. Three scorers were involved in the analysis of the DCA. Scorer A had more than 30 years of experience using the DCA, while scorers B and C had 6 months and 2 years, respectively. Within the laboratory, all new staff underwent a training programme that compared intra-laboratory performance in dicentric yields and dose estimates. In addition, inter-laboratory comparisons were tested with images from collaborative projects, e.g., [34–36]. Figure 2 shows that on average scorer B scored lower than A and C, but using ANOVA, this was only significant for total aberrations. The DCA data appear to indicate that all aberration endpoints increased over time and the significant difference between scorers was related to the progression of time. This can be explained as changes in staff during the study resulted in scorer B analysing more samples at the start than at the end of the project.

In common with the DCA, the yields of MN show an upward trend with the progression of time; although this cannot be related to inter-scorer difference. One possible factor influencing MN yields was the time the fixed sample were stored in the freezer in 3:1 methanol:acetic acid. Time constraints, such as staff and microscope availability during the project resulted in the fixed cells from the MNA samples being stored in a freezer at −20 °C for anything from 0 to 58 weeks before the slides were made, stained and analysed. Most of the later samples were stored at −20 °C for less time than the earlier samples and ANOVA indicated the time spent in the freezer had a significant effect on all the MNA endpoints ($p \leq 0.033$). Variable results in the automated MNA have also been reported by Depuydt et al. [37] with cells stored in fixative at 4 °C and −20 °C. One possibility is that the cells stored in fixative for long periods shrink or do not spread out well when dropped onto a slide. One of the parameters used by the MN classifier to detect bi-nucleated (BN) cells is based on size, hence different sub-sets of BN cells could be selected. Alternatively, fewer MN may be detected as a result of overlap with the main nuclei. When using automated analysis, all MNA samples should be stored and slides prepared in the same way as those used to train the MN classifier and produce dose–response curves.

For normal unexposed lymphocytes, the expected NDI values tend to be in the range from 1.30 to 2.20 [38]. Here, as shown in Figure 3, the range of NDI values was 1.05 to 1.50. These lower values probably reflect the fact that cells were delayed in their cell cycle after exposure to a 2 Gy genotoxic insult and that only the automated score of mono- and bi-nucleate cells were used to calculate the NDI. Figure 3 also shows that the range of values for the MN/cell (no cut off) is much wider than the MN/cell (cut off > 4 MN), 0.06–2.64 and 0.06–0.73, respectively, especially towards the latter part of the study. Previous work [25], suggests that many of the objects in BN cells automatically classified as containing more than four MN tend to be artefacts or debris. In addition, the cross-correlation analysis showed no correlation with NDI for MN (cut off > 4 MN), suggesting that when using automated scoring, cut off could be important.

A number of factors may influence the kinetics of foci formation/loss and small changes to reagents could affect staining quality [2,39]. Indeed, fluctuations in foci numbers were observed when new batches of gamma-H2AX antibody were used and may explain, or at least in part, the upward pattern of foci per cell that seems to repeat itself approximately every 5 months (see Figure 4). The GLM ANOVA showed the person staining the samples had a significant effect $p < 0.001$. All the samples were stained by one experienced person, except for one batch that was processed by a new less experienced member of staff. Batch normalisation, or the calculation of ratios for foci present at 24 vs. 0.5 h could be used to limit these effects when correlating this endpoint with, for example, clinical radiosensitivity.

5. Conclusions

Completing such a large scale study has provided some important points to consider for future studies. The experience of staff carrying out the assays is critical and laboratories involved in multi-partner studies must be very confident in their training/inter-comparison programmes. Moreover, if several laboratories undertake a joint study, the harmonisation of protocols and scoring would be essential. The cross endpoint correlation analysis of the present study showed that initial DNA damage, as measured by the FCA (0.5 Gy + 0.5 h), was significantly correlated with dicentrics/cell, that were the result of the mis-repair of double-strand breaks, but residual damage (FCA—4 Gy + 24 h) was not. Therefore, it is important to choose assays carefully as they do not all measure the same thing and a multi-parametric approach may be more useful, as developed in the EU MULTIBIODOSE project [40]. A multi-centre approach to such studies can also increase the amount of soring that could be performed and ensure that samples can be analysed promptly and not stored for long periods of time, as this seems to be important for the automated MNA. The RENEB network already undertakes training and harmonisation activities to strengthen radiation exposure assessment for a number of biological dosimetry assays [16] and is ideally placed to carry out large health effect studies.

Author Contributions: Conceptualization, K.R.; methodology, K.R., J.M. and S.B.; software, E.A.; validation, K.R., J.M., S.B. and E.A.; formal analysis, E.A.; investigation, J.M. and S.B.; resources, J.M. and S.B.; data curation, K.R., J.M. and E.A.; writing—original draft preparation, J.M.; writing—review and editing, J.M., K.R., S.B. and E.A.; visualization, K.R. and J.M.; supervision, K.R.; project administration, K.R. and J.M.; funding acquisition, K.R. All authors have read and agreed to the published version of the manuscript.

Funding: This research received funding from NIHR_CHPR (National Institute for Health Research_The Centre for Health Protection Research); project number 108299.

Acknowledgments: We thank all the patients and staff who participated in the study from the Royal Marsden NHS Foundation Trust, Royal Marsden Hospital, Sutton; the Brighton and Sussex University Hospital NHS Trust, Royal Sussex County Hospital, Brighton; the Torbay and South Devon NHS Foundation Trust, Torbay District General Hospital, Torquay; the Western Sussex Hospitals NHS Foundation Trust, Worthing Hospital, Worthing. The study was facilitated by John Yarnold, David Dearnaley, Sue Boyle and Lone Gothard of the Royal Marsden NHS Foundation Trust and The Institute of Cancer Research, Downs Road, Sutton SM2 5PT. UK. We also thank David Azria of the Centre Regional de Lutte Contre Le Cancer, Montpellier, France, for contributing to setting up the study. The authors are grateful to Jenna Al-hafidh and Clare Bricknell for their technical assistance and David Lloyd for his helpful comments on the manuscript.

Conflicts of Interest: The authors declare no conflict of interest.

References

1. Obe, G.; Natarajan, A.T. (Eds.) *Chromosome Aberrations*; Karger: Basel, Switzerland, 2004.
2. Rothkamm, K.; Barnard, S.; Moquet, J.; Ellender, M.; Rana, Z.; Burdak-Rothkamm, S. DNA damage foci Meaning and significance. *Environ. Mol. Mutagen.* **2015**, *56*, 491–504. [CrossRef]
3. International Atomic Energy Agency (IAEA). *Cytogenetic Dosimetry: Applications in Preparedness for and Response to Radiation Emergencies*; IAEA: Vienna, Austria, 2011.
4. Sun, M.; Moquet, J.E.; Barnard, S.; Lloyd, D.C.; Rothkamm, K.; Ainsbury, E.A. Doses in Radiation Accidents Investigated by Chromosomal Aberration Analysis XXV. Review of Cases Investigated, 2006–2015. PHE-CRCE-025. 2016; PHE Publication Gateway Number: 2015730. Available online: https://assets.publishing.service.gov.uk/government/uploads/system/uploads/attachment_data/file/515260/PHE-CRCE-025.pdf (accessed on 12 May 2016).
5. Sotnik, N.V.; Azizova, T.V.; Darroudi, F.; Ainsbury, E.A.; Moquet, J.E.; Fomina, J.; Lloyd, D.C.; Edwards, A.A. Verification by the FISH translocation assay of historic doses to Mayak workers from external gamma radiation. *Radiat. Environ. Biophys.* **2015**, *5494*, 445–451. [CrossRef]
6. Chua, M.L.K.; Rothkamm, K. Biomarkers of radiation exposure: Can they predict normal tissue radiosensitivity? *Clin. Oncol.* **2013**, *25*, 610–616. [CrossRef]
7. Rothkamm, K.; Lloyd, D. Established and emerging methods of biological dosimetry. In *Comprehensive Biomedical Physics*; Brahme, A., Ed.; Elsevier: Amsterdam, The Netherlands, 2014; Volume 7, pp. 289–310.
8. Borgmann, K.; Röper, B.; El-Awady, R.A.; Brackrock, S.; Bigalke, M.; Dörk, T.; Alberti, W.; Dikomey, E.; Dahm-Daphi, J. Indicators of late normal tissue response after radiotherapy for head and neck cancer: Fibroblasts, lymphocytes, genetics, DNA repair and chromosome aberrations. *Radiother. Oncol.* **2002**, *64*, 141–152. [CrossRef]
9. Chua, M.L.K.; Somaiah, N.; A'Hern, R.; Davies, S.; Gothard, L.; Yarnold, J.; Rothkamm, K. Residual DNA and chromosomal damage in ex vivo irradiated blood lymphocytes correlated with late normal tissue response to breast radiotherapy. *Radiother. Oncol.* **2011**, *99*, 362–366. [CrossRef]
10. Beaton, L.A.; Marro, L.; Samiee, S.; Malone, S.; Grimes, S.; Malone, K.; Wilkins, R.C. Investigating chromosome damage using fluorescent in situ hybridization to identify biomarkers of radiosensitivity in prostate cancer patients. *Int. J. Radiat. Biol.* **2013**, *89*, 1087–1093. [CrossRef]
11. Marková, E.; Somsedíková, A.; Vasilyev, S.; Pobijaková, M.; Lacková, A.; Lukačko, P.; Belyaev, I. DNA repair foci and late apoptosis/necrosis in peripheral blood lymphocytes of breast cancer patients undergoing radiotherapy. *Int. J. Radiat. Biol.* **2015**, *91*, 934–945.
12. Qvarnström, F.; Simonsson, M.; Nyman, J.; Hermansson, I.; Book, M.; Johansson, K.-A.; Turesson, I. Double strand break induction and kinetics indicate preserved hypersensitivity in keratinocytes to subtherapeutic doses for 7 weeks of radiotherapy. *Radiother. Oncol.* **2017**, *122*, 163–169. [CrossRef]
13. Talbot, C.J.; Veldwijk, M.R.; Azria, D.; Batini, C.; Bierbaum, M.; Brengues, M.; Chang-Claude, J.; Johnson, K.; Keller, A.; Smith, S.; et al. Multi-centre technical evaluation of the radiation-induced lymphocyte apoptosis assay as a predictive test for radiotherapy toxicity. *Clin. Transl. Radiat. Oncol.* **2019**, *18*, 1–8. [CrossRef]
14. Kulka, U.; Abend, M.; Ainsbury, E.; Badie, C.; Barquinero, J.F.; Barrios, L.; Beinke, C.; Bortolin, E.; Cucu, A.; De Amicis, A.; et al. RENEB–Running the European Network of biological dosimetry and physical retrospective dosimetry. *Int. J. Radiat. Biol.* **2017**, *93*, 2–14. [CrossRef]
15. RENEB Strategic Research Agenda. November 2015. Available online: http://www.reneb.net/wp-content/uploads/2017/10/reneb-sra_november-2015_2.pdf (accessed on 5 July 2016).
16. Gregoire, E.; Ainsbury, E.; Barrios, L.; Bassinet, C.; Fattibene, P.; Kulka, U.; Oestreicher, U.; Pantelias, G.; Terzoudi, G.; Trompier, F.; et al. The harmonization process to set up and maintain an operational biological and physical retrospective dosimetry network: QA QM applied to the RENEB network. *Int. J. Radiat. Biol.* **2017**, *93*, 81–86. [CrossRef]
17. Ainsbury, E.; Badie, C.; Barnard, S.; Manning, G.; Moquet, J.; Abend, M.; Antunes, A.C.; Barrios, L.; Bassinet, C.; Beinke, C.; et al. Integration of new biological and physical retrospective dosimetry methods into EU emergency response plans–joint RENEB and EURADOS inter-laboratory comparisons. *Int. J. Radiat. Biol.* **2017**, *93*, 99–109. [CrossRef]

18. FAST Trialists Group; Agrawal, R.K.; Alhasso, A.; Barrett-Lee, P.J.; Bliss, P.; Bloomfield, D.; Bowen, J.; Brunt, A.M.; Donovan, E.; Emson, M.; et al. First results of the randomised UK FAST Trial of radiotherapy hypofractionation for treatment of early breast cancer (CRUKE/04/015). *Radiother. Oncol.* **2011**, *100*, 93–100.
19. Dearnaley, D.; Syndikus, I.; Mossop, H.; Khoo, V.; Birtle, A.; Bloomfield, D.; Graham, J.; Kirkbride, P.; Logue, J.; Malik, Z.; et al. Conventional versus hypofractionated high-dose intensity-modulated radiotherapy for prostate cancer: 5-year outcomes of the randomised, non-inferiority, phase 3 CHHiP trial. *Lancet Oncol.* **2016**, *17*, 1047–1060. [CrossRef]
20. World Health Organisation. *Guidance on Regulations for the Transport of Infectious Substances*; 2009–2010 WHO/HSE/EPR/2008.10; WHO: Geneva, Switzerland, 2008.
21. Guogytė, K.; Plieskienė, A.; Ladygienė, R.; Vaisiūnas, Ž.; Sevriukova, O.; Janušonis, V.; Žilukas, J. Assessment of correlation between chromosomal radiosensitivity of peripheral blood lymphocytes after in vitro irradiation and normal tissue side effects for cancer patients undergoing radiotherapy. *Genome Integr.* **2017**, *8*, 1.
22. Rothkamm, K.; Barnard, S.; Ainsbury, E.A.; Al-Hafidh, J.; Barquinero, J.-F.; Lindholm, C.; Moquet, J.; Perälä, M.; Roch-Lefèvre, S.; Scherthan, H.; et al. Manual versus automated γ-H2AX foci analysis across five European laboratories: Can this assay be used for rapid biodosimetry in a large scale radiation accident? *Mutat. Res.* **2013**, *756*, 170–173. [CrossRef]
23. Horn, S.; Barnard, S.; Rothkamm, K. Gamma-H2AX-based dose estimation for whole and partial body radiation exposure. *PLoS ONE* **2011**, *6*, e25113. [CrossRef]
24. Lloyd, D.C.; Purrott, R.J.; Dolphin, G.W.; Bolton, D.; Edwards, A.A.; Corp, M.J. The relationship between chromosome aberrations and low LET radiation dose in human lymphocytes. *Int. J. Radiat. Biol.* **1975**, *28*, 75–90. [CrossRef]
25. Thierens, H.; Vral, A.; Vandevoorde, C.; Vandersickle, V.; de Gelder, V.; Romm, H.; Oestreicher, U.; Rothkamm, K.; Barnard, S.; Ainsbury, E.; et al. Is a semi-automated approach indicated in the application of the automated micronucleus assay for triage purposes? *Radiat. Prot. Dosimetry* **2014**, *159*, 87–94. [CrossRef]
26. Ainsbury, E.A.; Lloyd, D.C. Dose estimation software for radiation biodosimetry. *Health Phys.* **2010**, *98*, 290–295. [CrossRef]
27. Willems, P.; August, L.; Slabbert, J.; Romm, H.; Oestreicher, U.; Thierens, H.; Vral, A. Automated micronucleus (MN) scoring for population triage in case of large scale radiation events. *Int. J. Radiat. Biol.* **2010**, *86*, 2–11. [CrossRef]
28. Lloyd, D.C.; Edward, A.A.; Prosser, J.S. Chromosome aberrations induced in human lymphocytes by in-vitro acute X and gamma radiation. *Radiat. Prot. Dosimetry* **1986**, *15*, 83–88. [CrossRef]
29. Moquet, J.; Barnard, S.; Staynova, A.; Lindholm, C.; Monteiro Gil, O.; Martins, V.; Rößler, U.; Vral, A.; Vandevoorde, C.; Wojewódzka, M.; et al. The second gamma-H2AX assay inter-comparison exercise carried out in the framework of the European biodosimetry network (RENEB). *Int. J. Radiat. Biol.* **2017**, *93*, 58–64. [CrossRef]
30. Oestreicher, U.; Samaga, D.; Ainsbury, E.; Antunes, A.C.; Baeyens, A.; Barrios, L.; Beinke, C.; Beukes, P.; Blakely, W.F.; Cucu, A.; et al. RENEB intercomparisons applying the conventional dicentric chromosome assay (DCA). *Int. J. Radiat. Biol.* **2017**, *93*, 20–29. [CrossRef]
31. Lloyd, D.C.; Purrott, R.J.; Reeder, E.J. The incidence of unstable chromosomes aberrations in peripheral blood lymphocytes from unirradiated and occupationally exposed people. *Mutat. Res.* **1980**, *72*, 523–532. [CrossRef]
32. Hoffmann, G.R.; Sayer, A.M.; Littlefield, L.G. Higher frequency of chromosome aberrations in late-arising first-division metaphases than in early-arising metaphases after exposure of human lymphocytes to X-rays in G_0. *Int. J. Radiat. Biol.* **2002**, *78*, 765–772. [CrossRef]
33. Hone, P.A.; Edwards, A.A.; Lloyd, D.C.; Moquet, J.E. The yield of radiation-induced chromosomal aberrations in first division human lymphocytes depends on the culture time. *Int. J. Radiat. Biol.* **2005**, *81*, 523–529. [CrossRef]
34. Livingston, G.K.; Wilkins, R.C.; Ainsbury, E.A. Pilot website to support international collaboration for dose assessments in a radiation emergency. *Radiat. Meas.* **2011**, *46*, 912–915. [CrossRef]
35. Romm, H.; Ainsbury, E.; Bajinskis, A.; Barnard, S.; Barquinero, J.F.; Barrios, L.; Beinke, C.; Puig-Casanovas, R.; Deperas-Kaminska, M.; Gregoire, E.; et al. Web-based scoring of the dicentric assay, a collaborative biodosimetric scoring strategy for population triage in large scale radiation accidents. *Radiat. Environ. Biophys.* **2014**, *53*, 241–254. [CrossRef]
36. Romm, H.; Ainsbury, E.A.; Barquinero, J.F.; Barrios, L.; Beinke, C.; Cucu, A.; Moreno Domene, M.; Filippi, S.; Monteiro Gil, O.; Gregoire, E.; et al. Web based scoring is useful for validation and harmonisation of scoring criteria within RENEB. *Int. J. Radiat. Biol.* **2017**, *93*, 110–117. [CrossRef]

37. Depuydt, J.; Baeyens, A.; Barnard, S.; Beinke, C.; Benedek, A.; Beukes, P.; Buraczewska, I.; Darroudi, F.; De Sanctis, S.; Dominguez, I.; et al. RENEB intercomparison exercises analyzing micronuclei (Cytokinesis-block Micronucleus Assay). *Int. J. Radiat. Biol.* **2017**, *93*, 36–47. [CrossRef]
38. Fenech, M. Cytokinesis-block micronucleus cytome assay. *Nat. Protoc.* **2007**, *2*, 1084–1104. [CrossRef]
39. Rothkamm, K.; Horn, S. gamma-H2AX as protein biomarker for radiation exposure. *Ann. 1st Super Sanità.* **2009**, *45*, 265–271.
40. Ainsbury, E.A.; Al-Hafidh, J.; Bajinskis, A.; Barnard, S.; Barquinero, J.F.; Beinke, C.; de Gelder, V.; Gregoire, E.; Jaworska, A.; Lindholm, C.; et al. Inter- and intra-laboratory comparison of a multibiodosimetric approach to triage in a simulated, large scale radiation emergency. *Int. J. Radiat. Biol.* **2014**, *90*, 193–202. [CrossRef]

Publisher's Note: MDPI stays neutral with regard to jurisdictional claims in published maps and institutional affiliations.

Journal of *Personalized Medicine*

MDPI

Review

Ionizing Radiation Protein Biomarkers in Normal Tissue and Their Correlation to Radiosensitivity: Protocol for a Systematic Review

Anne Dietz, Maria Gomolka, Simone Moertl and Prabal Subedi *

Bundesamt für Strahlenschutz/Federal Office for Radiation Protection, Ingolstädter Landstraße 1, 85764 Oberschleissheim, Germany; adietz@bfs.de (A.D.); mgomolka@bfs.de (M.G.); smoertl@bfs.de (S.M.)
* Correspondence: psubedi@bfs.de; Tel.: +49-30183332244

Abstract: *Background:* Radiosensitivity is a significantly enhanced reaction of cells, tissues, organs or organisms to ionizing radiation (IR). During radiotherapy, surrounding normal tissue radiosensitivity often limits the radiation dose that can be applied to the tumour, resulting in suboptimal tumour control or adverse effects on the life quality of survivors. Predicting radiosensitivity is a component of personalized medicine, which will help medical professionals allocate radiation therapy decisions for effective tumour treatment. So far, there are no reviews of the current literature that explore the relationship between proteomic changes after IR exposure and normal tissue radiosensitivity systematically. *Objectives:* The main objective of this protocol is to specify the search and evaluation strategy for a forthcoming systematic review (SR) dealing with the effects of in vivo and in vitro IR exposure on the proteome of human normal tissue with focus on radiosensitivity. *Methods:* The SR framework has been developed following the guidelines established in the National Toxicology Program/Office of Health Assessment and Translation (NTP/OHAT) Handbook for Conducting a Literature-Based Health Assessment, which provides a standardised methodology to implement the Grading of Recommendations Assessment, Development and Evaluation (GRADE) approach to environmental health assessments. The protocol will be registered in PROSPERO, an open source protocol registration system, to guarantee transparency. *Eligibility criteria:* Only experimental studies, in vivo and in vitro, investigating effects of ionizing radiation on the proteome of human normal tissue correlated with radio sensitivity will be included. Eligible studies will include English peer reviewed articles with publication dates from 2011–2020 which are sources of primary data. *Information sources:* The search strings will be applied to the scientific literature databases PubMed and Web of Science. The reference lists of included studies will also be manually searched. *Data extraction and results:* Data will be extracted according to a pre-defined modality and compiled in a narrative report following guidelines presented as a "Synthesis without Meta-analyses" method. *Risk of bias:* The risk of bias will be assessed based on the NTP/OHAT risk of bias rating tool for human and animal studies (OHAT 2019). *Level of evidence rating*: A comprehensive assessment of the quality of evidence for both in vivo and in vitro studies will be followed, by assigning a confidence rating to the literature. This is followed by translation into a rating on the level of evidence (high, moderate, low, or inadequate) regarding the research question. Registration: PROSPERO Submission ID 220064.

Keywords: ionizing radiation; normal tissue; biomarker; radiotherapy; radiosensitivity; protein

Citation: Dietz, A.; Gomolka, M.; Moertl, S.; Subedi, P. Ionizing Radiation Protein Biomarkers in Normal Tissue and Their Correlation to Radiosensitivity: Protocol for a Systematic Review. *J. Pers. Med.* **2021**, *11*, 3. https://dx.doi.org/10.3390/jpm11010003

Received: 10 November 2020
Accepted: 18 December 2020
Published: 22 December 2020

1. Introduction

1.1. Background and Rationale

The International Agency for Research on Cancer (IARC) Global Cancer Observatory reports more than 18 million new cases of cancer in 2018 [1] and radiotherapy (RT) is used to treat 50–60% of cancers [2]. The delivered dose during standard RT is balanced between optimal tumor kill and avoidance of damage to surrounding tissues [3]. Depending on the tumor entity, up to 20% of patients show a moderate to severe detrimental response to ionizing radiation (IR) treatment [4]. Acute effects include erythema, inflammation and mucositis depending on cancer type while late effects are typically fibrosis, atrophy, vascular damage and neurocognitive and endocrine dysfunctions, especially for brain irradiated children [5–7]. These side effects limit radiation doses that can be applied to the tumor, often leading to suboptimal tumor control or to serious impairment of the quality of life of survivors. In a small subset of patients the severe reactions can be ascribed to known radiation hypersensitivity syndromes, such as Ataxia–Telangiectasia (A-T), Fanconi anemia (FA), or Nijmegen Breakage Syndrome (NBS) [8–10]. As late as 2010, children with AT mutations have succumbed to death following RT [11]. These genetic syndromes, however, only comprise about 1% of the patients demonstrating severe side effects [12]. Therefore, most of the normal tissue reactions cannot be explained by known genetic disorders and no clear guidelines exist for medical doctors to individually adapt their therapy scheme. This has led to an increased interest in predicting personalized radiosensitivity.

Radiosensitivity is any enhanced tissue or cell reaction after a subject has been exposed to IR when compared to the majority of other "normal" responding individuals [13,14]. The reactions include inflammation, fibrosis, cardiovascular illness, cataracts, and cognitive decline [15]. Individual radiosensitivity can be applied as component of personalized medicine in RT. Personalized medicine is not about finding out novel medications but sub-dividing individuals in various subgroups that vary in their response to treatment for a specific disease [16]. It is performed to tailor the treatment to the individual need. This implies that medical professionals can target cancer patients, who are radiosensitive, with lower doses and alternative treatment schedules, for example, chemotherapy rather than radiotherapy. On the other hand, patients who are less radiosensitive could be given higher doses of IR to maximize the likelihood of treatment success [14]. Moreover, although the potential for therapy using ionizing radiation is unparalleled, there is an increasing concern for the risks posed by low-dose occupational exposure among workers in nuclear industries and healthcare [17–19].

It was already established in the early twentieth century that individuals respond differently to IR [20] and the reason behind this is still under thorough investigation. Discovering breakthroughs in individualized radiosensitivity is difficult because the effect of IR is modified by age, gender, lifestyle, genetic predisposition, and the quality and quantity of IR dose these individuals receive [21]. Several conventional reviews that summarize IR-induced changes at a molecular level have been published over the years. For example, a compilation of cytogenetic damage, epigenomic alterations, induced and germline mutations, DNA and nucleotide pool damage, and transcriptomic and translational biomarkers of radiation exposure for epidemiological studies have been reported [22]. Similarly, DNA double stand break repairs, chromosomal aberrations and radiation-induced apoptosis in ex vivo irradiated blood lymphocytes as predictors of radiosensitivity have also been described [23]. A review of various proteomics approaches to investigate cancer radiotherapy in cancer and normal cell lines and in bio fluids of in vivo irradiated individuals has also been performed [24].

This review is different to conventional reviews—it is a systematic review (SR). Unlike conventional reviews, SR provides an unbiased selection of studies that include an objective and transparent evaluation of the evidence. [25,26]. SR begins with defining the terms PECO—population, exposure, comparators, and outcome, which helps to produce a well formulated research question for the SR. Each of the terms has an inclusion and exclusion criteria, which furthermore specifies which studies will be included. Each study is then evaluated for the relationship between exposure and outcome, as well as dissected based on questions that define selection, confounding, performance, attrition or exclusion, detection, and selective reporting risk of biases [27,28].

Out of 28,279 studies (PubMed search term: ionizing radiation [Title/Abstract], retrieval date 23 September 2020) there are no systematic reviews (SRs) that investigate proteomic changes after exposure to IR. Taking into consideration that the study of Pernot et al. [22] including protein biomarkers for IR exposure took place in 2012, we have compiled proteomic markers of radiosensitivity in normal tissues from the last 10 years (2011–2020). In this article we provide a protocol that determines our search and evaluation strategy for the actual systematic review.

Our planned review aims at presenting the status quo of IR-induced changes in protein expression in normal tissue that can be correlated to radiosensitivity, which can be used to further investigate the concept of individual radiosensitivity. This will help to personalize treatment strategies for cancer patients during radiotherapy (RT) or help to assist an individualized risk assessment process by identifying and protecting occupationally exposed persons l nuclear workers and radiologists. A future issue may be the protection of sensitive cosmonauts from harmful effects of cosmic radiation.

1.2. Objectives

The main objective of this SR is to evaluate the effects of ionizing radiation on the proteome of human normal tissue regarding radiosensitivity in experimental models (in vivo and in vitro).

Following sub-objectives will be taken into account:

1. Narrative presentation of the current status of knowledge obtained from experimental studies (in vivo, in vitro) evaluating the effect of ionizing radiation on the proteome of human normal tissue regarding radiosensitivity.
2. Evaluation of the quality of evidence using a confidence rating and establishing a level of evidence for the presence or absence of a biomarker for radio sensitivity in human normal tissue.

2. Methods

This structure for this systematic review, as presented in the graphical abstract, was adapted according to the National Toxicology Program/Office of Health Assessment and Translation NTP/OHAT handbook [27], which provides standard operating procedures for conducting a systematic review and integrating evidence [26,29]. To rate the quality of the scientific evidence, GRADE (Grading of Recommendations Assessment, Development and Evaluation) will be used. This is a formal process that is often used in systematic reviews, which is also applied to develop recommendations in guidelines that are as evidence-based as possible [25,29]. The selection of articles, data extraction and synthesis, as well as risk of bias assessment, will be performed manually. The synthesis of data will be performed narratively without meta-analysis, as explained by Campbell et al. [30]. This SR will adhere strictly to PRISMA (Preferred Reporting Items for Systematic Reviews and Meta-Analyses) guidelines [28,31], which provide an evidence-based minimum set of items that need to be reported for evaluation of randomized trials or can be used as a basis to judge other research types, e.g., evaluations of interventions. The protocol and the abstract will also be reported as described in PRISMA-P [32] and PRISMA-A [33] respectively.

The SR is registered in the International Prospective Register of Systematic Reviews on 10 November 2020 (submission ID 220064)

2.1. Eligibility Criteria

Studies that comply with elements of PECO (Population, Exposure, Comparators, and Outcome as outlined in Table 1) will be included in this SR.

2.1.1. Population

The population in this SR will include both in vivo and in vitro models.

In vivo models: This model will include humans or blood, biopsies, and body fluids taken from humans.

In vitro models: This model will include non-cancer tissue culture, primary human non-cancer cell lines, or non-cancer cell lines derived from humans.

This review will exclude non-human studies. This review will also exclude tumour cell lines, tumour tissue, and biopsies. The rationale behind excluding tumour data is that we focus on radiation induced effects in normal tissue. Although some mechanisms and pathways may overlap, there are also clear differences of radiation resistance and sensitivity mechanisms in tumour compared to normal tissue. The protein markers identified here should help to predict radiation sensitivity reactions of normal tissue of cancer patients and therefore assist a personalized radiation therapy treatment. In addition, identified markers can help in risk assessment of radiation exposed individuals, such as nuclear workers, accidentally exposed individuals, and individuals living in areas of higher background ionizing radiation.

Table 1. Population, exposure, comparators, and outcome (PECO) Statement with inclusion and exclusion criteria.

PECO		Inclusion Criteria	Exclusion Criteria
Population	In Vivo	Humans	Non-human
	In Vitro	Human tissues, primary human non-tumour cell line, derived human non-tumour cell line	Tumour cells and tissues, primary and secondary tumour cell lines
Exposure	In Vivo In vitro	Ionizing radiation (e.g., alpha and beta particles, X-Rays, Gamma rays, proton therapy)	Non-ionizing radiation (e.g., radio and microwaves, near infrared, ultraviolet, electromagnetic waves)
Comparators	In Vivo	Non-exposed humans, bio fluids before IR	Lacks control group
	In Vitro	Non-exposed cells or tissues	
Outcomes	In Vivo In vitro	Changes in protein expression correlated with radiosensitivity	Irrelevant outcome (e.g., changes in transcriptome, or protein changes not correlated to radiosensitivity)

2.1.2. Exposure

The exposure will be ionizing radiation (IR). The World Health Organization defines IR as radiation with enough energy that during an interaction with an atom, it can remove tightly bound electrons from atoms, which results in the atom being charged or ionized [34]. Therefore, this study will include all sources of IR: X-Ray, cosmic rays, gamma ray, alpha and beta particles, carbon and proton therapy, and all sources of natural background ionizing radiation. This review will exclude non-ionizing radiation (infrared, near-infrared, ultraviolet, microwaves, electromagnetic radiation or radio waves)

2.1.3. Comparators

Comparators in this study will be humans or in vitro models that have not been exposed to IR.

In case of studies including humans exposed to IR, material such as blood, before and after IR, taken from the same human, will be included. When tissue samples before and after irradiation are compared the localisation of the samples within the radiation field must be ensured and dose estimates should be provided.

In case of studies involving humans living in areas of higher-than-average natural background radiation, comparators will be humans that live in areas of average natural background radiation but from a similar demographic community.

Studies that do not have a comparator group will be excluded.

2.1.4. Outcomes

Outcomes of interest are changes in protein expression levels correlated to radiosensitivity. We have explained before that radiosensitivity could include inflammation, fibrosis, cardiovascular illness, and cognitive decline. Therefore, studies that have included information on such parameters will be included.

In Vivo models should report overall survival and in vitro models should mention survival, apoptosis, proliferation, colony formation or metabolic assays.

2.1.5. Exclusion criteria prioritisation

Studies will be excluded if they are:

- Not a primary study

- Irrelevant population: in vivo: not human data; in vitro: not human-derived cell lines, tumour cell lines, tumour tissues (or cell lines derived from tumour tissues)
- Irrelevant Exposure (not ionizing radiation)
- Irrelevant Outcome (not studies related to protein expression that correlates to radiosensitivity)
- Studies not in English, or no full text for the study is available
- Studies outside time frame (not within 2011–2020)

2.2. Search Strategy

2.2.1. Databases

The searches will be performed in NCBI PubMed [35] (https://pubmed.ncbi.nlm.nih.gov/) and ISI Web of Knowledge v.5.34 [36] (https://www.webofknowledge.com/). Any additional study might be added manually later. The references will be imported into Microsoft Excel and the duplicates removed. The search string for ISI Web of Knowledge is provided in Supplementary Information with this protocol.

2.2.2. Search Strings

The search strings will be a combination of population, exposure, and outcome elements from the PECO parameters. The population of interest are human and/or normal tissues, the exposure of interest is ionizing radiation, and the outcome of interest is 'radiosensitivity and the corresponding changes in protein expression'. Restriction for language and time period will be set where studies published between 2011 and 2020 in English will be considered. Search strings that were used in Web of Science are presented in Supplementary Information and the strings will be adapted and calibrated to be used in PubMed.

2.2.3. Study Selection

Studies will be subjected to a two-phase screening, which is also presented in the graphical abstract. As a Phase I screening, AD and PS will together cross-check the title, abstract, and the key words with the inclusion/exclusion criteria. Retained articles will be downloaded for a phase II full-text screening manually. Any article excluded in Phase II screening, along with the reason for exclusion, will be recorded and provided in the Supplementary Information. Any disagreements between the reviewers will be solved by consensus, involving MG or SM if necessary.

2.3. Data Extraction

Data extraction will be performed by PS and AD together and any discrepancies will be solved by consensus. Google sheets will be used to enter the data and the result will be finally reported in Microsoft Excel. The form for data extraction is provided in Supplementary Information.

2.4. Body of Evidence Structure

Evidence will be organised in outcome-related groups favouring data synthesis (proteins) and confidence rating at the health outcome level (radiation induced normal tissue radio sensitivity).

The criteria to determine the inclusion of specific studies or experiments in each outcome group will consider the evidence stream (i.e., in vivo, in vitro), health outcomes /endpoints or exposure regime (high or low dose, duration). Two outcomes, primary and secondary, have been defined. According to the literature, IR induces toxicity in normal tissue and in some cases shows a radio sensitive phenotype. This is the definition of primary outcome in this review. Secondary outcomes represent intermediary endpoints upstream of primary outcomes. Altered protein expression after exposure to IR, which may be grouped around specific signalling or functional pathways, has been defined as the secondary outcome.

2.5. *Internal Quality Assessment*

The included studies will be internally quality controlled using the Risk of Bias (RoB) tool developed by the Office of Health Assessment and Translation [27,37]. The RoB tool acts as an internal quality control in reviewing the articles included for the SR. Even though the studies follow a methodological flow, they might still have a bias, which might lead to an underestimation or an overestimation of the effect of the exposure. For example, if the population contains mainly older subjects and the comparator contains younger ones, the effect of the exposure might be overestimated. To critically evaluate the studies, the following questions will be asked:

2.5.1. Selection Bias

1. Was administered dose or exposure level adequately randomised?
2. Was allocation to study groups adequately concealed?
3. Did selection of study participants result in appropriate comparison groups?

2.5.2. Confounding Bias

4. Did the study design or analyses account for important confounding and modifying variables?

2.5.3. Performance Bias

5. Were experimental conditions identical across study groups?
6. Were the research personnel and human subjects blinded to the study group in the study?

2.5.4. Attrition/Exclusion Bias

7. Were outcome data complete without attrition or exclusion from analysis?

2.5.5. Detection Bias

8. Can we be confident in the exposure characterization?
9. Can we be confident in the outcome assessment?

2.5.6. Selective Reporting Bias

10. Were all measured outcomes reported?

2.5.7. Other Sources of Bias

11. Were there any other potential threats to internal validity (e.g., statistical methods were appropriate and researchers adhered to study protocol?)

Each question will be answered with 'definitely low risk of bias', 'probably low risk of bias', 'probably high risk of bias', or 'definitely high risk of bias'. Responses will be determined together by PS and AD. Considering the RoB responses of each question, the study will be categorized into three tiers, T1, T2 and T3, as proposed by the National Toxicology Program/Office for Health Assessment and Translation (NTP/OHAT). The tiers will be based on 'Key Questions', which are domains of randomization bias, outcome detection bias, and performance bias.

2.6. *Confidence Rating for Each Body of Evidence*

Extracted data from each study included will be considered as independent bodies of evidence. An assessment will be performed for each to define a confidence rating. The confidence rating reflects the reliability with which the study findings accurately depict a true effect of IR toxicity on normal tissue and linkage to radiosensitivity, as described in the NTP/OHAT handbook [27]. Each body of evidence is given an initial confidence rating that is downgraded or upgraded according to factors that decrease or increase confidence in the results.

Initial confidence rating is based on the presence or absence of four features. The features are (1) controlled exposure (2) exposure prior to outcome (3) individual outcome data and (4) use of comparison group

The ratings are as follow:

- High—4 features (++++)
- Moderate—3 features (+++)
- Low—2 features (++)
- Very Low—1 feature (+)

The initial confidence is then upgraded or downgraded depending on certain factors, and a confidence in the body of evidence is provided (Table 2). The factors increasing confidence are magnitude, dose response, and consistency across studies and the factors decreasing confidence are risk of bias, unexplained inconsistency, and imprecision.

Table 2. Accessing confidence in body of evidence.

Initial Confidence by Key Features of Study Design	Factors Decreasing Confidence	Factors Increasing Confidence	Confidence in the Body of Evidence
High (++++) 4 features	Risk of bias	Magnitude effect	High (++++)
Moderate (+++) 3 features	Unexplained inconsistency	Dose response	Moderate (+++)
Low (++) 2 features	Indirectness	Residual confounding	Low (++)
Very low (+) $\leq$1 feature	Imprecision	Consistency	Very low (+)

2.7. Translation of Confidence Rating Into Level of Evidence (for the Health Effect)

Ionizing radiation leads to toxicity in all living organisms, in both tumour and non-tumour cells. Therefore, the translation of confidence rating into levels of evidence will not be performed in the review. This SR aims to investigate proteomic changes in normal tissues and our population consists of in vitro studies of primary human material and immortalized cell lines as well as in vivo studies, on occupationally, naturally and accidentally exposed persons and on radiotherapy patients. The defined population in this SR are exposed to a broad range of radiation qualities, IR doses and dose-rates, and focusing on one particular type of dose and dose would hamper the objective of the study. Therefore, no preference for high or low-doses, respectively, or high or low-dose rates will be made. The different doses and dose-rates, however, will be provided for all selected studies in the final review.

2.8. Data Synthesis

Included data will likely comprise randomized and non-randomized trials. Moreover, clinical diversity is inevitable because of the defined PECO parameters as effects of IR on expression of different proteins being investigated. The secondary outcome is an altered protein expression after a population has been exposed to IR. It is highly probable that studies look at a diverse set of proteins, and studies will not have proteins in common that show an altered expression. Therefore, a meta-analyses might not be possible and in that case synthesis of results is performed in a narrative way or described textually. No reporting guidelines exist for narrative synthesis and although it provides a clear picture of the effects of exposure, such synthesis lacks transparency [38]. When methods other than meta-analyses are used to synthesize results, certain findings, such as reporting of synthesis structure and comparison grouping, standardised metric used for synthesis, synthesis method, presentation of data, and the summary of the synthesis finding, are left unreported. To counter these problems, data synthesis will be reported using the narrative synthesis without meta-analyses (SWiM) method, as presented by Campbell et al. [30].

2.9. Differences between Protocol and the Review

If there are any methodological deviations from this protocol in the review to be written, they will be mentioned in the 'Differences between protocol and review'.

2.10. Potential Applications of the Protocol/Review

The application or outcome of this protocol is the definition of parameters for the systematic evaluation of protein changes which are correlated with radiosensitivity in normal tissue. The primary outcome of the systematic review is the identification of these proteins. In the review article we will also discuss potential applications of these proteins in medical practice.

Supplementary Materials: The following are available online at https://www.mdpi.com/2075-4426/11/1/3/s1, data extraction form, Risk of bias questions, search algorithm for web of science and Prisma protocol checklist.

Author Contributions: Conceptualization, A.D., M.G., S.M., and P.S.; methodology, A.D., M.G., S.M., P.S.; formal analysis, A.D., M.G., S.M., P.S.; investigation, A.D., M.G., S.M., P.S.; resources, M.G., S.M.; writing—original draft preparation, A.D., P.S.; writing—review and editing, A.D., M.G., S.M., P.S.; supervision, M.G., S.M.; project administration, M.G., S.M.; funding acquisition, M.G., S.M. All authors have read and agreed to the published version of the manuscript.

Funding: This work was supported by the Bundesministerium für Bildung und Forschung (Germany) Grant 02NUK035D (AD) and Grant 02NUK047B (PS).

Acknowledgments: The authors would like to thank Bernd Henschenmacher and Elisa Pasqual for the guidance in writing this protocol and Lukas Duchrow for his help with statistics.

Conflicts of Interest: The authors declare no conflict of interest. The funders had no role in the design of the study; in the collection, analyses, or interpretation of data; in the writing of the manuscript, or in the decision to publish the results.

References

1. Global Cancer Observatory. Available online: https://gco.iarc.fr/ (accessed on 21 December 2020).
2. Rosenblatt, E.; Izewska, J.; Anacak, Y.; Pynda, Y.; Scalliet, P.; Boniol, M.; Autier, P. Radiotherapy capacity in European countries: An analysis of the Directory of Radiotherapy Centres (DIRAC) database. *Lancet Oncol.* **2013**, *14*, e79–e86. [CrossRef]
3. Lacombe, J.; Azria, D.; Mange, A.; Solassol, J. Proteomic approaches to identify biomarkers predictive of radiotherapy outcomes. *Expert Rev. Proteom.* **2013**, *10*, 33–42. [CrossRef] [PubMed]
4. Seibold, P.; Auvinen, A.; Averbeck, D.; Bourguignon, M.; Hartikainen, J.M.; Hoeschen, C.; Laurent, O.; Noël, G.; Sabatier, L.; Salomaa, S.; et al. Clinical and epidemiological observations on individual radiation sensitivity and susceptibility. *Int. J. Radiat. Biol.* **2019**, *96*, 324–339. [CrossRef] [PubMed]
5. Bledsoe, J.C. Effects of cranial radiation on structural and functional brain development in pediatric brain tumors. *J. Pediatric Neuropsychol.* **2015**, *2*, 3–13. [CrossRef]
6. Follin, C.; Erfurth, E.M. Long-term effect of cranial radiotherapy on pituitary-hypothalamus area in childhood acute lymphoblastic leukemia survivors. *Curr Treat. Options Oncol* **2016**, *17*, 50. [CrossRef]
7. Barnett, G.C.; West, C.M.; Dunning, A.M.; Elliott, R.M.; Coles, C.E.; Pharoah, P.D.; Burnet, N.G. Normal tissue reactions to radiotherapy: Towards tailoring treatment dose by genotype. *Nat. Rev. Cancer* **2009**, *9*, 134–142. [CrossRef]
8. Nakanishi, K.; Taniguchi, T.; Ranganathan, V.; New, H.V.; Moreau, L.A.; Stotsky, M.; Mathew, C.G.; Kastan, M.B.; Weaver, D.T.; D'Andrea, A.D. Interaction of FANCD2 and NBS1 in the DNA damage response. *Nat. Cell Biol.* **2002**, *4*, 913–920. [CrossRef]
9. Petrini, J.H. The mammalian Mre11-Rad50-nbs1 protein complex: Integration of functions in the cellular DNA-damage response. *Am. J. Hum. Genet.* **1999**, *64*, 1264–1269. [CrossRef]
10. Digweed, M. Human genetic instability syndromes: Single gene defects with increased risk of cancer. *Toxicol. Lett.* **1993**, *67*, 259–281. [CrossRef]
11. Pietrucha, B.M.; Heropolitanska-Pliszka, E.; Wakulinska, A.; Skopczynska, H.; Gatti, R.A.; Bernatowska, E. Ataxia-telangiectasia with hyper-IgM and Wilms tumor: Fatal reaction to irradiation. *J. Pediatr Hematol. Oncol.* **2010**, *32*, e28–e30. [CrossRef]
12. Mizutani, S.; Takagi, M. XCIND as a genetic disease of X-irradiation hypersensitivity and cancer susceptibility. *Int. J. Hematol.* **2013**, *97*, 37–42. [CrossRef] [PubMed]

13. Salomaa, S.; Jung, T. Roadmap for research on individual radiosensitivity and radiosusceptibility—The MELODI view on research needs. *Int. J. Radiat. Biol.* **2020**, *96*, 277–279. [CrossRef] [PubMed]
14. Gomolka, M.; Blyth, B.; Bourguignon, M.; Badie, C.; Schmitz, A.; Talbot, C.; Hoeschen, C.; Salomaa, S. Potential screening assays for individual radiation sensitivity and susceptibility and their current validation state. *Int. J. Radiat. Biol.* **2019**, *96*, 280–296. [CrossRef] [PubMed]
15. Averbeck, D.; Salomaa, S.; Bouffler, S.; Ottolenghi, A.; Smyth, V.; Sabatier, L. Progress in low dose health risk research: Novel effects and new concepts in low dose radiobiology. *Mutat. Res.* **2018**, *776*, 46–69. [CrossRef] [PubMed]
16. Mathur, S.; Sutton, J. Personalized medicine could transform healthcare. *Biomed. Rep.* **2017**, *7*, 3–5. [CrossRef] [PubMed]
17. Sakly, A.; Gaspar, J.F.; Kerkeni, E.; Silva, S.; Teixeira, J.P.; Chaari, N.; Ben Cheikh, H. Genotoxic damage in hospital workers exposed to ionizing radiation and metabolic gene polymorphisms. *J. Toxicol. Environ. Health A* **2012**, *75*, 934–946. [CrossRef] [PubMed]
18. Grellier, J.; Atkinson, W.; Berard, P.; Bingham, D.; Birchall, A.; Blanchardon, E.; Bull, R.; Guseva Canu, I.; Challeton-de Vathaire, C.; Cockerill, R.; et al. Risk of lung cancer mortality in nuclear workers from internal exposure to alpha particle-emitting radionuclides. *Epidemiology* **2017**, *28*, 675–684. [CrossRef]
19. Kneale, G.W.; Stewart, A.M. Factors affecting recognition of cancer risks of nuclear workers. *Occup. Environ. Med.* **1995**, *52*, 515–523. [CrossRef]
20. Bouchacourt, M.L. Sur la difference de sensibilite aux rayons de Roentgen de la peau des differents sujets, et, sur le meme sujet des differents regions du corps. *Sciences* **1911**, *94*, 942–947.
21. Habash, M.; Bohorquez, L.C.; Kyriakou, E.; Kron, T.; Martin, O.A.; Blyth, B.J. Clinical and functional assays of radiosensitivity and radiation-induced second cancer. *Cancers* **2017**, *9*, 147. [CrossRef]
22. Pernot, E.; Hall, J.; Baatout, S.; Benotmane, M.A.; Blanchardon, E.; Bouffler, S.; El Saghire, H.; Gomolka, M.; Guertler, A.; Harms-Ringdahl, M.; et al. Ionizing radiation biomarkers for potential use in epidemiological studies. *Mutat. Res.* **2012**, *751*, 258–286. [CrossRef] [PubMed]
23. Chua, M.L.; Rothkamm, K. Biomarkers of radiation exposure: Can they predict normal tissue radiosensitivity? *Clin. Oncol.* **2013**, *25*, 610–616. [CrossRef] [PubMed]
24. Azimzadeh, O.; Tapio, S. Proteomics approaches to investigate cancer radiotherapy outcome: Slow train coming. *Transl. Cancer Res.* **2017**, *6*, S779–S788. [CrossRef]
25. Rooney, A.A.; Cooper, G.S.; Jahnke, G.D.; Lam, J.; Morgan, R.L.; Boyles, A.L.; Ratcliffe, J.M.; Kraft, A.D.; Schunemann, H.J.; Schwingl, P.; et al. How credible are the study results? Evaluating and applying internal validity tools to literature-based assessments of environmental health hazards. *Environ. Int.* **2016**, *92–93*, 617–629. [CrossRef] [PubMed]
26. Higgins, J.P.T.; Thomas, J.; Chandler, J.; Cumpston, M.; Li, T.; Page, M.J.; Vivian, A.W. *Cochrane Handbook for Systematic Reviews of Interventions*, 2nd ed.; John Wiley & Sons: Chichester, UK, 2019.
27. National Toxicology Program; OHAT (Office of Health Assessment and Translation). *Handbook for Conducting a Literature-Based Health Assessment Using OHAT Approach for Systematic Review and Evidence Integration*; Services, United States Department of Health and Human Services: Washington, DC, USA, 2019.
28. Liberati, A.; Altman, D.G.; Tetzlaff, J.; Mulrow, C.; Gotzsche, P.C.; Ioannidis, J.P.; Clarke, M.; Devereaux, P.J.; Kleijnen, J.; Moher, D. The PRISMA statement for reporting systematic reviews and meta-analyses of studies that evaluate health care interventions: Explanation and elaboration. *PLoS Med.* **2009**, *6*, e1000100. [CrossRef]
29. Rooney, A.A.; Boyles, A.L.; Wolfe, M.S.; Bucher, J.R.; Thayer, K.A. Systematic review and evidence integration for literature-based environmental health science assessments. *Environ. Health Perspect.* **2014**, *122*, 711–718. [CrossRef]
30. Campbell, M.; McKenzie, J.E.; Sowden, A.; Katikireddi, S.V.; Brennan, S.E.; Ellis, S.; Hartmann-Boyce, J.; Ryan, R.; Shepperd, S.; Thomas, J.; et al. Synthesis without meta-analysis (SWiM) in systematic reviews: Reporting guideline. *BMJ* **2020**, *368*, l6890. [CrossRef]
31. Moher, D.; Liberati, A.; Tetzlaff, J.; Altman, D.G.; Group, P. Preferred reporting items for systematic reviews and meta-analyses: The PRISMA statement. *PLoS Med.* **2009**, *6*, e1000097. [CrossRef]
32. Shamseer, L.; Moher, D.; Clarke, M.; Ghersi, D.; Liberati, A.; Petticrew, M.; Shekelle, P.; Stewart, L.A.; Group, P.-P. Preferred reporting items for systematic review and meta-analysis protocols (PRISMA-P) 2015: Elaboration and explanation. *BMJ* **2015**, *350*, g7647. [CrossRef]
33. Beller, E.M.; Glasziou, P.P.; Altman, D.G.; Hopewell, S.; Bastian, H.; Chalmers, I.; Gotzsche, P.C.; Lasserson, T.; Tovey, D.; Group, P.F.A. PRISMA for abstracts: Reporting systematic reviews in journal and conference abstracts. *PLoS Med.* **2013**, *10*, e1001419. [CrossRef]
34. WHO. Ionizing Radiation. Available online: https://www.who.int/ionizing_radiation/about/what_is_ir/en/ (accessed on 15 October 2020).
35. National Library of Medicine. Pubmed. Available online: https://pubmed.ncbi.nlm.nih.gov/ (accessed on 15 October 2020).
36. Clarivate Analytics. Web of Science. Available online: https://apps.webofknowledge.com/ (accessed on 15 October 2020).
37. National Toxicology Program. *OHAT (Office of Health Assessment and Translation) Risk of Bias Rating Tool for Human and Animal Studies*; United States Department of Health and Human Services: Washington, DC, USA, 2015.
38. Campbell, M.; Katikireddi, S.V.; Sowden, A.; Thomson, H. Lack of transparency in reporting narrative synthesis of quantitative data: A methodological assessment of systematic reviews. *J. Clin. Epidemiol.* **2019**, *105*, 1–9. [CrossRef] [PubMed]

Journal of *Personalized Medicine*

MDPI

Systematic Review

Ionizing Radiation Protein Biomarkers in Normal Tissue and Their Correlation to Radiosensitivity: A Systematic Review

Prabal Subedi *, Maria Gomolka, Simone Moertl and Anne Dietz

Bundesamt für Strahlenschutz/Federal Office for Radiation Protection, Ingolstädter Landstraße 1, 85764 Oberschleissheim, Germany; mgomolka@bfs.de (M.G.); smoertl@bfs.de (S.M.); adietz@bfs.de (A.D.)
* Correspondence: psubedi@bfs.de; Tel.: +49-30183332244

Abstract: Background and objectives: Exposure to ionizing radiation (IR) has increased immensely over the past years, owing to diagnostic and therapeutic reasons. However, certain radiosensitive individuals show toxic enhanced reaction to IR, and it is necessary to specifically protect them from unwanted exposure. Although predicting radiosensitivity is the way forward in the field of personalised medicine, there is limited information on the potential biomarkers. The aim of this systematic review is to identify evidence from a range of literature in order to present the status quo of our knowledge of IR-induced changes in protein expression in normal tissues, which can be correlated to radiosensitivity. **Methods**: Studies were searched in NCBI Pubmed and in ISI Web of Science databases and field experts were consulted for relevant studies. Primary peer-reviewed studies in English language within the time-frame of 2011 to 2020 were considered. Human non-tumour tissues and human-derived non-tumour model systems that have been exposed to IR were considered if they reported changes in protein levels, which could be correlated to radiosensitivity. At least two reviewers screened the titles, keywords, and abstracts of the studies against the eligibility criteria at the first phase and full texts of potential studies at the second phase. Similarly, at least two reviewers manually extracted the data and accessed the risk of bias (National Toxicology Program/Office for Health Assessment and Translation—NTP/OHAT) for the included studies. Finally, the data were synthesised narratively in accordance to synthesis without meta analyses (SWiM) method. **Results**: In total, 28 studies were included in this review. Most of the records (16) demonstrated increased residual DNA damage in radiosensitive individuals compared to normo-sensitive individuals based on γH2AX and TP53BP1. Overall, 15 studies included proteins other than DNA repair foci, of which five proteins were selected, Vascular endothelial growth factor (VEGF), Caspase 3, $p16^{INK4A}$ (Cyclin-dependent kinase inhibitor 2A, CDKN2A), Interleukin-6, and Interleukin-1β, that were connected to radiosensitivity in normal tissue and were reported at least in two independent studies. **Conclusions and implication of key findings**: A majority of studies used repair foci as a tool to predict radiosensitivity. However, its correlation to outcome parameters such as repair deficient cell lines and patients, as well as an association to moderate and severe clinical radiation reactions, still remain contradictory. When IR-induced proteins reported in at least two studies were considered, a protein network was discovered, which provides a direction for further studies to elucidate the mechanisms of radiosensitivity. Although the identification of only a few of the commonly reported proteins might raise a concern, this could be because (i) our eligibility criteria were strict and (ii) radiosensitivity is influenced by multiple factors. **Registration**: PROSPERO (CRD42020220064).

Keywords: ionizing radiation; normal tissue; biomarker; radiotherapy; radiosensitivity; proteomics

Citation: Subedi, P.; Gomolka, M.; Moertl, S.; Dietz, A. Ionizing Radiation Protein Biomarkers in Normal Tissue and Their Correlation to Radiosensitivity: A Systematic Review. *J. Pers. Med.* **2021**, *11*, 140. https://doi.org/10.3390/jpm11020140

Academic Editors: Susan M. Bailey and Christophe Badie

Received: 30 December 2020
Accepted: 14 February 2021
Published: 19 February 2021

1. Introduction

1.1. Background and Rationale

Ionizing radiation is increasingly applied in medical therapy and diagnosis procedures. IARC Global Cancer Observatory reports more than 18 million new cases of cancer in 2018 (https://gco.iarc.fr/) [1] and radiotherapy (RT) is used to treat 50–60% of cancers [2].

For medical imaging and image-guided interventions, the total exposure in the USA has increased 6-fold since 1980 [3]. However, potential adverse health effects of radiation exposure for patients, as well as for medical staff, especially with a focus on individual differences in radiosensitivity, are poorly understood.

Radiosensitivity is a measure for the reactions of cells, tissues, or individuals to ionizing radiation (IR). Subjects with increased reactions are described as radiosensitive, when compared to a majority of other "normal" responding individuals [4–6]. The reactions include inflammation, fibrosis, cardiovascular illness, cataracts, and cognitive decline [7]. The occurrence and severity varies among individuals and may be affected by genetic as well as by life style factors. In 5–10% of patients the use of RT is limited by the occurrence of acute, clinically diverse, strong radiogenic side effects of normal tissue in the radiation field, leading to suboptimal tumour control or to serious impairment of the quality of life for patients [8–10]. A reliable, pre-therapeutic identification of radiosensitive patients would improve therapy because an individual dose adjustment could be applied. Furthermore, the identification of radiosensitive persons would be a valuable step in the protection of occupationally exposed persons. To foster research in this field, two radiation research platforms, Multidisciplinary European Low Dose Initiative (MELODI) and European Alliance Medical Radiation Protection Research (EURAMED), declared individual differences in radiation sensitivity as a key research priority.

In a small subset of patients the severe reactions can be ascribed to known radiation hypersensitivity syndromes, such as Ataxia–Telangiectasia (A–T), Fanconi anaemia (FA) or Nijmegen Breakage Syndrome (NBS) [11–13]. As late as 2010, children with A–T mutations have succumbed to death following RT [14]. These genetic syndromes, however, only comprise about 1% of the patients demonstrating severe side effects [15] and most of the enhanced tissue reactions cannot be explained by known genetic disorders.

Some further genetic associations were suggested by candidate gene approaches as well as by genome-wide association studies in radiotherapy patients. However, only a small proportion of radiosensitive individuals could be identified [16]. Additionally, functional assays such as DNA double stand break repair, induction of chromosomal aberrations, and radiation-induced apoptosis in ex vivo irradiated blood lymphocytes, have been described as predictors of radiosensitivity [17]. In parallel, a substantial number of IR-induced transcriptional and translational alterations were reported [18]. These studies benefit from recent technical developments in omics applications, which facilitate the cost effective quantification of numerous candidates, including posttranslational modifications of proteins. However, for most of the candidates, the potential correlation between IR-induced deregulation and radiosensitivity is under discussion.

Therefore, the purpose of this paper is to present the *status quo* of our knowledge of IR-induced changes in protein expression in normal tissue that can be correlated to radiosensitivity. We focus on proteins and protein modifications, as, due to posttranscriptional regulatory processes, the alterations in protein levels may describe the actual cell state, inclusive stress responses, more precisely than transcriptome changes [19]. The future goal will then be to establish protein biomarkers for the identification of radiosensitive or radio-resistant individuals. This will help to personalise treatment strategies to cancer patients during RT or help to assist an individualised risk assessment process by identifying and protecting occupationally radiation-exposed persons.

1.2. Objectives

The aim of this systematic review (SR) is to investigate the IR-induced changes, both in vivo and in vitro, in the human proteome that can be correlated to radiosensitivity.

2. Methods

2.1. Protocol and Registration

The review protocol [20] was registered to International Prospective Register of Systematic Reviews (PROSPERO) on 10.11.2020 (CRD42020220064).

2.2. Eligibility Criteria

Studies that comply with elements of Population, Exposure, Comparators, and Outcome (PECO) were eligible for this SR. The full description of PECO parameters was provided in the protocol [20]. In short, the population for this SR were primarily humans or human-derived non-tumour tissue and secondary non-tumour cell lines that were exposed to ionizing radiation. This population was compared to non-exposed individuals or *in vitro* cultures. Changes in expression of proteins after the exposure, which were associated with radiosensitivity, were defined as the outcome of this review. Only primary peer-reviewed published studies in English language were considered. As a study on ionizing radiation protein biomarkers for epidemiological studies was published in 2012 [21], studies between 2011 and 2020 were investigated in this SR.

2.3. Information Sources

Studies were identified using electronic databases and with consultations of field experts. The authors of the studies were not contacted for further studies or questions regarding the paper.

2.4. Search

NCBI PubMed (https://pubmed.ncbi.nlm.nih.gov/) [22] and ISI Web of Knowledge (v.5.34) (https://www.webofknowledge.com/) [23] were used to perform the searches. In addition, papers were also added manually. Search strings included a combination of population, exposure, and outcome elements and the applied search strings for ISI Web of Knowledge are provided in Supplementary Information 1. The Pubmed IDs of identified studies from manual as well as database searches were entered in Microsoft Excel and the duplicates (same studies in different databases) were removed using the built-in "Remove duplicate" tool.

2.5. Study Selection

A two-phase screening was performed by authors Dietz and Subedi in parallel. In phase I screening, title, abstract, and key words of all of the studies were cross-checked manually with the inclusion and exclusion criteria provided in the protocol [20]. The articles that were excluded after phase I screening are provided in Supplementary Information 2. A phase II screening (full-text screening) was performed on the remaining articles after phase I screening. The articles excluded after phase II screening, along with the reasons excluded are also given in Supplementary Information 2. Any disagreements between the reviewers was solved either in consensus, or by involving a third reviewer (Moertl or Gomolka) if necessary. The articles retained after phase II screening were used for Synthesis without Meta-analyses (SWiM).

2.6. Data Collection Process

The data collection was performed in Google Sheets by Subedi, Dietz, and Moertl, with one reviewer entering the data and the other person confirming it. The data were finally processed with Microsoft Excel. The form for data extraction is submitted in Supplementary Information 3, along with this review. Any disagreements were solved by consensus or by involving a third reviewer. In the case of missing information, the authors were not contacted and was denoted with 'nr'.

We extracted information about: the name of the protein; the fold change ratio after IR; bio fluids or cell lines being investigated; the method used to determine the fold change; the quality and quantity of IR; the characteristics of the donor(s) (age, sex, and diseased or healthy); eligibility criteria of the patients; the method used to quantify radiosensitivity (e.g., viability testing); the replicates performed for the experiment and the statistics to accompany the fold changes; the outcome of the change in protein expression; post-translational modification; and conflict of interest. The findings were summarised and the heterogeneity of the data was compared visually in form of tables.

2.7. Grouping Studies for Synthesis

This SR was performed to investigate the changes in protein expression in normal tissue after exposure to ionizing radiation. Therefore, the in vivo and in vitro studies were grouped together and no differences were made between the different radiation qualities. The doses are provided in Gray (Gy) and the dose-rates are provided in (Gy/min).

2.8. Standardised Metric and Transformation Used

The increase or decrease in protein expression after IR (fold changes, Equation (1)) was used as a measure of effect size of the exposure. The fold changes were not calculated in this manuscript but taken from the respective studies.

$$Fold\ change\ (protein) = \frac{Protein\ expression\ after\ IR}{Protein\ expression\ before\ IR} \quad (1)$$

2.9. Synthesis Methods

For each comparison, the null hypothesis represented by p-value, or in certain cases by an adjusted p-value resulting from multiple testing, was used as synthesis method for each outcome.

2.10. Certainity of Evidence

Studies which contained commonly deregulated proteins were pooled together. Studies were given an initial confidence rating of high, moderate, low, or very low based on the presence of features (controlled exposure, exposure prior to outcome, individual outcome data, and the use of comparison group). Following the OHAT method, which is based on Grading of Recommendations Assessment, Development and Evaluation (GRADE) working group guidelines, the studies were up- or downgraded. The factors increasing confidence were magnitude of the effect, dose response, residual confounding, and consistency, whereas the factors decreasing confidence were risk of bias, unexplained inconsistency, indirectness, and imprecision.

3. Results

After database searching and inclusion of manual sources, 2733 studies were identified. The records were screened for title, abstract, and key words, and 100 articles were selected for a full-text review. Finally, 28 articles were included for this SR (Figure 1). In the included articles, 13 studies examined solely DNA repair foci, 12 studies investigated proteins other than repair foci, with 3 studies also including repair foci.

3.1. Study Characteristics of the included Articles

The 16 studies that used repair foci to determine individual differences in radiosensitivity included 10 cohort studies (van Oorschot et al., 2014 [24], Vasireddy et al., 2010 [25], Bourton et al., 2011 [26], Mumbrekar et al., 2014 [27], Poulilou et al., 2015 [28], Lobachevsky et al., 2016 [29], Buchbinder et al., 2016 [30], Granzotto et al., 2016 [31], Djuzenova et al., 2013 [32], and Goutham et al., 2012 [33]) and 6 model system (Vandersickel et al., 2010 [34], Martin et al., 2014 [35], Martin et al., 2011, [36], Minafra et al., 2015 [37], Miyake et al., 2019 [38], and Nguyen et al., 2019 [39]). The detailed study characteristics of these studies is provided in Table 1a.

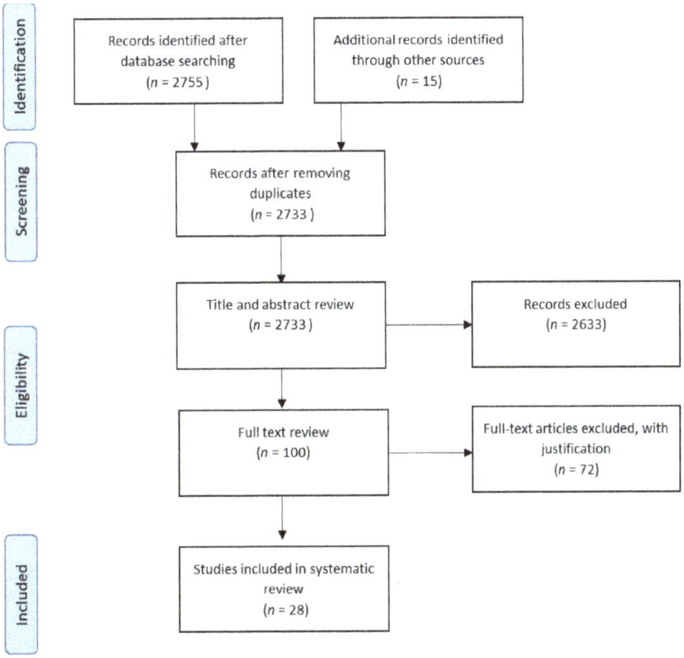

Figure 1. PRISMA flowchart that displays the number of records identified (2733), the number of records screened for a full-text review (100), and the number of records included in the review (28).

Amongst the studies, which investigated proteins other than repair foci, 15 studies were included: five cohort studies (Braicu et al., 2014 [40], Rodruiguez-Gil et al., 2014 [41], Skiöld et al., 2015 [42], Yu et al., 2018 [43], and Lacombe et al., 2019 [44]) and 10 studies on model systems (Cao et al., 2011 [45], Park et al., 2012 [46], Fekete et al., 2015 [47], Minafra et al., 2015 [37], Nishad and Ghosh, 2015 [48], Shimura et al., 2015 [49], Yim et al., 2017 [50], Miyake et al., 2019 [38], Nguyen et al., 2019 [39], Moertl at al., 2020 [51]). In total, 5 of these 10 studies were conducted with peripheral blood mononuclear cells (PBMCs) (Yu et al., 2018, Nguyen et al., 2019, Lacombe et al., 2019, Skiöld et al., 2015, and Nishad and Ghosh, 2015), and one with PBMCs-derived extracellular vesicles (Moertl et al., 2020). The detailed study characteristics are provided in Table 1b.

In total, the 28 included studies identified 76 proteins, which were correlated with normal tissue radiosensitivity. The results were prioritised so that the proteins identified in more than one study, regardless of the direction of regulation, along with their role in radiation response, were described further. Besides changes in repair foci (γH2AX and TP53BP1 quantities), the proteins were identified in more than one study are Vascular endothelial growth factor (VEGF), Caspase 3, p16^{INK4A} (Cyclin-dependent kinase inhibitor 2A, CDKN2A), Interleukin-6, and Interleukin-1B.

Table 1. (a) Study characteristics of included records concerning repair foci. (b) Study characteristics of included records containing proteins other than repair foci.

(a)								
Author, Date	**Title**	**Study Design**	**Sample-Size**	**Methods Used**	**Statistical Method**	**Repair Foci**	**Viability**	**Cell System**
Vasireddy, 2010 [25]	H2AX phosphorylation screen of cells from radiosensitive cancer patients reveals a novel DNA double-strand break repair cellular phenotype	Cohort	29	IF	nr	γH2AX	(RTOG)	lymphoblastoid cell lines (LCLs)
Bourton, 2011 [26]	Prolonged expression of the γ-H2AX DNA repair biomarker correlates with excess acute and chronic toxicity from radiotherapy treatment	Cohort	30	FACS	unpaired t-test	γH2AX	(RTOG)	lymphocytes
Goutham, 2012 [33]	DNA double-strand break analysis by γ-H2AX foci: a useful method for determining the overreactors to radiation-induced acute reactions among head-and-neck cancer patients	Cohort	54	IF	nr	γH2AX	(RTOG)	lymphocytes
Djuzenova, 2013 [32]	Radiosensitivity in breast cancer assessed by the histone γ-H2AX and 53BP1 foci	Cohort	69	IF	Student's t-test or one way ANOVA	γH2AX, 53BP1	(RTOG)	PBMCs
Mumbrekar, 2013 [27]	Influence of double-strand break repair on radiation therapy-induced acute skin reactions in breast cancer patients	Cohort	118	IF	t test, ANOVA followed by Tukey multiple comparison tests and Pearson correlation test	γH2AX	(RTOG)	lymphocytes

Table 1. *Cont.*

(a)

Author, Date	Title	Study Design	Sample-Size	Methods Used	Statistical Method	Repair Foci	Viability	Cell System
Oorschot, 2013 [24]	Reduced Activity of Double-Strand Break Repair Genes in Prostate Cancer Patients With Late Normal Tissue Radiation Toxicity	Cohort	61	IF	Continuous variables: Shapiro-Wilk test, normal distributed data: unpaired Student t test, non-normal distributed data: Mann–Whitney test	γH2AX	Late toxicity using EORTC	lymphocytes
Granzotto, 2015 [31]	Influence of Nucleoshuttling of the ATM Protein in the Healthy Tissues Response to Radiation Therapy: Toward a Molecular Classification of Human Radiosensitivity	Cohort	117	IF	ANOVA	γH2AX, pATM	Common Terminology CTCAE, RTOG	fibroblasts
Poulilιou, 2015 [28]	Survival Fraction at 2 Gy and γH2AX Expression Kinetics in Peripheral Blood Lymphocytes From Cancer Patients: Relationship With Acute Radiation-Induced Toxicities	Cohort	89	WB	nr	γH2AX	Common Terminology CTCAE, Trypan Blue assay	PBMCs
Lobachevsky, 2016 [29]	Compromised DNA repair as a basis for identification of cancer radiotherapy patients with extreme radiosensitivity	Cohort	28	IF	Unpaired t-test, Mann–Whitney test	γH2AX	(RTOG)	lymphocytes, hair follicles
Buchbinder, 2018 [30]	Application of a radiosensitivity flow assay in a patient with DNA ligase 4 deficiency	Cohort	11	IF	nr	γH2AX	known sensitivity LIG4-SCID	T cells

Table 1. *Cont.*

(a)

Author, Date	Title	Study Design	Sample-Size	Methods Used	Statistical Method	Repair Foci	Viability	Cell System
Vandersickel, 2010 [34]	Early Increase in Radiation-induced γH2AX Foci in a HumanKu70/80 Knockdown Cell Line Characterised by an Enhanced Radiosensitivity	model system	1	IF	nr	γH2AX	known sensitivity Ku70i	LVTHM cells synchronised in the G0–G1 phase, Ku70i cells synchronised in the G0–G1 phase
Martin, 2011 [36]	Assessing 'radiosensitivity' with kinetic profiles of γ-H2AX, 53BP1 and BRCA1 foci	model system	15	IF	unpaired t test	γH2AX, 53BP1	clonogenic survival	LCL
Martin, 2014 [35]	Homozygous mutation of MTPAP causes cellular radiosensitivity and persistent DNA double-strand breaks	model system	4	IF	Student's t-test	γH2AX	clonogenic survival	LCL
Minafra, 2015 [37]	Gene Expression Profiling of MCF10A Breast Epithelial Cells Exposed to IOERT	model system	1	IF	nr	γH2AX	clonogenic survival	MCF10A
Miyake, 2019 [38]	DNA Damage Response After Ionizing Radiation Exposure in Skin Keratinocytes Derived from Human-Induced Pluripotent Stem Cells	model system	1	IF	Student's t test (1-tailed)	γH2AX, 53BP1	Cell survival WST-8 assay; TUNEL assay	Normal human skin fibroblast NB1RGB, iPSCs NB1RGB C2, NB1RGB KCs 1stP, NB1RGB KCs 2ndP, NB1RGB KCs 3rdP
Nguyen, 2019 [39]	Human CCR6+ Th17 Lymphocytes Are Highly Sensitive to Radiation-Induced Senescence and Are a Potential Target for Prevention of Radiation-Induced Toxicity	model system	32	IF	two-tailed Mann–Whitney U-test, Kruskal–Wallis test	γH2AX	Annexin V-FITC; Senescence-associated β-Galactosidase	Treg, CCR6+Th17, CCR6negTh

Table 1. *Cont.*

(b)

Author, Date	Title	Study Design	Sample-Size	Methods Used	Statistical Method	Results (Protein Name)	Viability	Cell System
Braicu, 2014 [40]	Role of serum VEGFA, TIMP2, MMP2, and MMP9 in Monitoring Response to Adjuvant Radiochemotherapy in Patients with Primary Cervical Cancer – Results of a Companion Protocol of the Randomised NOGGO-AGO Phase III Clinical Trial	Cohort	72	ELISA	Fisher's exact test	VEGFA, TIMP2, MMP2, MMP9	overall survival	Serum
Rodriguez-Gil, 2014 [41]	Inflammatory Biomarker C-Reactive Protein and Radiotherapy-Induced Early Adverse Skin Reactions in Patients with Breast Cancer	Cohort	159	ELISA	two-sided Student's t-test	C-reactive protein (CRP)	EASR	plasma
Skiöld, 2014 [42]	Unique proteomic signature for radiation sensitive patients; a comparative study between normo-sensitive and radiation sensitive breast cancer patients	Cohort	17	LC-MS/MS	Student's t-test	8-oxo-dG, BLVRB, PRDX2, SOD1, CA1, PARK7, SH3BGRL3	RTOG	blood/leukocytes (RTOG 0), blood/leukocytes (RTOG 4)
Yu, 2018 [43]	Cofilin-2 Acts as a Marker for Predicting Radiotherapy Response and Is a Potential Therapeutic Target in Nasopharyngeal Carcinoma	Cohort	70	ELISA	Wilcoxon rank-sum test, t test or one-way analysis of variance (ANOVA)	Cofilin-2	Patients were divided into radiosensitivity and radio-resistance groups according to therapeutic effects	Serum
Lacombe, 2019 [44]	Quantitative proteomic analysis reveals AK2 as potential biomarker for late normal tissue radiotoxicity	Cohort	5	WB	Mann–Whitney test	adenylate kinase 2 (AK2), annexin A1 (ANXA1), isocitrate dehydrogenase 2 (IDH2), HSPA8, Nox4	RILA	T lymphocytes (Grade > 2 breast fibrosis+), T lymphocytes (Grade < 2 breast fibrosis+)

Table 1. *Cont.*

(b)

Author, Date	Title	Study Design	Sample-Size	Methods Used	Statistical Method	Results (Protein Name)	Viability	Cell System
Cao, 2011 [45]	Different radiosensitivity of CD4+CD25+ regulatory T cells and effector T cells to low dose gamma irradiation in vitro	model system	5	FACS, Luminex	Wilcoxon's signed rank test	Caspase 3, Bax, IL-1 Beta, IL-2, IL-4, IL-6, IL-10, Interferon Gamma, TNF alpha	Annexin V-FITC	CD4+CD25+ regulatory T cells and effector T cells
Park, 2012 [46]	Radio-sensitivities and angiogenic signaling pathways of irradiated normal endothelial cells derived from diverse human organs	model system	1	ELISA	Student's t-test	angiostatin	clonogenic survival	HHSEC, HDMEC
Fekete, 2015 [47]	Effect of High-Dose Irradiation on Human Bone-Marrow-Derived Mesenchymal Stromal Cells	model system	nr	Luminex	unpaired, two sided Student's t-test	PDGF-AA, PDGF-AB/BB, GRO, IL-6, VEGF	CyQUANT Cell Proliferation Assay, Trypan blue staining, colony formation	MSCs
Minafra, 2015 [37]	Gene Expression Profiling of MCF10A Breast Epithelial Cells Exposed to IOERT	model system	1	WB	nr	PARP, FAS, Pro-Caspase 8, PLK1, P53, p-EGFR, EGFR, c-MYC,	clonogenic survival	MCF10A cell line
Nishad, 2015 [48]	Dynamic changes in the proteome of human peripheral blood mononuclear cells with low dose ionizing radiation Radiotherapy-Induced Early Adverse Skin Reactions in	model system	8	2DE-MS, WB	Student's t-test	GRP78, HSP90, PDIA3, PRDX6	trypan blue, PI Staining, alkaline comet assay	PBMCs

Table 1. *Cont.*

(b)

Author, Date	Title	Study Design	Sample-Size	Methods Used	Statistical Method	Results (Protein Name)	Viability	Cell System
Shimura, 2015 [49]	Nuclear accumulation of cyclin D1 following long-term fractionated exposures to low-dose ionizing radiation in normal human diploid cells	model system	1	WB	Student's t-test	cyclin D1	cell growth assay	WI-38 (detergent insoluble fraction)
Yim, 2017 [50]	Phosphoprotein profiles of candidate markers for early cellular responses to low-dose γ-radiation in normal human fibroblast cells	model system	1	WB, antibody microarray	Student's t-test	Phospho-Gab2 (Tyr643), Phospho-P95/NBS (Ser343), Phospho-BTK (Tyr550), Phospho-Elk1 (Ser383), Phospho-ETK (Tyr40), Phospho-CaMK4 (Thr196/200), Phospho-MEK1 (Thr298), Phospho-PLCG1 (Tyr1253), Phospho-IRS-1 (Ser612), Phospho-TFII-I (Tyr248), Phospho-IKK-alpha/beta (Ser176/177), Phospho-MEK1 (Thr286), Phospho-Pyk2 (Tyr580), Phospho-Keratin 8 (Ser431), Phospho-ERK3 (Ser189), Phospho-Chk1 (Ser296), Phospho-CBL (Tyr700), Phospho-BTK (Tyr550), Phospho-LIMK1/2 (Thr508/505), p-BTK(Tyr550)/BTK, p-Gab2(Tyr643)/Gab2, p-BTK(Tyr550)/BTK, p-Gab2(Tyr643)/Gab2,	MTT	MRC5, NHDF

Table 1. *Cont.*

(b)

Author, Date	Title	Study Design	Sample-Size	Methods Used	Statistical Method	Results (Protein Name)	Viability	Cell System
Miyake, 2019 [38]	DNA Damage Response After Ionizing Radiation Exposure in Skin Keratinocytes Derived from Human-Induced Pluripotent Stem Cells	model system	1	IF	Student's t test (1-tailed)	p16	Cell survival WST-8 assay, TUNEL assay	Skin keratinocytes were derived from iPSCs
Nguyen, 2019 [39]	Human CCR6+Th17 lymphocytes are highly sensitive to radiation-induced senescence and are a potential target for prevention of radiation-induced toxicity	model system	32	IF, Luminex	two-tailed Mann–Whitney U-test, Kruskal–Wallis test	Caspase 3, p16Ink4a, p21Cdkn1a, IL-1 Beta, VEGF-A, IL-8, H2A.J	Annexin V-FITC, Senescence-associated β-Galactosidase	CCR6+Th17 lymphocytes
Moertl, 2020 [51]	Radiation Exposure of Peripheral Mononuclear Blood Cells Alters the Composition and Function of Secreted Extracellular Vesicles	model system	5	LC-MS/MS	two-sided Student's t-test	hemopexin (HPX), syntaxin-binding protein 3 (STXBP3), proteasome subunit alpha type-6 (PSMA6)	sub-G1 fraction, Caspase 3 activity	PBMC-derived EVs

Abbreviations: (a) Criteria for adverse events (CTCAE), European organisation for research and treatment of cancer (EORTC), Fluorescence-activated cell sorting (FACS), Immunofluorescence (IF), not reported (nr), Peripheral blood mononuclear cell (PBMC), Radiation therapy oncology group (RTOG), Western Blot WB). (b) Two-dimensional gel electrophoresis (2-DE), Enzyme-linked immunosorbent assay (ELISA), Immunofluorescence (IF), Liquid chromatography (LC), Mass spectrometry (MS), not reported (nr), radiation-induced lymphocyte apoptosis (RILA), Radiation therapy oncology group (RTOG), Western blot (WB).

3.2. IR-Induced Changes in Repair Foci Proteins

H2AX, a variant of the histone protein H2A, is located in the nucleus and its functions include chromatin organisation and DNA damage response. In case of DNA double strand break damage, its phosphorylation by PI3 kinases ATM, ATR, and DNAPKcs signals the damaged site, and recruits downstream DNA repair proteins [52–55]. The phosphorylated isoform on serine 139 is termed as γH2AX [52,53]. The initial γH2AX signal develops and expands within the first hour after DNA damage induction. With subsequent repair of the damaged sites, the signal decreases again. Depending on the amount and the complexity of the DNA damage and on DNA repair capacity, the differences in DNA repair kinetic and residual foci level are observed [56]. In addition to γH2AX, another component of the DNA double strand break repair machinery, TP53BP1 (Tumour Protein P53 Binding Protein 1) [32,36], was also identified as a target candidate to predict radiation sensitivity. TP53BP1 plays an essential role in the canonical non-homologous end joining (NHEJ) repair of DNA double strand breaks (DSB), which is the main repair pathway of DSB in G0–G1 cell cycle phase, e.g., in peripheral blood lymphocytes [57]. TP53BP1 clusters appears during radiation response and disappears in a similar time dependent kinetic as γH2AX foci do. γH2AX and TP53BP1 quantities were measured by immunofluorescence microscopy in most of the studies except for Bourton et al. and Poulilíou et al. In their studies, γH2AX expression was analysed by fluorescence-activated cell sorting (FACS) and western blot, respectively. The IR-induced alterations of γH2AX and TP53BP1 expressions are presented in detail in Supplementary Information 4.

In all studies, irradiation was performed with gamma or X-ray radiation at a high dose rate and doses from 0.5 2.0 Gy. Studies were performed in different cell lines (fibroblast, lymphoblastoid, epithelial cell lines) harbouring DNA repair defects, or in primary cells (blood cells, hair follicle) from cancer patients. From all parameters investigated, such as basal foci level, radiation induced foci and residual foci at later repair time points, elevated levels of residual γH2AX or TP53BP1 foci appear to be robust to identify radiosensitive cells or individuals.

DNA repair deficient individuals demonstrate delayed development of the initial DNA damage or delayed DNA repair, resulting in an increased level of residual damage after 24 hours [35,36]. Therefore γH2AX is considered as a putative predictive biomarker to detect radiation sensitive individuals harbouring DNA repair defects by performing an *in vitro* challenging assay and investigating signal development and disappearance [26,56,58]. Promising studies demonstrating a positive association of increased residual damage in ATM [35,36,59], Ligase IV deficient radiation sensitive individuals [30,36], and in cancer patients experiencing strong acute or late side effects from the radiation treatment [24–29,32] are presented. However, the literature overview has shown multiple factors, such as high variability of the assay itself, the lack of a standardized protocol including a fixed in vitro exposure dose, repair time point to analyse residual foci, and comparator group, bias the results. Therefore, correlation to outcome parameters such as genetically defined repair deficient cell lines and patients, as well as association to clinical radiation sensitivity, still remain contradictory [5,34,60]. Our systematic review and others show that although γH2AX and TP53BP1 expressions have the potential to predict an in vitro radiation response in a number of patients; large cohorts need to be analysed by standardised protocols to improve the robustness and sensitivity of the assay, and to decipher the subgroups of patients for which the assay is a meaningful tool to predict detrimental radiation reactions [5,18,61].

3.3. IR-Induced Deregulated Proteins Excluding Repair Foci and Risk of Biases

An aim of our SR is to discover new feasible markers on protein levels that are associated with radiosensitivity, besides repair foci proteins. To provide a rich reflection of evidence for the reader, we included both significantly deregulated and not deregulated proteins in Supplementary Information 5. There is comparatively little evidence published on this topic within the inclusion parameters specified (especially the correlation to radiosensitivity). Therefore, if the studies included experiments that depict cell survival, the paper was incorporated to the synthesis, irrespective of a direct correlation of the outcome to radiosensitivity. Table 2 presents the evaluation of studies containing proteins, other than repair foci, on all applicable risk of bias (RoB) questions as developed by the Office of Health Assessment and Translation (OHAT) [62]. The questions concerning the RoB tools and the criteria to judge the different biases are provided in the protocol [20] and in Supplementary Information 6. Although a set of 11 questions was used to evaluate the studies, the studies were categorised into three tiers (T1, T2, or T3) primarily based on the responses to the following key questions (Supplementary Information 7)

1. Can we be confident in the exposure assessment?
2. Can we be confident in the outcome assessment?
3. Did the study design or analyses account for important confounding and modifying variables?

None of the studies were categorised in T1, one study (Park, 2012) was categorised into T3, and the rest were categorised as T2. The RoB questions are suited to cohort and human clinical trials compared to model systems. Concealment, randomisation, and blinding in most studies on model systems are not performed because (i) it is usually a single person that performs the studies and (ii) it is not a common practice to conceal the study groups from the researcher. Therefore, most studies received a 'probably high risk of bias' assessment in randomisation, concealment, and blinding domains. Although randomisation is performed during the accessing of outcomes, for example, when performing mass spectrometric analyses or measuring γH2AX quantities on coded slides, more often than not, it is not reported to ensure brevity during publication. Based on the results from this SR, we can recommend that studies on model systems should take care of randomisation, concealing of study groups, blinding the accessors, and, most important, reporting them.

Table 2. Accessing risk of bias for studies that included proteins other than repair foci.

	Risk of Bias Domains and Ratings	Miyake, 2019	Cao, 2011	Nguyen, 2019	Minafra, 2015	Yim, 2017	Braicu, 2014	Park, 2012	Fekete, 2015	Shumura, 2015	Lacombe, 2019	Skiöld, 2014	Nishad, 2015	Rodruiguez-Gil, 2014	Moertl, 2020	Granzotto, 2016	Yu, 2018
Key criteria	Can we be confident in the exposure characterisation?	–	+	+	++	++	–	–	-	+	-	+	+	-	++	+	–
	Can we be confident in the outcome assessment?	-	–	-	-	+	+	-	+	+	++	+	+	++	-	+	++
	Did the study design or analyses account for important confounding and modifying variables?	+	-	++	+	++	–	-	+	-	+	-	-	++	-	-	+
Other RoB criterion	Was administered dose or exposure level adequately randomised?	-	-	-	-	-	-	-	-	-	–	-	+	-	-	-	+
	Was allocation to study groups adequately concealed?	-	-	-	-	-	-	-	-	-	-	-	-	-	-	-	-
	Did selection of study participants result in appropriate comparison groups?	++	++	-	++	++	++	+	+	-	+	-	+	++	++	-	+
	Were experimental conditions identical across study groups?	-	++	-	-	-	-	-	-	–	-	+	++	-	++	-	++
	Were the research personnel and human subjects blinded to the study group in the study?	-	-	-	-	-	-	-	-	-	-	-	-	-	-	-	-
	Were outcome data complete without attrition or exclusion from analysis?	-	+	+	++	-	++	+	++	++	++	++	++	++	++	-	++
	Were all the measured outcomes reported?	+	++	++	++	++	++	++	++	-	++	++	++	++	++	++	++
	Were there no other potential threat to internal validity (e.g., statistical methods were appropriate and researchers adhered to study protocol?	–	-	++	-	+	-	-	++	+	++	-	+	+	++	+	++
	Final Category	T2	T2	T2	T2	T2	T2	T3	T2	T2	T2	T2	T2	T2	T2	T2	T2

Definitely high risk of bias (–), probably high risk of bias (-), probably low risk of bias (+), definitely low risk of bias (++).

The proteins that were reported in at least two studies (Table 3) are explained further:

Table 3. List of proteins identified in at least two studies, not concerning repair foci.

Priority Group	Author, Date	Marker	Outcome	Cell System
1	Braicu, 2014	VEGFA	decrease in VEGFA concentration leads to increase in survival, >500 pg/mL negative influence on survival	Serum
	Fekete, 2015	VEGFA	nr	MSCs
	Nguyen, 2019	VEGFA	resistant compared to Treg	CCR6 + Th17
2	Cao, 2011	Caspase 3 #	radiosensitive	CD4 + CD25 + Treg cells
	Nguyen, 2019	Caspase 3	resistant compared to Treg	CCR6 + Th17
2	Miyake, 2019	p16	resistant compared to primary fibroblasts (IR-induced senescence)	NB1RGB KCs 1stP, 2ndP and 3rdP
	Nguyen, 2019	p16	resistant compared to Treg (IR-induced senescence)	CCR6 + Th17
2	Cao, 2011	IL-6	radiosensitive	CD4 + CD25 + Treg cells
	Fekete, 2015	IL-6	nr	MSCs
2	Cao, 2011	IL-1Beta	radiosensitive	CD4 + CD25 + Treg cells
	Nguyen, 2019	IL-1Beta	sensitive compared to CCR6 + Th17	CCR6negTh

higher increase in sensitive cells, proteins upregulated post-IR shown in orange, downregulation in blue, and no change in black.

3.3.1. Vascular Endothelial Growth Factor (VEGF)

VEGF induces endothelial cell proliferation, promotes cell migration, inhibits apoptosis, and induces permeabilization of blood vessels [63,64]. Furthermore VEGF is associated with autophagy, a conserved and essential mechanism for both protecting and killing cells during stress response [65]. Autophagy is carried out by lysosomal degradation of macroproteins or even whole organelles [66,67] and is thought to contribute to normal tissue and tumour radio-resistance [68–70].

Nguyen et al. reported an increase in VEGF secretion 48 h after exposure to 2 Gy IR (^{137}Cs, dose rate 2.7 Gy/min) in CCR6+Th17 T cells, which are highly sensitive to IR-induced senescence. This may contribute to IR-induced normal tissue damage and might facilitate tumour recurrence and metastasis after radiotherapy [39]. Braicu et al. investigated VEGF levels in the serum of patients with locally advanced FIGO stage Ib–IIb cervical cancer before and after chemoradiotherapy (6 MV photon linear acceleration). They demonstrated that a decrease in VEGFA concentration leads to an increase in overall survival; an increase of more than 500 pg/mL VEGF in serum negatively influenced the overall survival due to the resistance to chemoradiotherapy [40]. Fekete et al. described an increase in VEGF levels in non-irradiated MSCs (Bone-Marrow-Derived Mesenchymal Stromal Cells), whereas no significant change was observed in irradiated MSCs (30 Gy, 7, 14, 21, and 28 d post IR with ^{137}Cs) [47].

VEGF is a key mediator of neovascularisation and is highly expressed in cancer cells and tumour-associated stromal cells [71]. In a meta-analysis conducted to evaluate the relationship between serum VEGF expression and radiosensitivity in Asian non-small cell lung cancer (NSCLC) patients, it was established that lower expression of VEGF led to a longer overall survival and could be a useful biomarker to predict radiosensitivity and prognosis of NSCLC patients [72]. Hu et al. reported IR-induced increased VEGF expression in HeLa cells in vivo and in vitro and a knockdown of VEGF expression in HeLa cells indicated increased cellular sensitivity to radiation [73].

The effect of radiation exposure on VEGF seems to be cell type dependent. However, first in vitro and in vivo studies suggest its importance for normal tissue radiosensitivity. Therefore, it is a promising candidate marker to study radiosensitivity in future projects.

3.3.2. Caspase 3

Caspase 3 is involved in the activation cascade of several caspases responsible for apoptosis by proteolytically cleaving poly(ADP-ribose) polymerase (PARP). Furthermore it cleaves and activates Caspase-6, -7, and -9 [74].

Both, Cao et al. [45] and Nguyen et al. [39] conducted their studies on ^{137}Cs irradiated T cells (dose rate 2.7 and 4.8 Gy/min, respectively) and observed a radiation induced increase in Caspase 3 concentration, where Cao et al. reported a higher increase in radiosensitive CD4+CD25+ Treg cells compared to normo-sensitive CD4+CD25- T cells after overnight incubation post 0.94, 1.875, and 7.5 Gy. Nguyen et al. described a greater Caspase 3 activation (48 h post 2 Gy) in CCR6negTh cells compared to CCR6+Th17 that are rather prone to IR-induced senescence than to apoptosis. When lymphocytes from healthy donors were irradiated with 1, 2, or 4 Gy (^{60}Co), a dose-dependent increase in active Caspase 3 was observed that included high intra-individual variability [75]. This suggests that Caspase 3 could effectively be used as a tool to detect individual differences in radiosensitivity, which could be used on patients before they undergo radiotherapy. In a study conducted in MCF-7 breast cancer cells, it was discovered that Caspase 3 plays a critical role in radiotherapy-induced apoptosis, and this suggests that Caspase 3 deficiency may contribute to the radio-resistance of breast cancers [76]. Although an activation of Caspase 3 seems to be a potential candidate to define radiosensitive cells, due to limited numbers of donors (5 and 32), the results needs to be validated in further studies.

3.3.3. p16^{INK4A} (Cyclin-Dependent Kinase Inhibitor 2A, CDKN2A)

p16 acts as a negative regulator of normal cell proliferation by inhibiting CDK 4 and CDK 6 interaction with cyclin D and the phosphorylation of retinoblastoma protein, prohibiting progression from G1 phase to S phase [77,78]. p16 is a known marker for senescence through its contribution to the repression of proliferation-associated genes. High-Mobility Group A proteins act together with p16 to promote senescence-associated heterochromatic foci (SAHF) formation () and proliferative arrest [79].

Miyake et al. observed that an increase in p16 expression in keratinocytes (passage 1, 2, and 3), was characterised as radio-resistant but not in fibroblasts or induced pluripotent stem cells (iPSCs) 72 h after 2 Gy ^{60}Co γ irradiation (dose rate 2.7 Gy/min) [38]. Nguyen et al. showed that p16 expression was higher in CCR6+Th17 cells (radio-resistant compared to Treg cells) 48 h after 2 Gy ^{137}Cs with a dose rate of 2.7 Gy/min IR and led to IR-induced senescence [39]. In contrast, studies have shown that p16 expression leads to radio-sensitisation in cancer cell lines [80–82]. Since p16 is known to be a marker for senescence and the study results between tumour cell and normal cells are controversial, p16 is not a promising marker to determine individual differences in radiosensitivity.

3.3.4. Interleukin-6 (IL-6)

The pleiotropic cytokine IL-6 comprises a wide variety of biological functions including immunity, tissue regeneration, and metabolism [83]. It is a potent inducer of the acute phase response and a rapid production of IL-6 contributes to host defence during infection or injury. IL-6 expression is tightly regulated, both transcriptionally and post-transcriptionally and its immoderate production causes severe inflammatory diseases.

Cao et al. reported that IL-6 is significantly downregulated in response to 0.94 and 1.87 Gy (^{137} Cs, dose rate 4.8 Gy/min) in radiosensitive Treg cells, but not in T cells showing a normal sensitivity [45]. The study of Fekete et al. found increased IL-6 levels during culture of both exposed and non-exposed MSCs (bone-marrow-derived mesenchymal stromal cells) 7, 14, 21, and 28 d post IR with ^{137} Cs [47].

Chen et al. showed that irradiation-induced IL-6 and the subsequent recruitment of myeloid-derived suppressor cells could be responsible for tumour regrowth [84]. Several clinical observations have documented increased IL-6 levels in plasma from patients with therapy-resistant metastatic disease compared to patients with earlier stages of the disease and healthy individuals. Higher levels of IL-6 in body fluids were associated with poor prognosis and survival [85–90]. These findings fit to the results of Cao et al. showing that downregulation of IL-6 enhances radiosensitivity. Concerning normal tissue, more evidence is needed to confirm these findings.

3.3.5. Interleukin-1 Beta (IL-1β)

IL-1β is a proinflammatory cytokine and works in coaction with interleukin-12 and induces interferon gamma synthesis from T-helper 1 cells [91]. By inducing VEGF production synergistically with TNF and IL-6, IL-1β is involved in angiogenesis [92].

Like for IL-6, Cao et al found a significantly downregulated IL-1β in response to 0.94 and 1.87 Gy ^{137}Cs irradiation, delivered with a dose rate of 4.8 Gy/min in radiosensitive Treg cells, but not in normal sensitive T cells [45]. Secretion of IL-1β was increased only in CCR6negTh and not in CCR6+Th17 cells 48 h after 2 Gy (^{137}Cs, dose rate 2.7 Gy/min) irradiation according to Nguyen et al. [39]. Chen et al. reported a significant overexpression of IL-1 beta in cancer specimens compared to non-malignant tissues. By blocking IL-1 β, tumour growth, invasion ability, and treatment resistance were attenuated [93]. Regarding the diverse observations of Cao et al. and Nguyen et al., IL-1β does not seem to be a favourable biomarker.

The studies that contained the previous markers were further evaluated based on a Grading of Recommendations Assessment, Development and Evaluation (GRADE) approach (Table 4). Each study received an initial confidence rating based on the presence or absence of four features, which were (1) controlled exposure, (2) exposure prior to outcome, (3) individual outcome data, and (4) use of comparison group. The studies that received the same initial confidence were pooled together and either up-graded depending on magnitude effect, dose response, residual confounding, consistency, or downgraded based on risk of bias, unexplained inconsistency indirectness, or imprecision. The factors that decreased confidence were risk of bias, unexplained consistency, and indirectness. The detailed information is provided in the protocol [20].

Table 4. Accessing confidence in body of evidence in selected studies.

Author, Date	Initial Confidence by Features of Study Design				Initial Confidence Rating	Factors Decreasing Confidence	Factors Increasing Confidence	Final Confidence
	Controlled Exposure	Exposure Prior to Outcome	Individual Outcome Data	Use of Comparison Groups				
Fekete, 2015	×	√	×	×	Very low	Risk of bias Unexplained consistency Indirectness Imprecision	Magnitude effect Dose Response Residual Confounding Consistency	Very low
Braicu, 2014	×	√	√	√	Moderate			Low
Nguyen, 2019	√	√	√	×	Moderate			Moderate
Cao, 2011	√	√	√	√	High			High
Miyake, 2019	×	√	√	×	Low			Low

Significant interactions for aforementioned proteins, TP53BP1, and γH2AX (Figure 2), were identified when an in silico protein enrichment was performed on the STRING 11 database [94,95]. The generated network consisted of 7 nodes that are connected via

15 edges, whereas only 7 edges would be expected when using only 7 proteins for analysis. The interactions suggest that the proteins are likely to be biologically connected.

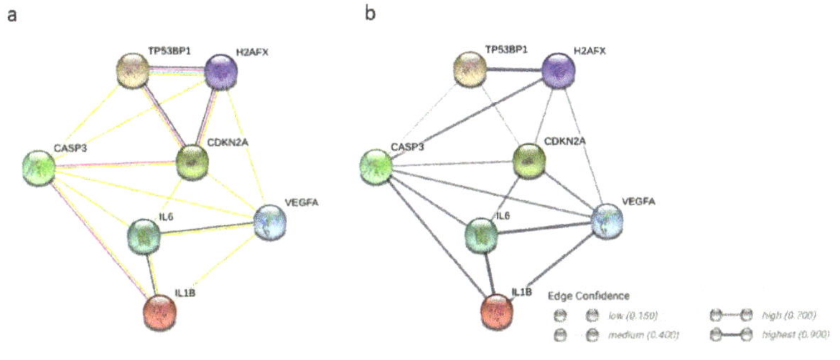

Figure 2. Protein-protein interaction enrichment network generated in STRING 11.0 using proteins identified in at least two studies: p16 (CDKN2A), VEGFA, IL6, IL-1β, CASP3, TP53BP1, and γH2AX: (**a**) The lines represent protein–protein association where pink lines are known experimentally determined interactions, blue from curated databases, green are from text-mining, and black represents co-expression; (**b**) The thickness of the edges display the confidence in interaction: medium (0.400), high (0.700), and highest (0.900) in this network.

4. Outlook

First of all, it is important to understand the proteomic landscape of normal tissues. Different tissues and cell types harbour divergent baseline protein expression [96]. Most of the studies are focused on blood or blood cell-derived changes, but normal tissue reaction post IR is multifaceted and dependent on tissue types. Therefore more mechanistic studies are required to identify the tissue-specific impact of proteins on radiosensitivity. In this regard the validation of proteins for different dose rates will be an important point in future studies, because new developments in radiotherapy, such as ultra-high dose radiotherapy (FLASH) use much higher dose rates which may affect radiosensitivity differentially.

Second, radiosensitivity is a complex issue as many risk factors modify the radiation reaction, thus determining each predictor's overall impact is difficult to characterise. Some of the factors that influence radiosensitivity and complicate the discovery of a ubiquitous applicable biomarker are specified in this section.

There are several known hereditary hyper-radiosensitive disorders arising from rare mutations in DNA repair genes of large effect. All belong to XCIND syndromes, named after distinct hypersensitivity to ionizing radiation (X-ray), cancer susceptibility, immunodeficiency, neurological abnormality, and double-strand DNA breakage. Examples of such syndromes are Ataxia telangiectasia, Fanconi anemia, Ligase IV syndrome, Radiosensitive severe combined immunodeficiency disease (RS-SCID), Radiosensitivity, immunodeficiency, dysmorphic features, and learning difficulties (RIDDLE) syndrome, or ataxia telangiectasia and Rad3-related protein (ATR)-Seckel syndrome [15,97–99]. Polymorphic variants, as well as mutations in multiple genes that lead to similar or different DNA damage response pathways, will contribute to genetically defined radiosensitivity in a complex manner.

Age and gender are crucial factors influencing individual differences in radiosensitivity. Children aged 0–5 years are expected to be the most sensitive group concerning radiation-induced leukaemia, as well as skin, breast, thyroid, and brain cancer for both high and low dose radiation exposures [100–105]. Sex influences the radiation response and the radiation-induced cancer risk [106]. Epidemiological studies from the Chernobyl disaster in 1986 and the Hiroshima and Nagasaki atomic bomb survivors provide evidence that females possess a greater risk for solid cancers [107–109] mainly due to cancer of reproductive tissue [110] and thyroid and brain cancer [106,111].

The anatomical structure (organ size, body mass index), as well as breathing rates, and individual metabolism of exposed individuals alter radiation doses received by organs and tissues, which leads to inter-individual variations [112–116]. Lifestyle is another aspect that affects individual cancer susceptibility when radiation exposure is considered. Although smoking and ionizing radiation exposure are the most studied influences, other co-exposures such as heavy metals, medication, alcohol consumption, dietary habits, and combined exposure to other radiation qualities such as radon needs to be taken into account [117–119]. Additionally, already diseased individuals cope poorly to radiation exposure compared to healthy ones. [120,121].

5. Conclusions

The fact that there is a clear evidence that not all individuals share the same radiation-induced risk of adverse health outcomes is also backed by the reports from the advisory group on ionizing radiation (UK) [122] and International Commission on Radiological Protection (ICRP) [123]. Radiosensitivity represents a complex phenotype and this is perhaps why we identified few IR-induced proteins (γH2AX, TP53BP1, VEGF, CASP3, CDKN2A, IL-6, and IL-1B), that correlated to radiosensitivity, when common markers in at least two studies were considered. These candidate proteins and their possible interaction partners should be investigated further, to discover biomarkers that can properly define radiation sensitivity.

The need to discover biomarkers for disease risk or susceptibility of radiation related risks for individuals or population subgroups is vital and also stressed by MELODI platform [124]. Not only would patients benefit by an individualised cancer treatment but also individualised risk assessment and prevention measurements can protect at-risk occupationally exposed individuals more efficiently. This systematic review highlights the fact that there is a lack of basic studies with a focus on normal tissue in contrast to tumour tissues. More studies based on functional assays are needed to survey the role of specific proteins in different normal tissues. In addition, the frequently statistically underpowered studies do strengthen the need to use large cohorts, as well as very sensitive methods for the biomarker search, as well as focusing on functional tests of potential markers in different accessible normal tissue (lymphocytes, fibroblasts, keratinocytes, and body fluids).

6. Differences between Protocol and the Review

The GRADE tool to up- or downgrade studies was not performed on all studies but only on studies that included proteins, other than repair foci, reported in at least two studies.

Supplementary Materials: The following are available online at https://www.mdpi.com/2075-4426/11/2/140/s1: Supplementary Information 1 (Search algorithm for ISI Web of Science), Supplementary Information 2 (List of rejected articles), Supplementary Information 3 (Data extraction sheet), Supplementary Information 4 (IR-induced changes in repair foci proteins), Supplementary Information 5 (IR-induced changes in non-repair foci proteins), Supplementary Information 6 (Risk of bias questions), Supplementary Information 7 (Risk of bias categorisation into T1, T2, and T3, PRISMA and SWiM checklist.

Author Contributions: Conceptualisation, A.D., M.G., S.M., and P.S.; methodology, A.D., M.G., S.M., P.S.; formal analysis, A.D., M.G., S.M., P.S.; investigation, A.D., M.G., S.M., P.S.; resources, M.G., S.M.; writing—original draft preparation, A.D., M.G., S.M., P.S.; writing—review and editing, A.D., M.G., S.M., P.S.; supervision, M.G., S.M.; project administration, M.G., S.M.; funding acquisition, M.G., S.M. All authors have read and agreed to the published version of the manuscript.

Funding: A.D. is funded by the Bundesministeriums für Bildung und Forschung (BMBF, Germany) within the "ReparaturFoci (RF) project (02NUK035D)" and P.S. is funded by the BMBF within the project "Zielstrukturen der individuellen Strahlenempfindlichkeit (ZISStrans) (02NUK047B)".

Institutional Review Board Statement: Not applicable.

Informed Consent Statement: Not applicable.

Data Availability Statement: Data is provided in the manuscript.

Acknowledgments: The authors would like to thank Bernd Henschenmacher and Elisa Pasqual for the guidance in writing this review and Lukas Duchrow and David Endesfelder for their help with statistics. Felix Kästle helped organise the table for the list of rejected articles.

Conflicts of Interest: The authors declare no conflict of interest. The funders had no role in the design of the study; in the collection, analyses, or interpretation of data; in the writing of the manuscript, or in the decision to publish the results.

References

1. Global Cancer Observatory. Available online: https://gco.iarc.fr/today/data/factsheets/cancers/39-All-cancers-fact-sheet.pdf (accessed on 11 December 2020).
2. Rosenblatt, E.; Izewska, J.; Anacak, Y.; Pynda, Y.; Scalliet, P.; Boniol, M.; Autier, P. Radiotherapy capacity in European countries: An analysis of the Directory of Radiotherapy Centres (DIRAC) database. *Lancet Oncol.* **2013**, *14*, e79–e86. [CrossRef]
3. Fazel, R.; Gerber, T.C.; Balter, S.; Brenner, D.J.; Carr, J.J.; Cerqueira, M.D.; Chen, J.; Einstein, A.J.; Krumholz, H.M.; Mahesh, M.; et al. Approaches to enhancing radiation safety in cardiovascular imaging: A scientific statement from the American Heart Association. *Circulation* **2014**, *130*, 1730–1748. [CrossRef]
4. Salomaa, S.; Jung, T. Roadmap for research on individual radiosensitivity and radiosusceptibility—The MELODI view on research needs. *Int. J. Radiat. Biol.* **2020**, *96*, 277–279. [CrossRef]
5. Gomolka, M.; Blyth, B.; Bourguignon, M.; Badie, C.; Schmitz, A.; Talbot, C.; Hoeschen, C.; Salomaa, S. Potential screening assays for individual radiation sensitivity and susceptibility and their current validation state. *Int. J. Radiat. Biol.* **2019**, *96*, 280–296. [CrossRef]
6. Wojcik, A.; Bouffler, S.; Hauptmann, M.; Rajaraman, P. Considerations on the use of the terms radiosensitivity and radiosusceptibility. *J. Radiol. Prot.* **2018**, *38*, N25–N29. [CrossRef]
7. Averbeck, D.; Salomaa, S.; Bouffler, S.; Ottolenghi, A.; Smyth, V.; Sabatier, L. Progress in low dose health risk research: Novel effects and new concepts in low dose radiobiology. *Mutat. Res.* **2018**, *776*, 46–69. [CrossRef]
8. Hoeller, U.; Borgmann, K.; Bonacker, M.; Kuhlmey, A.; Bajrovic, A.; Jung, H.; Alberti, W.; Dikomey, E. Individual radiosensitivity measured with lymphocytes may be used to predict the risk of fibrosis after radiotherapy for breast cancer. *Radiother. Oncol.* **2003**, *69*, 137–144. [CrossRef] [PubMed]
9. Heemsbergen, W.D.; Peeters, S.T.; Koper, P.C.; Hoogeman, M.S.; Lebesque, J.V. Acute and late gastrointestinal toxicity after radiotherapy in prostate cancer patients: Consequential late damage. *Int. J. Radiat. Oncol. Biol. Phys.* **2006**, *66*, 3–10. [CrossRef] [PubMed]
10. Pollack, A.; Zagars, G.K.; Antolak, J.A.; Kuban, D.A.; Rosen, I.I. Prostate biopsy status and PSA nadir level as early surrogates for treatment failure: Analysis of a prostate cancer randomized radiation dose escalation trial. *Int. J. Radiat. Oncol. Biol. Phys.* **2002**, *54*, 677–685. [CrossRef]
11. Nakanishi, K.; Taniguchi, T.; Ranganathan, V.; New, H.V.; Moreau, L.A.; Stotsky, M.; Mathew, C.G.; Kastan, M.B.; Weaver, D.T.; D'Andrea, A.D. Interaction of FANCD2 and NBS1 in the DNA damage response. *Nat. Cell Biol.* **2002**, *4*, 913–920. [CrossRef] [PubMed]
12. Petrini, J.H. The mammalian Mre11-Rad50-nbs1 protein complex: Integration of functions in the cellular DNA-damage response. *Am. J. Hum. Genet.* **1999**, *64*, 1264–1269. [CrossRef]
13. Digweed, M. Human genetic instability syndromes: Single gene defects with increased risk of cancer. *Toxicol. Lett.* **1993**, *67*, 259–281. [CrossRef]
14. Pietrucha, B.M.; Heropolitanska-Pliszka, E.; Wakulinska, A.; Skopczynska, H.; Gatti, R.A.; Bernatowska, E. Ataxia-telangiectasia with hyper-IgM and Wilms tumor: Fatal reaction to irradiation. *J. Pediatr. Hematol. Oncol.* **2010**, *32*, e28–e30. [CrossRef]
15. Mizutani, S.; Takagi, M. XCIND as a genetic disease of X-irradiation hypersensitivity and cancer susceptibility. *Int. J. Hematol.* **2013**, *97*, 37–42. [CrossRef]
16. Andreassen, C.N.; Schack, L.M.; Laursen, L.V.; Alsner, J. Radiogenomics—Current status, challenges and future directions. *Cancer Lett.* **2016**, *382*, 127–136. [CrossRef]
17. Chua, M.L.; Rothkamm, K. Biomarkers of radiation exposure: Can they predict normal tissue radiosensitivity? *Clin. Oncol.* **2013**, *25*, 610–616. [CrossRef] [PubMed]
18. Hall, J.; Jeggo, P.A.; West, C.; Gomolka, M.; Quintens, R.; Badie, C.; Laurent, O.; Aerts, A.; Anastasov, N.; Azimzadeh, O.; et al. Ionizing radiation biomarkers in epidemiological studies—An update. *Mutat. Res.* **2017**, *771*, 59–84. [CrossRef]
19. Tebaldi, T.; Re, A.; Viero, G.; Pegoretti, I.; Passerini, A.; Blanzieri, E.; Quattrone, A. Widespread uncoupling between transcriptome and translatome variations after a stimulus in mammalian cells. *BMC Genomics* **2012**, *13*, 220. [CrossRef] [PubMed]
20. Dietz, A.; Gomolka, M.; Moertl, S.; Subedi, P. Ionizing Radiation Protein Biomarkers in Normal Tissue and Their Correlation to Radiosensitivity: Protocol for a Systematic Review. *J. Pers. Med.* **2020**, *11*, 3. [CrossRef]

21. Pernot, E.; Hall, J.; Baatout, S.; Benotmane, M.A.; Blanchardon, E.; Bouffler, S.; El Saghire, H.; Gomolka, M.; Guertler, A.; Harms-Ringdahl, M.; et al. Ionizing radiation biomarkers for potential use in epidemiological studies. *Mutat. Res.* **2012**, *751*, 258–286. [CrossRef]
22. National Library of Medicine, Pubmed. Available online: https://pubmed.ncbi.nlm.nih.gov/ (accessed on 28 December 2020).
23. Clarivate Analytics, Web of Science. Available online: https://apps.webofknowledge.com/ (accessed on 28 December 2020).
24. Van Oorschot, B.; Hovingh, S.E.; Moerland, P.D.; Medema, J.P.; Stalpers, L.J.; Vrieling, H.; Franken, N.A. Reduced activity of double-strand break repair genes in prostate cancer patients with late normal tissue radiation toxicity. *Int. J. Radiat. Oncol. Biol. Phys.* **2014**, *88*, 664–670. [CrossRef]
25. Vasireddy, R.S.; Sprung, C.N.; Cempaka, N.L.; Chao, M.; McKay, M.J. H2AX phosphorylation screen of cells from radiosensitive cancer patients reveals a novel DNA double-strand break repair cellular phenotype. *Br. J. Cancer* **2010**, *102*, 1511–1518. [CrossRef] [PubMed]
26. Bourton, E.C.; Plowman, P.N.; Smith, D.; Arlett, C.F.; Parris, C.N. Prolonged expression of the gamma-H2AX DNA repair biomarker correlates with excess acute and chronic toxicity from radiotherapy treatment. *Int. J. Cancer* **2011**, *129*, 2928–2934. [CrossRef]
27. Mumbrekar, K.D.; Fernandes, D.J.; Goutham, H.V.; Sharan, K.; Vadhiraja, B.M.; Satyamoorthy, K.; Bola Sadashiva, S.R. Influence of double-strand break repair on radiation therapy-induced acute skin reactions in breast cancer patients. *Int. J. Radiat. Oncol. Biol. Phys.* **2014**, *88*, 671–676. [CrossRef]
28. Pouliliou, S.E.; Lialiaris, T.S.; Dimitriou, T.; Giatromanolaki, A.; Papazoglou, D.; Pappa, A.; Pistevou, K.; Kalamida, D.; Koukourakis, M.I. Survival Fraction at 2 Gy and gammaH2AX Expression Kinetics in Peripheral Blood Lymphocytes From Cancer Patients: Relationship With Acute Radiation-Induced Toxicities. *Int. J. Radiat. Oncol. Biol. Phys.* **2015**, *92*, 667–674. [CrossRef] [PubMed]
29. Lobachevsky, P.; Leong, T.; Daly, P.; Smith, J.; Best, N.; Tomaszewski, J.; Thompson, E.R.; Li, N.; Campbell, I.G.; Martin, R.F.; et al. Compromized DNA repair as a basis for identification of cancer radiotherapy patients with extreme radiosensitivity. *Cancer Lett.* **2016**, *383*, 212–219. [CrossRef]
30. Buchbinder, D.; Smith, M.J.; Kawahara, M.; Cowan, M.J.; Buzby, J.S.; Abraham, R.S. Application of a radiosensitivity flow assay in a patient with DNA ligase 4 deficiency. *Blood Adv.* **2018**, *2*, 1828–1832. [CrossRef]
31. COPERNIC Project Investigators; Granzotto, A.; Benadjaoud, M.A.; Vogin, G.; Devic, C.; Ferlazzo, M.L.; Bodgi, L.; Pereira, S.; Sonzogni, L.; Forcheron, F.; et al. Influence of Nucleoshuttling of the ATM Protein in the Healthy Tissues Response to Radiation Therapy: Toward a Molecular Classification of Human Radiosensitivity. *Int. J. Radiat. Oncol. Biol. Phys.* **2016**, *94*, 450–460. [CrossRef]
32. Djuzenova, C.S.; Elsner, I.; Katzer, A.; Worschech, E.; Distel, L.V.; Flentje, M.; Polat, B. Radiosensitivity in breast cancer assessed by the histone gamma-H2AX and 53BP1 foci. *Radiat. Oncol.* **2013**, *8*, 98. [CrossRef]
33. Goutham, H.V.; Mumbrekar, K.D.; Vadhiraja, B.M.; Fernandes, D.J.; Sharan, K.; Kanive Parashiva, G.; Kapaettu, S.; Bola Sadashiva, S.R. DNA double-strand break analysis by gamma-H2AX foci: A useful method for determining the overreactors to radiation-induced acute reactions among head-and-neck cancer patients. *Int. J. Radiat. Oncol. Biol. Phys.* **2012**, *84*, e607–e612. [CrossRef]
34. Vandersickel, V.; Depuydt, J.; Van Bockstaele, B.; Perletti, G.; Philippe, J.; Thierens, H.; Vral, A. Early increase of radiation-induced gammaH2AX foci in a human Ku70/80 knockdown cell line characterized by an enhanced radiosensitivity. *J. Radiat. Res.* **2010**, *51*, 633–641. [CrossRef]
35. Martin, N.T.; Nakamura, K.; Paila, U.; Woo, J.; Brown, C.; Wright, J.A.; Teraoka, S.N.; Haghayegh, S.; McCurdy, D.; Schneider, M.; et al. Homozygous mutation of MTPAP causes cellular radiosensitivity and persistent DNA double-strand breaks. *Cell Death Dis.* **2014**, *5*, e1130. [CrossRef]
36. Martin, N.T.; Nahas, S.A.; Tunuguntla, R.; Fike, F.; Gatti, R.A. Assessing 'radiosensitivity' with kinetic profiles of gamma-H2AX, 53BP1 and BRCA1 foci. *Radiother. Oncol.* **2011**, *101*, 35–38. [CrossRef]
37. Minafra, L.; Bravatà, V.; Russo, G.; Forte, G.I.; Cammarata, F.P.; Ripamonti, M.; Candiano, G.; Cervello, M.; Giallongo, A.; Perconti, G.; et al. Gene Expression Profiling of MCF10A Breast Epithelial Cells Exposed to IOERT. *Anticancer Res.* **2015**, *35*, 3223–3234.
38. Miyake, T.; Shimada, M.; Matsumoto, Y.; Okino, A. DNA Damage Response After Ionizing Radiation Exposure in Skin Keratinocytes Derived from Human-Induced Pluripotent Stem Cells. *Int. J. Radiat. Oncol. Biol. Phys.* **2019**, *105*, 193–205. [CrossRef]
39. Nguyen, H.Q.; Belkacemi, Y.; Mann, C.; Hoffschir, F.; Kerbrat, S.; Surenaud, M.; Zadigue, P.; de La Taille, A.; Romeo, P.H.; Le Gouvello, S. Human CCR6+ Th17 Lymphocytes Are Highly Sensitive to Radiation-Induced Senescence and Are a Potential Target for Prevention of Radiation-Induced Toxicity. *Int. J. Radiat. Oncol. Biol. Phys.* **2020**, *108*, 314–325. [CrossRef] [PubMed]
40. Braicu, E.I.; Gasimli, K.; Richter, R.; Nassir, M.; Kümmel, S.; Blohmer, J.-U.; Yalcinkaya, I.; Chekerov, R.; Ignat, I.; Ionescu, A.; et al. Role of serum VEGFA, TIMP2, MMP2 and MMP9 in Monitoring Response to Adjuvant Radiochemotherapy in Patients with Primary Cervical Cancer—Results of a Companion Protocol of the Randomized NOGGO-AGO Phase III Clinical Trial. *Anticancer Res.* **2014**, *34*, 385–391.
41. Rodriguez-Gil, J.L.; Takita, C.; Wright, J.; Reis, I.M.; Zhao, W.; Lally, B.E.; Hu, J.J. Inflammatory biomarker C-reactive protein and radiotherapy-induced early adverse skin reactions in patients with breast cancer. *Cancer Epidemiol. Biomark. Prev.* **2014**, *23*, 1873–1883. [CrossRef]

42. Skiold, S.; Azimzadeh, O.; Merl-Pham, J.; Naslund, I.; Wersall, P.; Lidbrink, E.; Tapio, S.; Harms-Ringdahl, M.; Haghdoost, S. Unique proteomic signature for radiation sensitive patients; a comparative study between normo-sensitive and radiation sensitive breast cancer patients. *Mutat. Res.* **2015**, *776*, 128–135. [CrossRef]
43. Yu, B.B.; Lin, G.X.; Li, L.; Qu, S.; Liang, Z.G.; Chen, K.H.; Zhou, L.; Lu, Q.T.; Sun, Y.C.; Zhu, X.D. Cofilin-2 Acts as a Marker for Predicting Radiotherapy Response and Is a Potential Therapeutic Target in Nasopharyngeal Carcinoma. *Med. Sci. Monit.* **2018**, *24*, 2317–2329. [CrossRef] [PubMed]
44. Lacombe, J.; Brengues, M.; Mange, A.; Bourgier, C.; Gourgou, S.; Pelegrin, A.; Ozsahin, M.; Solassol, J.; Azria, D. Quantitative proteomic analysis reveals AK2 as potential biomarker for late normal tissue radiotoxicity. *Radiat. Oncol.* **2019**, *14*, 142. [CrossRef]
45. Cao, M.; Cabrera, R.; Xu, Y.; Liu, C.; Nelson, D. Different radiosensitivity of CD4(+)CD25(+) regulatory T cells and effector T cells to low dose gamma irradiation in vitro. *Int. J. Radiat. Biol.* **2011**, *87*, 71–80. [CrossRef]
46. Park, M.T.; Oh, E.T.; Song, M.J.; Lee, H.; Park, H.J. Radio-sensitivities and angiogenic signaling pathways of irradiated normal endothelial cells derived from diverse human organs. *J. Radiat. Res.* **2012**, *53*, 570–580. [CrossRef]
47. Fekete, N.; Erle, A.; Amann, E.M.; Furst, D.; Rojewski, M.T.; Langonne, A.; Sensebe, L.; Schrezenmeier, H.; Schmidtke-Schrezenmeier, G. Effect of high-dose irradiation on human bone-marrow-derived mesenchymal stromal cells. *Tissue Eng. Part C Methods* **2015**, *21*, 112–122. [CrossRef]
48. Nishad, S.; Ghosh, A. Dynamic changes in the proteome of human peripheral blood mononuclear cells with low dose ionizing radiation. *Mutat. Res. Genet. Toxicol. Environ. Mutagen.* **2016**, *797*, 9–20. [CrossRef]
49. Shimura, T.; Hamada, N.; Sasatani, M.; Kamiya, K.; Kunugita, N. Nuclear accumulation of cyclin D1 following long-term fractionated exposures to low-dose ionizing radiation in normal human diploid cells. *Cell Cycle* **2014**, *13*, 1248–1255. [CrossRef]
50. Yim, J.H.; Yun, J.M.; Kim, J.Y.; Lee, I.K.; Nam, S.Y.; Kim, C.S. Phosphoprotein profiles of candidate markers for early cellular responses to low-dose gamma-radiation in normal human fibroblast cells. *J. Radiat. Res.* **2017**, *58*, 329–340. [CrossRef] [PubMed]
51. Moertl, S.; Buschmann, D.; Azimzadeh, O.; Schneider, M.; Kell, R.; Winkler, K.; Tapio, S.; Hornhardt, S.; Merl-Pham, J.; Pfaffl, M.W.; et al. Radiation Exposure of Peripheral Mononuclear Blood Cells Alters the Composition and Function of Secreted Extracellular Vesicles. *Int. J. Mol. Sci.* **2020**, *21*, 2336. [CrossRef]
52. Rogakou, E.P.; Pilch, D.R.; Orr, A.H.; Ivanova, V.S.; Bonner, W.M. DNA double-stranded breaks induce histone H2AX phosphorylation on serine 139. *J. Biol. Chem.* **1998**, *273*, 5858–5868. [CrossRef]
53. Rogakou, E.P.; Boon, C.; Redon, C.; Bonner, W.M. Megabase chromatin domains involved in DNA double-strand breaks in vivo. *J. Cell Biol.* **1999**, *146*, 905–916. [CrossRef]
54. Paull, T.T.; Rogakou, E.P.; Yamazaki, V.; Kirchgessner, C.U.; Gellert, M.; Bonner, W.M. A critical role for histone H2AX in recruitment of repair factors to nuclear foci after DNA damage. *Curr. Biol.* **2000**, *10*, 886–895. [CrossRef]
55. Burma, S.; Chen, D.J. Role of DNA-PK in the cellular response to DNA double-strand breaks. *DNA Repair* **2004**, *3*, 909–918. [CrossRef]
56. Lobrich, M.; Shibata, A.; Beucher, A.; Fisher, A.; Ensminger, M.; Goodarzi, A.A.; Barton, O.; Jeggo, P.A. gammaH2AX foci analysis for monitoring DNA double-strand break repair: Strengths, limitations and optimization. *Cell Cycle* **2010**, *9*, 662–669. [CrossRef]
57. Panier, S.; Boulton, S.J. Double-strand break repair: 53BP1 comes into focus. *Nat. Rev. Mol. Cell. Biol.* **2014**, *15*, 7–18. [CrossRef]
58. Bourton, E.C.; Plowman, P.N.; Zahir, S.A.; Senguloglu, G.U.; Serrai, H.; Bottley, G.; Parris, C.N. Multispectral imaging flow cytometry reveals distinct frequencies of gamma-H2AX foci induction in DNA double strand break repair defective human cell lines. *Cytom. A* **2012**, *81*, 130–137. [CrossRef] [PubMed]
59. Kuhne, M.; Riballo, E.; Rief, N.; Rothkamm, K.; Jeggo, P.A.; Lobrich, M. A double-strand break repair defect in ATM-deficient cells contributes to radiosensitivity. *Cancer Res.* **2004**, *64*, 500–508. [CrossRef]
60. Valdiglesias, V.; Giunta, S.; Fenech, M.; Neri, M.; Bonassi, S. gammaH2AX as a marker of DNA double strand breaks and genomic instability in human population studies. *Mutat. Res.* **2013**, *753*, 24–40. [CrossRef]
61. Vandevoorde, C.; Gomolka, M.; Roessler, U.; Samaga, D.; Lindholm, C.; Fernet, M.; Hall, J.; Pernot, E.; El-Saghire, H.; Baatout, S.; et al. EPI-CT: In vitro assessment of the applicability of the gamma-H2AX-foci assay as cellular biomarker for exposure in a multicentre study of children in diagnostic radiology. *Int. J. Radiat. Biol.* **2015**, *91*, 653–663. [CrossRef]
62. National Toxicology Program. *Handbook for Conducting a Literature-Based Health Assessment Using OHAT Approach for Systematic Review and Evidence Integration*; U.S. Department of Health and Human Services; National Toxicology Program: Washington, DC, USA, 2019.
63. Murphy, J.F.; Fitzgerald, D.J. Vascular endothelial growth factor induces cyclooxygenase-dependent proliferation of endothelial cells via the VEGF-2 receptor. *FASEB J.* **2001**, *15*, 1667–1669. [CrossRef]
64. Dixelius, J.; Olsson, A.K.; Thulin, A.; Lee, C.; Johansson, I.; Claesson-Welsh, L. Minimal active domain and mechanism of action of the angiogenesis inhibitor histidine-rich glycoprotein. *Cancer Res.* **2006**, *66*, 2089–2097. [CrossRef]
65. Yu, L.; Chen, Y.; Tooze, S.A. Autophagy pathway: Cellular and molecular mechanisms. *Autophagy* **2018**, *14*, 207–215. [CrossRef]
66. Shintani, T.; Klionsky, D.J. Autophagy in health and disease: A double-edged sword. *Science* **2004**, *306*, 990–995. [CrossRef]
67. Mizushima, N.; Levine, B.; Cuervo, A.M.; Klionsky, D.J. Autophagy fights disease through cellular self-digestion. *Nature* **2008**, *451*, 1069–1075. [CrossRef]
68. Yuan, X.; Du, J.; Hua, S.; Zhang, H.; Gu, C.; Wang, J.; Yang, L.; Huang, J.; Yu, J.; Liu, F. Suppression of autophagy augments the radiosensitizing effects of STAT3 inhibition on human glioma cells. *Exp. Cell Res.* **2015**, *330*, 267–276. [CrossRef] [PubMed]

69. Chang, L.; Graham, P.H.; Hao, J.; Ni, J.; Bucci, J.; Cozzi, P.J.; Kearsley, J.H.; Li, Y. PI3K/Akt/mTOR pathway inhibitors enhance radiosensitivity in radioresistant prostate cancer cells through inducing apoptosis, reducing autophagy, suppressing NHEJ and HR repair pathways. *Cell Death Dis.* **2014**, *5*, e1437. [CrossRef]
70. Zois, C.E.; Koukourakis, M.I. Radiation-induced autophagy in normal and cancer cells: Towards novel cytoprotection and radio-sensitization policies? *Autophagy* **2009**, *5*, 442–450. [CrossRef]
71. Ferrara, N.; Gerber, H.P.; LeCouter, J. The biology of VEGF and its receptors. *Nat. Med.* **2003**, *9*, 669–676. [CrossRef]
72. Fu, Z.Z.; Sun, X.D.; Li, P.; Zhang, Z.; Li, G.Z.; Gu, T.; Shao, S.S. Relationship between serum VEGF level and radiosensitivity of patients with nonsmall cell lung cancer among asians: A meta-analysis. *DNA Cell Biol.* **2014**, *33*, 426–437. [CrossRef] [PubMed]
73. Hu, X.; Xing, L.; Wei, X.; Liu, X.; Pang, R.; Qi, L.; Song, S. Nonangiogenic function of VEGF and enhanced radiosensitivity of HeLa cells by inhibition of VEGF expression. *Oncol. Res.* **2012**, *20*, 93–101. [CrossRef] [PubMed]
74. Nicholson, D.W.; Ali, A.; Thornberry, N.A.; Vaillancourt, J.P.; Ding, C.K.; Gallant, M.; Gareau, Y.; Griffin, P.R.; Labelle, M.; Lazebnik, Y.A.; et al. Identification and inhibition of the ICE/CED-3 protease necessary for mammalian apoptosis. *Nature* **1995**, *376*, 37–43. [CrossRef]
75. Santos, N.; Silva, R.F.; Pinto, M.; Silva, E.B.D.; Tasat, D.R.; Amaral, A. Active caspase-3 expression levels as bioindicator of individual radiosensitivity. *Acad. Bras. Cienc.* **2017**, *89*, 649–659. [CrossRef] [PubMed]
76. Yang, X.H.; Edgerton, S.; Thor, A.D. Reconstitution of caspase-3 sensitizes MCF-7 breast cancer cells to radiation therapy. *Int. J. Oncol.* **2005**, *26*, 1675–1680. [CrossRef] [PubMed]
77. Okamoto, A.; Demetrick, D.J.; Spillare, E.A.; Hagiwara, K.; Hussain, S.P.; Bennett, W.P.; Forrester, K.; Gerwin, B.; Serrano, M.; Beach, D.H.; et al. Mutations and altered expression of p16INK4 in human cancer. *Proc. Natl. Acad. Sci. USA* **1994**, *91*, 11045–11049. [CrossRef]
78. Bockstaele, L.; Kooken, H.; Libert, F.; Paternot, S.; Dumont, J.E.; de Launoit, Y.; Roger, P.P.; Coulonval, K. Regulated activating Thr172 phosphorylation of cyclin-dependent kinase 4(CDK4): Its relationship with cyclins and CDK "inhibitors". *Mol. Cell Biol.* **2006**, *26*, 5070–5085. [CrossRef]
79. Narita, M.; Narita, M.; Krizhanovsky, V.; Nunez, S.; Chicas, A.; Hearn, S.A.; Myers, M.P.; Lowe, S.W. A novel role for high-mobility group a proteins in cellular senescence and heterochromatin formation. *Cell* **2006**, *126*, 503–514. [CrossRef] [PubMed]
80. Matsumura, Y.; Yamagishi, N.; Miyakoshi, J.; Imamura, S.; Takebe, H. Increase in radiation sensitivity of human malignant melanoma cells by expression of wild-type p16 gene. *Cancer Lett.* **1997**, *115*, 91–96. [CrossRef]
81. Lee, A.W.; Li, J.H.; Shi, W.; Li, A.; Ng, E.; Liu, T.J.; Klamut, H.J.; Liu, F.F. p16 gene therapy: A potentially efficacious modality for nasopharyngeal carcinoma. *Mol. Cancer* **2003**, *2*, 961–969.
82. Dok, R.; Kalev, P.; Van Limbergen, E.J.; Asbagh, L.A.; Vazquez, I.; Hauben, E.; Sablina, A.; Nuyts, S. p16INK4a impairs homologous recombination-mediated DNA repair in human papillomavirus-positive head and neck tumors. *Cancer Res.* **2014**, *74*, 1739–1751. [CrossRef] [PubMed]
83. Kang, S.; Tanaka, T.; Narazaki, M.; Kishimoto, T. Targeting Interleukin-6 Signaling in Clinic. *Immunity* **2019**, *50*, 1007–1023. [CrossRef]
84. Chen, M.F.; Hsieh, C.C.; Chen, W.C.; Lai, C.H. Role of interleukin-6 in the radiation response of liver tumors. *Int. J. Radiat. Oncol. Biol. Phys.* **2012**, *84*, e621–e630. [CrossRef]
85. Twillie, D.A.; Eisenberger, M.A.; Carducci, M.A.; Hseih, W.-S.; Kim, W.Y.; Simons, J.W. Interleukin-6: A candidate mediator of human prostate cancer morbidity. *Urology* **1995**, *45*, 542–549. [CrossRef]
86. Shariat, S.F.; Andrews, B.; Kattan, M.W.; Kim, J.; Wheeler, T.M.; Slawin, K.M. Plasma levels of interleukin-6 and its soluble receptor are associated with prostate cancer progression and metastasis. *Urology* **2001**, *58*, 1008–1015. [CrossRef]
87. George, D.J.; Halabi, S.; Shepard, T.F.; Sanford, B.; Vogelzang, N.J.; Small, E.J.; Kantoff, P.W. The prognostic significance of plasma interleukin-6 levels in patients with metastatic hormone-refractory prostate cancer: Results from cancer and leukemia group B 9480. *Clin. Cancer Res.* **2005**, *11*, 1815–1820. [CrossRef] [PubMed]
88. Choi, Y.S.; Kim, S.; Oh, Y.S.; Cho, S.; Hoon Kim, S. Elevated serum interleukin-32 levels in patients with endometriosis: A cross-sectional study. *Am. J. Reprod. Immunol.* **2019**, *82*, e13149. [CrossRef]
89. Berek, J.S.; Chung, C.; Kaldi, K.; Watson, J.M.; Knox, R.M.; Martínez-Maza, O. Serum interleukin-6 levels correlate with disease status in patients with epithelial ovarian cancer. *Am. J. Obstet. Gynecol.* **1991**, *164*, 1038–1043. [CrossRef]
90. Scambia, G.; Testa, U.; Benedetti Panici, P.; Foti, E.; Martucci, R.; Gadducci, A.; Perillo, A.; Facchini, V.; Peschle, C.; Mancuso, S. Prognostic significance of interleukin 6 serum levels in patients with ovarian cancer. *Br. J. Cancer* **1995**, *71*, 354–356. [CrossRef] [PubMed]
91. Tominaga, K.; Yoshimoto, T.; Torigoe, K.; Kurimoto, M.; Matsui, K.; Hada, T.; Okamura, H.; Nakanishi, K. IL-12 synergizes with IL-18 or IL-1beta for IFN-gamma production from human T cells. *Int. Immunol.* **2000**, *12*, 151–160. [CrossRef] [PubMed]
92. Nakahara, H.; Song, J.; Sugimoto, M.; Hagihara, K.; Kishimoto, T.; Yoshizaki, K.; Nishimoto, N. Anti-interleukin-6 receptor antibody therapy reduces vascular endothelial growth factor production in rheumatoid arthritis. *Arthritis Rheum.* **2003**, *48*, 1521–1529. [CrossRef]
93. Chen, M.F.; Lu, M.S.; Chen, P.T.; Chen, W.C.; Lin, P.Y.; Lee, K.D. Role of interleukin 1 beta in esophageal squamous cell carcinoma. *J. Mol. Med.* **2012**, *90*, 89–100. [CrossRef] [PubMed]

94. Szklarczyk, D.; Franceschini, A.; Wyder, S.; Forslund, K.; Heller, D.; Huerta-Cepas, J.; Simonovic, M.; Roth, A.; Santos, A.; Tsafou, K.P.; et al. STRING v10: Protein-protein interaction networks, integrated over the tree of life. *Nucleic Acids Res.* **2015**, *43*, D447–D452. [CrossRef] [PubMed]
95. Szklarczyk, D.; Gable, A.L.; Lyon, D.; Junge, A.; Wyder, S.; Huerta-Cepas, J.; Simonovic, M.; Doncheva, N.T.; Morris, J.H.; Bork, P.; et al. STRING v11: Protein-protein association networks with increased coverage, supporting functional discovery in genome-wide experimental datasets. *Nucleic Acids Res.* **2019**, *47*, D607–D613. [CrossRef]
96. Wilhelm, M.; Schlegl, J.; Hahne, H.; Gholami, A.M.; Lieberenz, M.; Savitski, M.M.; Ziegler, E.; Butzmann, L.; Gessulat, S.; Marx, H.; et al. Mass-spectrometry-based draft of the human proteome. *Nature* **2014**, *509*, 582–587. [CrossRef]
97. Gatti, R.A.; Boder, E.; Good, R.A. Immunodeficiency, radiosensitivity, and the XCIND syndrome. *Immunol. Res.* **2007**, *38*, 87–101. [CrossRef]
98. Nahas, S.A.; Gatti, R.A. DNA double strand break repair defects, primary immunodeficiency disorders, and 'radiosensitivity'. *Curr. Opin. Allergy Clin. Immunol.* **2009**, *9*, 510–516. [CrossRef]
99. O'Driscoll, M.; Gennery, A.R.; Seidel, J.; Concannon, P.; Jeggo, P.A. An overview of three new disorders associated with genetic instability: LIG4 syndrome, RS-SCID and ATR-Seckel syndrome. *DNA Repair* **2004**, *3*, 1227–1235. [CrossRef]
100. Royal, H.D. Effects of low level radiation-what's new? *Semin. Nucl. Med.* **2008**, *38*, 392–402. [CrossRef] [PubMed]
101. Preston, R.J. Children as a sensitive subpopulation for the risk assessment process. *Toxicol. Appl. Pharm.* **2004**, *199*, 132–141. [CrossRef] [PubMed]
102. Kleinerman, R.A. Cancer risks following diagnostic and therapeutic radiation exposure in children. *Pediatr. Radiol.* **2006**, *36* (Suppl. 2), 121–125. [CrossRef] [PubMed]
103. Pearce, M.S.; Salotti, J.A.; Little, M.P.; McHugh, K.; Lee, C.; Kim, K.P.; Howe, N.L.; Ronckers, C.M.; Rajaraman, P.; Craft, A.W.; et al. Radiation exposure from CT scans in childhood and subsequent risk of leukaemia and brain tumours: A retrospective cohort study. *Lancet* **2012**, *380*, 499–505. [CrossRef]
104. Mathews, J.D.; Forsythe, A.V.; Brady, Z.; Butler, M.W.; Goergen, S.K.; Byrnes, G.B.; Giles, G.G.; Wallace, A.B.; Anderson, P.R.; Guiver, T.A.; et al. Cancer risk in 680,000 people exposed to computed tomography scans in childhood or adolescence: Data linkage study of 11 million Australians. *BMJ* **2013**, *346*, f2360. [CrossRef]
105. Brenner, D.J.; Doll, R.; Goodhead, D.T.; Hall, E.J.; Land, C.E.; Little, J.B.; Lubin, J.H.; Preston, D.L.; Preston, R.J.; Puskin, J.S.; et al. Cancer risks attributable to low doses of ionizing radiation: Assessing what we really know. *Proc. Natl. Acad. Sci. USA* **2003**, *100*, 13761–13766. [CrossRef]
106. Narendran, N.; Luzhna, L.; Kovalchuk, O. Sex Difference of Radiation Response in Occupational and Accidental Exposure. *Front. Genet.* **2019**, *10*, 260. [CrossRef] [PubMed]
107. Grant, E.J.; Brenner, A.; Sugiyama, H.; Sakata, R.; Sadakane, A.; Utada, M.; Cahoon, E.K.; Milder, C.M.; Soda, M.; Cullings, H.M.; et al. Solid Cancer Incidence among the Life Span Study of Atomic Bomb Survivors: 1958–2009. *Radiat. Res.* **2017**, *187*, 513–537. [CrossRef]
108. Wakeford, R. Radiation effects: Modulating factors and risk assessment—An overview. *Ann. ICRP* **2012**, *41*, 98–107. [CrossRef] [PubMed]
109. Preston, D.L.; Ron, E.; Tokuoka, S.; Funamoto, S.; Nishi, N.; Soda, M.; Mabuchi, K.; Kodama, K. Solid cancer incidence in atomic bomb survivors: 1958–1998. *Radiat. Res.* **2007**, *168*, 1–64. [CrossRef]
110. Dreicer, M. Chernobyl: Consequences of the Catastrophe for People and the Environment. *Environ. Health Perspect.* **2010**, *118*, A500.
111. Schmitz-Feuerhake, I.; Busby, C.; Pflugbeil, S. Genetic radiation risks: A neglected topic in the low dose debate. *Environ. Health Toxicol.* **2016**, *31*, e2016001. [CrossRef] [PubMed]
112. Bentzen, S.M.; Overgaard, J. Patient-to-Patient Variability in the Expression of Radiation-Induced Normal Tissue Injury. *Semin. Radiat. Oncol.* **1994**, *4*, 68–80. [CrossRef]
113. Fekrmandi, F.; Panzarella, T.; Dinniwell, R.E.; Helou, J.; Levin, W. Predictive factors for persistent and late radiation complications in breast cancer survivors. *Clin. Transl. Oncol.* **2020**, *22*, 360–369. [CrossRef] [PubMed]
114. Barnett, G.C.; West, C.M.; Dunning, A.M.; Elliott, R.M.; Coles, C.E.; Pharoah, P.D.; Burnet, N.G. Normal tissue reactions to radiotherapy: Towards tailoring treatment dose by genotype. *Nat. Rev. Cancer* **2009**, *9*, 134–142. [CrossRef] [PubMed]
115. Marsh, J.W.; Harrison, J.D.; Laurier, D.; Birchall, A.; Blanchardon, E.; Paquet, F.; Tirmarche, M. Doses and lung cancer risks from exposure to radon and plutonium. *Int. J. Radiat. Biol.* **2014**, *90*, 1080–1087. [CrossRef]
116. Cardis, E.; Kesminiene, A.; Ivanov, V.; Malakhova, I.; Shibata, Y.; Khrouch, V.; Drozdovitch, V.; Maceika, E.; Zvonova, I.; Vlassov, O.; et al. Risk of thyroid cancer after exposure to 131I in childhood. *J. Natl. Cancer Inst.* **2005**, *97*, 724–732. [CrossRef]
117. Belli, M.; Ottolenghi, A.; Weiss, W. The European strategy on low dose risk research and the role of radiation quality according to the recommendations of the "ad hoc" High Level and Expert Group (HLEG). *Radiat. Environ. Biophys.* **2010**, *49*, 463–468. [CrossRef] [PubMed]
118. Kreuzer, M.; Auvinen, A.; Cardis, E.; Durante, M.; Harms-Ringdahl, M.; Jourdain, J.R.; Madas, B.G.; Ottolenghi, A.; Pazzaglia, S.; Prise, K.M.; et al. Multidisciplinary European Low Dose Initiative (MELODI): Strategic research agenda for low dose radiation risk research. *Radiat. Environ. Biophys.* **2018**, *57*, 5–15. [CrossRef] [PubMed]
119. Kreuzer, M.; Sobotzki, C.; Schnelzer, M.; Fenske, N. Factors Modifying the Radon-Related Lung Cancer Risk at Low Exposures and Exposure Rates among German Uranium Miners. *Radiat. Res.* **2018**, *189*, 165–176. [CrossRef] [PubMed]

120. Bassi, C.; Xavier, D.; Palomino, G.; Nicolucci, P.; Soares, C.; Sakamoto-Hojo, E.; Donadi, E. Efficiency of the DNA repair and polymorphisms of the XRCC1, XRCC3 and XRCC4 DNA repair genes in systemic lupus erythematosus. *Lupus* **2008**, *17*, 988–995. [CrossRef] [PubMed]
121. Bashir, S.; Harris, G.; Denman, M.A.; Blake, D.R.; Winyard, P.G. Oxidative DNA damage and cellular sensitivity to oxidative stress in human autoimmune diseases. *Ann. Rheum Dis.* **1993**, *52*, 659–666. [CrossRef]
122. Health Protection Agency. Human Radiosensitivity. Report of the Independent Advisory Group on Ionising Radiation. Available online: https://assets.publishing.service.gov.uk/government/uploads/system/uploads/attachment_data/file/333058/RCE-21_v2_for_website.pdf (accessed on 17 December 2020).
123. Genetic susceptibility to cancer. International Commission on Radiological Protection (ICRP) publication 79. Approved by the Commission in May 1997. International Commission on Radiological Protection. *Ann. ICRP* **1998**, *28*, 1–157.
124. Seibold, P.; Auvinen, A.; Averbeck, D.; Bourguignon, M.; Hartikainen, J.M.; Hoeschen, C.; Laurent, O.; Noël, G.; Sabatier, L.; Salomaa, S.; et al. Clinical and epidemiological observations on individual radiation sensitivity and susceptibility. *Int. J. Radiat. Biol.* **2019**, *96*, 324–339. [CrossRef]

Journal of
Personalized
Medicine

MDPI

Review

Markers Useful in Monitoring Radiation-Induced Lung Injury in Lung Cancer Patients: A Review

Mariola Śliwińska-Mossoń [1], Katarzyna Wadowska [1,*], Łukasz Trembecki [2,3] and Iwona Bil-Lula [1]

[1] Department of Medical Laboratory Diagnostics, Division of Clinical Chemistry and Laboratory Haematology, Wroclaw Medical University, ul. Borowska 211A, 50-556 Wroclaw, Poland; mariola.sliwinska-mosson@umed.wroc.pl (M.Ś.-M.); iwona.bil-lula@umed.wroc.pl (I.B.-L.)

[2] Department of Radiation Oncology, Lower Silesian Oncology Center, pl. Hirszfelda 12, 53-413 Wroclaw, Poland; lukasz.trembecki@umed.wroc.pl

[3] Department of Oncology, Faculty of Medicine, Wroclaw Medical University, pl. Hirszfelda 12, 53-413 Wroclaw, Poland

* Correspondence: katarzyna.wadowska@student.umed.wroc.pl

Received: 9 June 2020; Accepted: 22 July 2020; Published: 26 July 2020

check for updates

Abstract: In 2018, lung cancer was the most common cancer and the most common cause of cancer death, accounting for a 1.76 million deaths. Radiotherapy (RT) is a widely used and effective non-surgical cancer treatment that induces remission in, and even cures, patients with lung cancer. However, RT faces some restrictions linked to the radioresistance and treatment toxicity, manifesting in radiation-induced lung injury (RILI). About 30–40% of lung cancer patients will develop RILI, which next to the local recurrence and distant metastasis is a substantial challenge to the successful management of lung cancer treatment. These data indicate an urgent need of looking for novel, precise biomarkers of individual response and risk of side effects in the course of RT. The aim of this review was to summarize both preclinical and clinical approaches in RILI monitoring that could be brought into clinical practice. Next to transforming growth factor-β1 (TGFβ1) that was reported as one of the most important growth factors expressed in the tissues after ionizing radiation (IR), there is a group of novel, potential biomarkers—microRNAs—that may be used as predictive biomarkers in therapy response and disease prognosis.

Keywords: lung cancer; radiotherapy; radiotherapy monitoring; radiation-induced lung injury; RILI; pneumonitis; radiation-induced lung fibrosis; RILF; circulating biomarkers; microRNA

---

1. Introduction

According to the WHO (2018), cancer is a leading cause of death worldwide, accounting for an estimated 9.6 million deaths. Lung cancer, which was rare before 1900 with fewer than 400 cases described in the medical literature, now is the most common cancer, accounting for an 2.09 million cases in 2018, and the most common cause of cancer death (1.76 million deaths) [1–3]. Lung cancer is regarded as any tumor of the respiratory epithelium or pneumocytes, whose main risk factors are exposure to environmental carcinogens, irradiation, and genetic disorders [4,5]. Clinical classification distinguishes two main groups of lung cancer, small cell lung carcinoma (SCLC, 15% of all lung cancers) and non-small cell lung carcinoma (NSCLC, 85% of all lung cancers), which are additionally subcategorized into adenocarcinoma, squamous cell carcinoma (SCC), and large cell carcinoma [6–8]. The distinction between adenocarcinoma and SCC is crucial for therapeutic decision making. The most significant dividing line is between patients who are candidates for surgical lung cancer resection and inoperable patients who will benefit from chemotherapy, radiotherapy (RT) or both [3]. The management of therapeutic strategies depends on lung cancer stage at the time of its diagnosis and is listed in Table 1.

RT has a potential role in all stages of NSCLC, and it can be used either as definitive or palliative therapy. RT should be provided for all patients with stage III NSCLC and in patients with stage IV disease who may benefit from local therapy. Uses of RT for NSCLC include (1) definitive therapy for locally advanced NSCLC, generally combined with chemotherapy; (2) definitive therapy in patients with early-stage disease, who are medically inoperable, who refuse surgery, or who are high-risk surgical candidates; (3) preoperative or postoperative therapy for selected patients treated with surgery; (4) therapy for limited recurrences and metastases; and (5) palliative therapy for patients with incurable NSCLC [9–13]. The main restrictions of RT are tumor hypoxia, repopulation, DNA damage repair, and molecular mechanisms linked to RT resistance and treatment toxicity, manifesting in radiation-induced lung injury (RILI). RILI, next to the local recurrence and distant metastasis are substantial challenges to the successful management of lung cancer [2,13–16].

Contrary to the increase in number of lung cancer cases over the last few decades, the 5-year overall survival (OS) of lung cancer patients has not changed appreciably. Despite recent advances in understanding the molecular biology of lung cancer and the introduction of new therapeutic agents in the treatment, the 5-year OS rate is less than 16% [12,13,17]. These data indicate an urgent need for the development of novel, more personalized therapeutic approaches and more precise markers (molecular biomarkers for radiosensitivity, immune host markers, fuller imaging analysis like radiomics) of individual response and risk of side effects. Improvement of the RT's efficacy requires maximization of tumor control and minimization of RT treatment toxicity [9,11,14].

Table 1. Therapeutic strategies in non-small cell lung carcinoma (NSCLC) based upon the stages of lung cancer adapted from the 8th Edition of TNM [3,18].

Eight Edition TNM Staging System				Treatment Options
Stage IA1	T1a	N0	M0	surgery alone
Stage IA2	T1b	N0	M0	
Stage IA3	T1c	N0	M0	
Stage IB	T2a	N0	M0	<4 cm surgery alone >4 cm surgery followed by adjuvant chemotherapy
Stage IIA	T2b	N0	M0	Surgery followed by adjuvant chemotherapy There is no role of postoperative radiation therapy in patients following resection of stage I or II NSCLC with negative margins
Stage IIB	T1a-T2b	N1	M0	Patients with stage I and II disease who refuse or are not suitable candidates for surgery should be considered for radiation therapy with curative intent
	T3	N0	M0	
Stage IIIA	T1-2b	N2	M0	N0 or N1 nodes—Surgery followed by adjuvant chemotherapy N2 or N3 nodes—No surgery, treatment with combined chemoradiation therapy
	T3	N1	M0	
	T4	N0/N1	M0	
Stage IIIB	T1-2b	N3	M0	The optimal treatment strategy has not been clearly defined; despite many potential treatment options, none yields a very high probability of cure; stage III is highly heterogeneous, and no single treatment approach can be recommended for all patients
	T3/T4	N0/N1	M0	
	T3/T4	N3	M0	
Stage IVA	Any T	Any N	M1a/M1b	Use of pain medications and the appropriate use of radiotherapy and systemic therapy, which may compromise of traditional cytotoxic chemotherapy, targeted therapy, and immunotherapy depending on the specific diagnosis and molecular subtype
Stage IVB	Any T	Any N	M1c	

TNM—TNM Classification of Malignant Tumors (tumor-lymph nodes-metastasis); T1—≤3 cm surrounded by lung/visceral pleura, not involving main bronchus; T1a—primary tumor ≤ 1 cm; T1b—>1 to ≤2 cm; T1c—>2 to ≤3 cm; T2—>3 to ≤5 cm or involvement of main bronchus without carina, regardless of distance from carina or invasion visceral pleural or atelectasis or post-obstructive pneumonitis extending to hilum; T2a—>3 to ≤4 cm; T2b—>4 to ≤5 cm; T3—>5 to ≤7 cm in greatest dimension or tumor of any size that involves chest wall, pericardium, phrenic nerve or satellite nodules in the same lobe; T4—>7 cm in greatest dimension or any tumor with invasion of mediastinum, diaphragm, heart, great vessels, recurrent laryngeal nerve, carina, trachea, esophagus, spine or separate tumor in different lobe of ipsilateral lung; N0—no lymph nodes metastasis; N1—ipsilateral peribronchial and/or hilar nodes and intrapulmonary nodes; N2—ipsilateral mediastinal and/or subcarinal nodes; N3—contralateral mediastinal or hilar; ipsilateral/contralateral scalene/supraclavicular; M0—no distant metastasis; M1—distant metastasis; M1a—tumor in contralateral lung or pleural/pericardial nodule/malignant effusion; M1b—single extrathoracic metastasis, including single non-regional lymph node; M1c—multiple extrathoracic metastases in one or more organs.

Regardless of a vast number of cytokines, growth factors and circulating markers representing potential culprit biological processes that are involved in radiotherapy response, there are no blood-based biomarkers in clinical practice that would enable assessment of their relationship with radiotherapy response and toxicity. Current data in preclinical practice report a possible application of microRNA as radiosensitizing biomarkers in RT response and prognosis [13,19].

In this study, we provide an overview of possible markers useful in monitoring RILI in lung cancer patients, starting with circulating cytokines pro- and anti-inflammatory and ending with the molecular approaches in the diagnostics.

2. Radiation-Induced Lung Injury

Generally, RT is a low-toxic treatment; however, the lung is a radiosensitive organ and tends to be easily damaged by radiation beams. Depending on the assessment methods, it is estimated that about 5% to nearly 40% of lung cancer patients will develop RILI [2,15,20]. Some of the direct and indirect radiation-induced pulmonary effects may begin within nanoseconds after radiation exposure through induction of free radicals, leading to synthetization and secretion of growth factor between a few hours and days following irradiation. The tissue undergoes progressive and dysregulated processes, i.e., inflammation-induced depletion of alveolar surface cells, infiltration of inflammatory cells into the interstitial space, exudative response, and fibrotic changes [2,21–23]. Radiation-induced lung disease (RILD) following radiotherapy is separated into two phases—an acute phase (lung infections and inflammations, pneumonitis) during the first 6-months and a permanent phase (pulmonary fibrosis) >6-months post-RT, but in spite of that, RILD is a dynamic process, and it is still unclear how the acute and chronic phases relate to each other [24]. The acute phase is characterized by infiltration and accumulation of inflammatory immune cells in the lung alveoli from the vascular side, loss of type I pneumocytes, and increased capillary permeability, resulting in an interstitial and alveolar edema [15,16,25]. The late phase of RILI is characterized by endothelial damage, fibrin proliferation, and disproportionate extracellular matrix development, leading to impaired gas exchange [26,27].

Radiation-induced pneumonitis (RP) is considered to be the most serious dose-limiting complication of RT. The severity of RP depends on multiple factors, including treatment factors (dosimetric parameters—total radiation dose, number of fractions, volume of irradiated parenchyma), physiologic factors (age, gender), and genetic factors (genetic variants that confer radiosensitivity) [2,15,25,28]. Typical symptoms of RILI include dry cough, dyspnea, low-grade fever, shortness of breath, chest pain and discomfort, the radiologic findings on chest X-ray and computed tomography (CT) scan are typical symptoms of RILI [29]. Clinical research showed that interleukin (Il)-1, Il-6, tumor necrosis factor (TNF)-α, transforming growth factor (TGF)-β and platelet-derived growth factor (PDGF) are associated with the occurrence of radiation pneumonitis [30].

Radiation-induced lung fibrosis (RILF), i.e., the late phase of RILI, is characterized by a tissue repair response triggered by chronic inflammation that is a culprit of excessive free radical production and chronic changes in immunological mediators. Long term upregulation of TGFβ, Il-1, or TNFα and continuous free radical production are leading to the formation of morphological changes in the structure of inter/intracellular spaces. These changes are characterized by fibroblast replication with excessive extracellular matrix deposition and are resulting in reduced lung compliance and increased work of breathing [31]. The clinical symptoms include progressive dyspnea, deterioration of pulmonary function, and interstitial fluid accumulation, leading to the respiratory failure and even a death. Pulmonary fibrosis may be divided into three specific phases. The first phase usually occurs in a few days to 3–4 weeks, sometimes up to 2–3 months after the RT, and it is characterized by pneumocytes type II damage, with the release of significant amounts of surfactant. Usually, the first phase is not detected in histopathological or radiological examination. The next phase, i.e., exudative phase, occurs between 3 to 6 months after RT. Histopathological analysis of the lung alveoli reveals the leukocyte–macrophage reactions and thickening of the intercellular space due to the fibrin fibers deposition. Characteristic physical symptoms of this phase are cough, shortness of breath, chest pains, a mild fever, and tachycardia. The third phase, acute pulmonary fibrosis, occurs a few months after radiotherapy. Lung fibrosis is characterized by the increasing inflammation, fibroblasts migration, and collagen deposition in pulmonary tissue. These changes reduce lung capacity and lead to a significant impairment of gas exchange [32–34].

Post-radiation side effects are correlated with chronic inflammatory diseases and are characterized by common, epigenetic pathogenesis basis. Histone acetylation regulates activation and inhibition of inflammatory genes known to play crucial roles in chronic inflammatory diseases [31]. The BET (bromodomain and extraterminal domain) family proteins are epigenetic reader proteins that recognize acetylated chromatin (the histone acetylation code of epigenetic modifications). These proteins are involved in the regulation of inflammatory cytokine genes expression in macrophages and take a part in cancer development [31,35]. Modulation of the BET proteins genes expression may drive the inhibition of proinflammatory responses, so BET proteins inhibition via JQ1 targeting is a novel therapeutic strategy in fibrosis treatment. In patients treated with combination of RT and JQ1, significant attenuation of the interstitial septal thickening, inflammatory infiltration, and fibrotic nodules in the alveolar structures and pulmonary parenchyma were observed. Moreover, decreased expression of collagen I and TGFβ indicates a radioprotective role of JQ1 [31].

Tissue injury induces inflammatory and repair responses that involve myriad interactions in epithelial-mesenchymal communication. Epithelial and inflammatory cells release profibrotic mediators such as TGFβ, PDGF, Il-1β and TNFα [7]. Ionizing radiation (IR) leads to massive free radical production and DNA damage that triggers cell death through apoptosis or necrosis. In case of cell death, pro- and anti-inflammatory cytokines and chemokines are secreted, and their overproduction generates reactive oxygen species (ROS) and nitric oxygen (NO). Chronic oxidative damage stimulates collagen production, leading to the tissue stiffness observed in RILF [16]. Cytokines such as Il-1, Il-4, Il-6, Il-8, Il-13, Il-33, TNFα, or TGFβ can be used to monitor the course and effectiveness of RT, as well as to determine the risk of side effects occurrence. There are a number of potential, specific markers, characteristic for pulmonary alveoli damage.

Other obstacles in the course of RT treatment are diverse radiosensitivity and radioresistance. However, there is substantial evidence pointing at microRNAs' (miRNAs) involvement in the RT response. miRNAs are a class of small, single-stranded, non-coding RNAs that post-transcriptionally regulate gene expression and influence signaling pathways that could alter a series of cellular functions, including the response to IR [36–38]. miRNAs may be an appropriate tool to (1) profile the tumor's radioresistance before treatment delivery; (2) monitor the response in the course of treatment and, on this basis, select intensification strategies; and (3) define the final response to the therapy along with risks of recurrence or metastization [36].

3. Promising Circulating Biomarkers in Radiotherapy Monitoring

3.1. Pro- and Anti-Inflammatory Cytokines

3.1.1. Transforming Growth Factor-β

The TGFβ family is a group of pleiotropic growth factors (TGFβ isoforms, anti-Mullerian hormone, bone morphogenic proteins—BMPs) that activate the signal transduction cascade involved in carcinogenesis and tumor progression. These cytokines are a master regulator of lung development, inflammation, and injury-repair processes, and their role depends largely on their expression [10,39]. In mammalians, there are three isoforms present—TGFβ1, TGFβ2, and TGFβ3, all of which activate the same receptors and share some functions [40]. The human TGFβ1 gene is located on chromosome 19q13.1-13.39. There is an association between rs1800469 (C-509T) and rs1800470 (T869C) polymorphisms and susceptibility of radiation pneumonitis. rs1800469 polymorphism is associated with higher TGFβ production and is more prevalent in smokers [7,41].

The TGFβ is a polypeptide synthesized as a large latent precursor molecule, activated by interactions with integrins after the injury of pulmonary epithelium or endothelium. Integrin αvβ6-mediated activation is the most recognized and studied mechanism in pulmonary fibrosis. Furthermore, the TGFβ may be activated by matrix metalloproteinases (MMPs), plasmin, thrombospondin, extracellular matrix (ECM) proteins such as VCAN (versican) and ED-A-FN (extradomain-A fibronectin) or by extracellular acidification and ROS [7,42]. TGFβ's active form binds to a complex consisting of two Type I (TGFβRI) and two Type II (TGFβR2) TGFβ receptors, which initiates an intracellular signaling cascade. TGFβ's signaling goes through phosphorylation and activation of the intracellular receptor-regulated R-Smad (Smad2 and Smad3) proteins in fibroblasts. Activated Smads translocate to the nucleus, where activate transcription of the genes involved in fibroblast differentiation and matrix synthesis [7,31,39].

The TGFβ1 mediates cellular processes, including growth, differentiation, cell migration, chemotaxis, and apoptosis, and its expression is elevated in the airway epithelium, alveoli macrophages, airway smooth muscle cells, and fibroblasts in various pulmonary disease entities. TGFβ1 was reported as one of the most important growth factors among the molecules expressed in tissues following IR exposure. TGFβ1 is also associated with the incidence of RP and may serve as a sensitive marker of fibrinolytic changes that stimulate the differentiation of fibroblasts into myofibroblasts [10,39,43,44]. Myofibroblasts drive the cycle of increased epithelial injury (especially alveolar type II cells) and boost collagen synthesis. TGFβ1 also promotes goblet cell hyperplasia, subepithelial fibrosis, epithelial damage, and airway smooth muscle hypertrophy [39]. TGFβ1 is the most commonly used marker in the course of RILI. In the study by Wang et al. (2017), it has been shown that higher TGF-β1 2w/pre ratio (the ratio between TGFβ1 plasma level before and two weeks after radiotherapy) is associated with higher risk of RILI, and the TGFβ1 may predict RILI at 2 weeks during radiotherapy [45]. TGFβ1's evaluation before, during, and after RT may estimate the risk of complications. The elevated levels of TGFβ1, before the implementation of the therapy, do not mean that the patient will develop RP and subsequent fibrosis; however, the persistent high level of TGFβ1 after therapy suggests the probability of radiation-induced inflammation occurrence [44,46,47].

Modulation of TGFβ1 signaling can be a future direction in treatment. Animal studies have revealed that anti-TGFβ antibodies can attenuate RILI and reduce inflammation by decreasing the level of TGFβ1. A radioprotective effect of JQ1 was also showed, which through suppressing intracellular signaling pathways, leads to weakening of RILF and collagen production reduction [31].

3.1.2. Interleukins

Increased neutrophils and macrophages accumulation is observed in irradiated lung tissues and in the later RILF. Macrophages migrate from the bone marrow to the alveolar space and act as a source of numerous cytokines, including interleukin. The main proinflammatory interleukins of acute lung response are Il-1α and Il-6 [25].

Interleukins are synthesized by a large variety of cells, including monocytes, alveolar macrophages, type II pneumocytes, fibroblasts, and T lymphocytes. Interleukins may also be released from the damaged tumor cells, which have a crucial role in the immune system host defense and tumorigenic processes [15,48].

For instance, Il-6 holds effects on cellular function regulation, i.e., growth, proliferation, differentiation, metabolism, the acute-phase reaction, angiogenesis, hematopoiesis, and apoptosis. The elevated levels of Il-6 before and after RT are connected with the development of inflammation. Overproduction of Il-6 has been described in the acute radiation-induced processes, and it may be linked to the risk and occurrence of severe RP. The data suggest that Il-6 can be used as a predictive tool in the RP development. However, Il-6, similarly to other cytokines, is pleiotropic and non-specific for the radiation injury [15,43,44,46,48].

Il-8 produced by NSCLC cells plays an important role as a neutrophil-, basophil-, and T-lymphocyte-activator and chemoattractant. Data from the animal studies showed that Il-8 induces collagen synthesis and cell proliferation. Despite this, it was found that Il-8 has anti-inflammatory effect in humans [13,45,48]. Evaluation of Il-8 before RT has revealed 4 times higher levels of Il-8 in patients without inflammatory symptoms in comparison with the group of patients with symptoms [46,49]. In the study by Wang et al. (2017), lower baseline level of Il-8 was associated with higher risk of RILT. These data suggest that Il-8 may be a good predictor of the post-RT complications risk [45].

Another anti-inflammatory cytokine is Il-10, produced by macrophages and monocytes. Its main function is inflammation restraint by the inhibition of pro-inflammatory cytokines production and reduction of the antigen-presenting cells activity. Low Il-10's concentration in the course of RT is connected with inflammation development. In the study by Arpin et al. (2005), Il-10 levels remained low in patients with RP throughout the treatment. Simultaneously, there was a consistent increase of circulating Il-10 at 2 weeks of treatment in patients without radiation pneumonitis [50].

Il-17 also has an important role in processes of lung injury induced by RT. High serum Il-17 levels at baseline of RT may indicate an increased vulnerability to RP. The study by Guo et al. (2017) was focused on the observation of Il-17's expression levels throughout RT. Cytokine's level peaked at 4 weeks and subsequently declined at 8 weeks after RT. There are data that suggest that treatment with IL-17 antibody alleviated RP and subsequent fibrosis, improving patients' OS [30].

Il-4, -13, and -18 may induce inflammatory disorders as well, playing a key role in the development of RILI and fibrosis. Such circulating interleukins may be a good predictors of RT side effects and a risk of RILI. However, single determinations are not reliable, and the best option is to identify several parameters simultaneously, several times during the course of irradiation [16,48].

3.1.3. Tumor Necrosis Factor-α

TNFα, pro-inflammatory cytokine produced by activated macrophages, triggers the production of other pro-inflammatory cytokines, growth factors, and acute-phase proteins [51,52]. TNFα's immunoregulatory effects stimulate fibroblasts growth, secretion of ECM proteins, and production of collagenases and activates the cascades of other pro-inflammatory cytokines (IL-1, IL-6, and IFN). Early release of TNFα is a critical factor after lung irradiation [43,53,54]. In the study by Zhang et al. (2008), it was shown that mouse's lungs can be protected from RILI through TNFα signaling blocking, either via knockdown or by using antisense oligonucleotides against the TNFα receptor [55]. In another study, treatment with a recombinant TNFα receptor resulted in the fibrinolytic lesions regression within damaged lungs [43]. Data points to the TNFα participation in the initial phase of RP and to a correlation between TNFα level and the occurrence of RILT [56]. However, there is no evidence on whether TNFα may be used as the predicting factor of RILT before the treatment with RT.

3.2. Indicators of Pneumocytes Damage

3.2.1. Protein A and D of the Surfactant

Type II pneumocytes are responsible for the secretion of pulmonary surfactant. Surfactant reduces surface tension in the alveoli and facilitates alveolar expansion, permitting in this way normal gas exchange. Furthermore, surfactants regulate lung immune response and clearance of foreign particles, debris, and inflammatory material [57]. Alveolar type II pneumocytes are highly sensitive to IR injury. RILI is characterized by decreased endogenous surfactant production by type II pneumocytes and its increased degradation [58]. Surfactant insufficiency leads to the alveolar collapse and so to poor health outcomes.

Surfactant, also called surface-active agent, consists of phospholipids, carbohydrates, and proteins such as surfactant protein (SP)-A and -D. SP-D reduces surface tension at the pulmonary air-liquid interface and enhances defense as the first line of innate pulmonary immunity. Surfactant proteins stimulate macrophages to produce pro-inflammatory cytokines (TGFβ, interleukins) and ROS. Radiation-induced degradation of type II pneumocytes leads to the release of SP-A and SP-D and hence to inflammation progression. Increased permeability of pulmonary epithelial cells results in facilitated passage of SP-A and SP-D to the systemic circulation and to increased levels of circulating SPs. SP-D is a more sensitive marker of the pulmonary pathological changes than SP-A [46,59–61].

Numerous studies revealed elevated serum and plasma levels of SP-D in patients with RP. Sasaki et al. (2001) hypothesized that serum SP-D monitoring is a practical and useful method for the early detection of RP [62]. However, there are some limitations in patients with normal SP-D serum levels before RT [46].

3.2.2. Glycoprotein Krebs von den Lugen 6

A mucin-like glycoprotein Krebs von den Lugen 6 (KL-6) is another indicator of type II pneumocytes damage and may be used in RT monitoring [63]. KL-6 antigen, also called sialylated carbohydrate antigen-6, is a high-molecular-weight glycoprotein classified as "cluster 9" according to the Third International Workshop on Lung Tumor and Differentiation Antigens. Anti-KL-6 monoclonal antibody (mAb) is considered to recognize the specific MUC1 glycopeptide sequence, which makes it a potential diagnostic and therapeutic agent. However, the precise glycan structure of the epitope recognized by anti-KL-6 mAb remains unclear [64,65].

According to immunohistochemistry and cytometry, KL-6 has been classified in the MUC1 group [66–68]. KL-6 is strongly expressed by type II pneumocytes and bronchiolar epithelial cells. Damaged pulmonary cells release KL-6, which makes KL-6 an indicator of interstitial lung diseases and acute lung injury. KL-6 demonstrates proliferative and anti-apoptotic effects, aiding with TGFβ1 effects, which indicates its contribution in pulmonary fibrotic processes. Therefore, at the clinical level, KL-6 is considered as useful biomarker in the determination of pulmonary fibrosis activity [59,66,69]. KL-6's increase of at least 1.5 values on the upper limit of the reference range before RT is a marker of a high risk of complications. [46,66,68]. Serum levels of KL-6 and SP-D are good markers, with a high sensitivity for the detection of patients with a high risk of RP and RP's severity monitoring [70]. Furthermore, serum KL-6 level significantly correlates with severity and responses to therapy in pulmonary fibrosis [63]. At this point, KL-6 is not used routinely in clinical practice, but its use is expected to increase in the future. All above described markers, their functions and usage in monitoring of radiotherapy are collected in Table 2.

Table 2. Featured biological markers, their functions and usage in monitoring of radiotherapy.

Biological Marker	Function in Radiation-Induced Lung Injury (RILI)	Research Studies	Conclusions	Reference
TGFβ1	TGFβ stimulates the differentiation of fibroblasts into myofibroblasts and promotes goblet cell hyperplasia, subepithelial fibrosis, epithelial damage, and airway smooth muscle hypertrophy	Higher TGF-β 2w/pre ratio (the ratio between TGFβ plasma level before and two weeks after RT) is associated with higher risk of RILI; the persistent high level of TGFβ after therapy suggests the occurrence of symptoms of radiation-induced inflammation	TGFβ plasma levels may identify individuals at high risk for the development of RILI	[39,43–47]
Il-6	Il-6 holds effects on the regulation of cellular functions such as growth, proliferation, differentiation, metabolism, the acute-phase reaction, angiogenesis, hematopoiesis, and apoptosis	Higher concentrations of Il-6, before and after treatment, are connected with the development of inflammation; overproduction of Il-6 in the acute radiation-induced process is associated with the risk and occurrence of severe RP	Il-6 can be used as a predictive marker of the RP development	[15,43,44,46,48]
Il-8	Il-8 is a neutrophil-, basophil-, and T-lymphocyte-activator and chemoattractant; Il-8 induces collagen synthesis and cell proliferation and has an anti-inflammatory effect	Lower baseline level of Il-8 is associated with higher risk of RILI (patients without inflammatory symptoms have about 4 times higher levels of Il-8 than the group of patients with the presence of symptoms)	The evaluation of Il-8 before therapy can be a good predictor for the risk of complications	[13,45,46,48,49]
Il-10	Il-10 downregulates inflammation by inhibiting the production of pro-inflammatory cytokines and reducing the activity of antigen-presenting cells	Levels of Il-10 are remained low in patients with RP throughout the treatment; a consistent increase of circulating Il-10 is observed at 2 weeks of treatment in patients without RP	The evaluation of Il-10 throughout the treatment may be a good predictor of RP	[50]
TNFα	TNFα stimulates the fibroblasts growth, secretion of ECM proteins, production of collagenases, and activation of cascades of other pro-inflammatory cytokines (IL-1, IL-6, IFN)	The early release of TNFα is a critical factor after lung irradiation; blocking of TNFα signaling via knockdown or using antisense oligonucleotides against the TNFα receptor can protect mouse lung from radiation injury; treatment with a recombinant TNFα receptor results in the regression of fibrinolytic lesions within damaged lungs	TNFα may indicate RP in its initial phase; correlation between the occurrence of RILI and the level of TNFα	[43,53–56]
SP-A and SP-D	Degradation of type II pneumocytes results in facilitated passage of SP-A and SP-D to the systemic circulation and increased levels of circulating SPs; SPs stimulate macrophages to production of pro-inflammatory cytokines (TGFβ, interleukins) and ROS	Serum and plasma levels of SP-D are elevated in patients with RP	Serum SP-D monitoring is a practical and useful method for the early detection of RP	[46,59–62]

Table 2. *Cont.*

Biological Marker	Function in Radiation-Induced Lung Injury (RILI)	Research Studies	Conclusions	Reference
KL-6	KL-6 demonstrates proliferative and anti-apoptotic effects and contributes in pulmonary fibrotic processes	An increased level of KL-6 at least 1.5 values of the upper limit of the reference range before radiotherapy correlates with a high risk of complications; serum KL-6 level correlates with severity and response to therapy in pulmonary fibrosis	Monitoring of the severity of RP; useful biomarker of pulmonary fibrosis activity	[46,59,66,68–70]

TGFβ—transforming growth factor β; Il—interleukin; TNFα—tumor necrosis factor α; SP—surfactant protein; KL-6—Krebs von den Lugen-6; RILI—radiation-induced lung injury; ECM—extracellular matrix; IFN—interferon; ROS—reactive oxygen species; RT—radiotherapy; RP—radiation-induced pneumonitis.

4. MicroRNAs in Radiotherapy

microRNAs (miRNAs) are the subject of interest in various medical fields, both as a diagnostic tool and therapeutic targets. Some of the miRNAs have already passed through the phases I and II of clinical trials. Multiple studies are concerned with the radiosensitizing and radioprotective role of miRNAs in patients' response to RT treatment [19,37]. First reports point out microRNAs' potential as predictive biomarkers in therapy response and disease prognosis. microRNAs represent ideal markers because of their (1) specificity for the administered treatment; (2) stability in tissues, and body fluids; and (3) fast, robust, and economic expression detection [19,71].

microRNAs activity affects the response to IR by their involvement in the regulatory mechanisms of the DNA damage response (DDR), at the different levels and through (1) signaling pathways, (2) checkpoints in the cell cycle, and (3) specific repair processes that restore the single- or double-strand break (SSB, DSB) [36]. In Table 3 are presented microRNAs and their involvement in the above mentioned regulatory mechanisms. Findings of Li-Peng Jiang et al. (2017) [72] provide strong evidence that miR-21 may inhibit PD-CD4 expression and activate phosphoinositide 3-kinase (PI3K)/AKT/mTOR signaling pathways, affecting the radiosensitivity of NSCLC cells. On the contrary, the study by Yin et al. (2017) [73] has revealed that disturbance of the let-7/LIN28 double-negative feedback loop is involved in the regulation of radioresistance. Assessment of let-7 expression and its target gene—LIN28 may be used as predictive biomarkers of response to RT in NSCLC patients. Weidhaas et al. (2017) [74] reported that both of the lung cell lines (normal tissue -CLR2741-, and tumor tissue -A549-) reacted after the exposition to IR, characterizing a downregulation of all miRNAs, with one exception, let-7g, which was conversely upregulated. At the same time, down regulation of miR-9 and let-7g play a critical role in activation of NF-κB1 [75]. In addition, miR-210 appears to be a component of the radioresistance of hypoxic cancer cells. miR-210 could stabilize hypoxia-inducible factor (HIF) to promote DNA repair and activate Notch signaling pathway in angiogenesis [12,76,77]. Angiogenesis is an important factor contributing to the radioresistance of lung cancer. However, the associated mechanisms underlying radiotherapy-induced proangiogenesis are unclear.

Many studies focus on demonstrating the role of specific miRNAs in radiosensitivity and the processes standing behind it. Sun et al. (2020) [78] showed that miR-125a level varies in NSCLC cell lines with different radiosensitivities. Additionally, the authors demonstrated that miR-125a-5p upregulates apoptosis in lung cancer cells, increasing their radiosensitivity. Moreover, the expression of miR-125 is regulated by a single-nucleotide polymorphism (SNP), rs12976445, which is associated with the risk of RP [79]. Liu et al. (2013) [80] showed that inhibition of miR-21 significantly enhances the sensitivity of NSCLC cells to chemotherapeutic agents (cisplatin and docetaxel) and irradiation. In this study, authors demonstrated that overexpression of miR-21 may downregulate the expression of PTEN (tumor suppressor gene, an essential regulator of cell proliferation, differentiation, growth, and apoptosis) in NSCLC cells, making it a rational therapeutic strategy for the treatment of NSCLC in the future [80,81]. Another study revealed that miR-21 overexpression is correlated with collagen production at the radiation injury site, accompanied by the significant downregulation of several miR-21 targets, including Smad7. These findings suggest that increased miR-21 contributes to fibrotic responses observed in mesenchymal cells at the injury site through the potentiation of TGF-β signaling. Moreover, local targeting of miR-21 at the injured area may have potential therapeutic utility in mitigating RILF [82].

Table 3. Pathways and mechanisms of response to radiation damage regulated by miRNAs.

MicroRNA	Effects	Reference
	PI3K/AKT and MAPK signaling pathways	
miR-21 let-7 family	• overexpression of miR-21 is associated with radiation efficacy attenuation and shorter median of OS in NSCLC patients • underexpression of let-7 and overexpression of LIN28 regulates proliferative capability of NSCLC cells and hence promotes resistance to RT or cisplatin treatment • overexpression of let-7a decreases expression of K-Ras and is related to A549 cells radiosensitization	[72–74,83]
	Cell-cycle progression checkpoints	
miR-21 miR-34b miR-138	• underexpression of miR-21 inhibits proliferation and cell cycle progression of A549 cells; it also promotes A549 cells' apoptosis after exposure to irradiation • overexpression of miR-34b increases radio sensitivity of the p53 wild type-, and KRAS mutated-cells of NSCLC, even at low doses of RT • miR-138 expression in irradiated lung cancer cell decreases the SENP1 expression, resulting in cell cycle arrest in the G1/G0 phase	[84–86]
	Double-strand break repair	
miR-101 miR-182	• miR-101 acts as radiosensitizer, its overexpression reduces the levels of DNA-PKcs and ATM, thus increasing the radiosensitivity of tumor cells • knockdown of miR-182 suppresses cell proliferation and increases cell apoptosis after irradiation; unrepaired DNA damage in miR-182 knockdown cells results in cell cycle arrest	[87,88]
	HIF-dependent transcriptional regulation	
miR-210	• hypoxic cells are resistant to radiotherapy and chemotherapy; miR-210 is a component of the radioresistance of hypoxic cancer cells that induces and stabilizes HIF-1 through a positive regulatory loop	[76]
	Inhibition of NFκB1	
miR-9	• overexpression of miR-9 and let-7h inhibits NFκB1, leading to the increase of RT efficiency in lung cancer treatment	[75]

PI3K—phosphoinositide 3-kinase; MAPK—mitogen-activated protein kinase; OS—overall survival; NSCLC—non-small cell lung carcinoma; RT—radiotherapy; K-ras—Kirsten rat sarcoma; A549—culture of human lung carcinoma cell line; SENP1—sentrin-specific protease 1; G1/G0—gap 1/gap 0; DNA-PKcs—DNA-protein kinase catalytic subunit; HIF—hypoxia-inducible factor; NFκB1—nuclear factor κB1.

5. Future Perspective

There is little information on the predictive value of functional and biological indicators for predicting post-radiation effects, including lung inflammation in lung cancer patients treated with RT. Therefore, in the future, the introduction of markers useful in monitoring RILI is a chance to improve the clinical outcomes in patients treated with RT.

6. Executive Summary

RT as one of the main treatment approaches in lung cancer patients should be effective but also safe. Unfortunately, it is impossible to completely eliminate the risk side effects such as acute inflammation or lung fibrosis. Therefore, various markers, both biochemical and genetic, may be used to monitor RT. These include determination of KL-6 and SP-A and -D concentrations, which provide information about the integrity of the blood–air barrier. Elevation of their concentrations indicates type II pneumocytes damage, characteristic of the first phase of RILI and pulmonary fibrosis. Surfactant proteins are sensitive and early markers of post-radiation lung injury, which makes them good predictive parameters.

Determination of proinflammatory cytokines like TGFβ, TNFα and interleukins is also helpful in such cases. Exposure to IR leads to relatively quick appearance of proinflammatory factors in the patient's circulating system. Cytokines multiple determinations before, during, and after RT may be useful in the prediction of complications risk level. Monitoring the course of RT is extremely important in effective treatment and for improving patients' conditions.

Another determinant of the therapy's effectiveness is the assessment of microRNAs expressions, which are great indicators of both radioresistance and radiosensitivity. The data indicate possibilities of microRNAs application in the RT monitoring. However, they have not been moved to the clinical setting yet.

Author Contributions: Conceptualization, M.Ś.-M., Ł.T.; resources, M.Ś.-M. and K.W.; writing—original draft preparation, M.Ś.-M. and K.W.; writing—review and editing, M.Ś.-M., K.W., and I.B.-L.; visualization, K.W. and I.B.-L.; supervision, M.Ś.-M.; project administration, M.Ś.-M., Ł.T. and I.B.-L. All authors have read and agreed to the published version of the manuscript.

Funding: The publication was prepared under the project financed from the funds granted by the Ministry of Science and Higher Education in the "Regional Initiative of Excellence" programme for the years 2019–2022, project number 016/RID/2018/19, amount of funding 11 998 121.30 PLN.

Conflicts of Interest: The authors declare no conflicts of interest.

Abbreviations

A549	culture of human lung carcinoma cell line
BET	bromodomain and extraterminal domain
BMP	bone marrow protein
CT	computed tomography
DDR	DNA damage response
DNA	deoxyribonucleic acid
DNA-PKcs	DNA-protein kinase catalytic subunit
DSB	double-strand break
ECM	extracellular matrix
ED-A-FN	extradomain-A fibronectin
G0/G1	gap 0/gap 1
HIF	hypoxia-inducible factor
IFN	interferon
Il	interleukin
IR	ionizing radiation
KL-6	glycoprotein Krebs von den Lugen-6
K-ras	Kirsten rat sarcoma
MAPK	mitogen-activated protein kinase
MMP	matrix metalloproteinases
MUC1	mucin 1
NFκB1	nuclear factor κB1
NK	natural killer
NO	nitric oxygen
NSCLC	non-small cell lung carcinoma
OS	overall survival
PDGF	platelet-derived growth factor
PI3K	phosphoinositide 3-kinase
RILD	radiation-induced lung disease
RILF	radiation-induced lung fibrosis
RILI	radiation-induced lung injury
ROS	reactive oxygen species
RP	radiation-induced pneumonitis

RT	radiotherapy
SCC	squamous cell carcinoma
SCLC	small cell lung carcinoma
SENP1	sentrin-specific protease 1
SNP	single nucleotide polymorphism
SP	surfactant protein
SSB	single-strand break
surfactant	surface-active agent
TGFβ	transforming growth factor β
TNFα	tumor necrosis factor α
TNM	TNM Classification of Malignant Tumors (tumor-lymph nodes-metastasis
VCAN	versican
WHO	World Health Organization

References

1. Cancer. Available online: http://archive.today/2020.07.03-074914/https://www.who.int/news-room/fact-sheets/detail/cancer (accessed on 29 June 2020).
2. Du, L.; Ma, N.; Dai, X.; Yu, W.; Huang, X.; Xu, S.; Liu, F.; He, Q.; Liu, Y.; Wang, Q.; et al. Precise prediction of the radiation pneumonitis in lung cancer: An explorative preliminary mathematical model using genotype information. *J. Cancer* **2020**, *11*, 2329–2338. [CrossRef] [PubMed]
3. Horn, L.; Lovly, C.M. Neoplasms of the lung. In *Harrison's Principles of Internal Medicine*, 20th ed.; Jameson, J., Fauci, A.S., Kasper, D.L., Hauser, S.L., Longo, D.L., Loscalzo, J., Eds.; McGraw-Hill: New York, NY, USA, 2018.
4. Woodworth, A.L.; Schuler, E. The respiratory system. In *Laposata's Laboratory Medicine: Diagnosis of Disease in the Clinical Laboratory*, 3th ed.; Laposata, M., Ed.; McGraw-Hill: New York, NY, USA, 2019.
5. Stoeckel, D.A.; Matuschak, G.M. Lung cancer. In *Respiratory: An. Integrated Approach to Disease*; Lechner, A.J., Matuschak, G.M., Brink, D.S., Eds.; McGraw-Hill: New York, NY, USA, 2012.
6. Inamura, K. Lung Cancer: Understanding Its Molecular Pathology and the 2015 WHO Classification. *Front. Oncol.* **2017**, *7*, 193. [CrossRef] [PubMed]
7. Kulkarni, T.; O'Reilly, P.; Antony, V.B.; Gaggar, A.; Thannickal, V.J. Matrix Remodeling in Pulmonary Fibrosis and Emphysema. *Am. J. Respir. Cell Mol. Biol.* **2016**, *54*, 751–760. [CrossRef] [PubMed]
8. Starek, A.; Podolak, I. Carcinogenic effect of tobacco smoke. *Rocz. Panstw. Zakl. Hig.* **2009**, *60*, 299–310. [PubMed]
9. NCCN. National Comprehensive Cancer Network Guidelines, NSCLC, Principles of Radiation Therapy. Available online: http://archive.today/2020.07.03-083935/https://www.nccn.org/professionals/physician_gls/default.aspx (accessed on 30 June 2020).
10. Lu, Z.; Tang, Y.; Luo, J.; Zhang, S.; Zhou, X.; Fu, L. Advances in targeting the transforming growth factor β1 signaling pathway in lung cancer radiotherapy (Review). *Oncol. Lett.* **2017**, *14*, 5681–5687. [CrossRef]
11. Long, L.; Zhang, X.; Bai, J.; Li, Y.; Wang, X.; Zhou, Y. Tissue-specific and exosomal miRNAs in lung cancer radiotherapy: From regulatory mechanisms to clinical implications. *Cancer Manag. Res.* **2019**, *11*, 413–4424. [CrossRef]
12. Xu, Y.; Liao, X.; Chen, X.; Li, D.; Sun, J.; Liao, R. Regulation of miRNAs affects radiobiological response of lung cancer stem cells. *Biomed. Res. Int.* **2015**, *2015*, 851841. [CrossRef]
13. Salem, A.; Mistry, H.; Backen, A.; Hodgson, C.; Koh, P.; Dean, E.; Priest, L.; Haslett, K.; Trigonis, I.; Jackson, A.; et al. Cell Death, Inflammation, Tumor Burden, and Proliferation Blood Biomarkers Predict Lung Cancer Radiotherapy Response and Correlate With Tumor Volume and Proliferation Imaging. *Clin. Lung Cancer* **2018**, *19*, 239–248.e7. [CrossRef]
14. Walls, G.; Hanna, G.; Qi, F.; Zhao, S.; Xia, J.; Ansari, M.; Landau, D. Predicting outcomes from radical radiotherapy for non-small cell lung cancer: A systematic review of the existing literature. *Front. Oncol.* **2018**, *8*, 433. [CrossRef]
15. Fu, Z.Z.; Peng, Y.; Cao, L.Y.; Chen, Y.S.; Li, K.; Fu, B.H. Correlations Between Serum IL-6 Levels and Radiation Pneumonitis in Lung Cancer Patients: A Meta-Analysis. *J. Clin. Lab. Anal.* **2016**, *30*, 145–154. [CrossRef]
16. Amini, P.; Saffar, H.; Nourani, M.R.; Motevaseli, E.; Najafi, M.; Ali Taheri, R.; Qazvini, A. Curcumin Mitigates Radiation-induced Lung Pneumonitis and Fibrosis in Rats. *Int. J. Mol. Cell Med.* **2018**, *7*, 212–219. [PubMed]

17. He, X.; Yang, A.; Mcdonald, D.; Riemer, E.; Vanek, K.; Schulte, B.; Wang, G. MiR-34a modulates ionizing radiation-induced senescence in lung cancer cells. *Oncotarget* **2017**, *8*, 69797–69807. [CrossRef] [PubMed]
18. Mets, O.; Smthuis, R. Lung—Cancer TNM 8th Edition. Available online: http://archive.today/2020.07.03-083910/https://radiologyassistant.nl/chest/lung-cancer-tnm-8th-edition (accessed on 29 June 2020).
19. Moertl, S.; Mutschelknaus, L.; Heider, T.; Atkinson, M.J. MicroRNAs as novel elements in personalized radiotherapy. *Transl. Cancer Res.* **2016**, *5* (Suppl. 6), S1262–S1269. [CrossRef]
20. Yu, H.M.; Liu, Y.F.; Cheng, Y.F.; Hu, L.K.; Hou, M. Effects of Rhubarb Extract on Radiation-Induced Lung Toxicity Via Decreasing Transforming Growth Factor-β1 and Interleukin-6 in Lung Cancer Patients Treated with Radiotherapy. *Lung Cancer* **2008**, *59*, 219–226. [CrossRef] [PubMed]
21. Jain, V.; Berman, A.T. Radiation Pneumonitis: Old Problem, New Tricks. *Cancers* **2018**, *10*, 222. [CrossRef] [PubMed]
22. Deng, G.; Liang, N.; Xie, J.; Luo, H.; Qiao, L.; Zhang, J.; Wang, D.; Zhang, J. Pulmonary toxicity generated from radiotherapeutic treatment of thoracic malignancies. *Oncol. Lett.* **2017**, *14*, 501–511. [CrossRef]
23. Jackson, I.L.; Zhang, Y.; Bentzen, S.M.; Hu, J.; Zhang, A.; Vujaskovic, Z. Pathophysiological mechanisms underlying phenotypic differences in pulmonary radioresponse. *Sci. Rep.* **2016**, *6*, 36579. [CrossRef]
24. Veiga, C.; Chandy, E.; Jacob, J.; Yip, N.; Szmul, A.; Landau, D.; McClelland, J. Investigation of the evolution of radiation-induced lung damage using serial CT imaging and pulmonary function tests. *Radiother. Oncol.* **2020**, *148*, 89–96. [CrossRef]
25. Yu, H.H.; Chengchuan Ko, E.; Chang, C.L.; Yuan, K.S.; Wu, A.; Shan, Y.S.; Wu, S.Y. Fucoidan Inhibits Radiation-Induced Pneumonitis and Lung Fibrosis by Reducing Inflammatory Cytokine Expression in Lung Tissues. *Mar. Drugs* **2018**, *16*, 392. [CrossRef]
26. Krawczuk-Rybak, M. Late effects of treatment of childhood cancer—On the basis of the literature and own experience. *Med. Wieku Rozwoj.* **2013**, *17*, 130–136.
27. Larici, A.R.; Del Ciello, A.; Maggi, F.; Immacolata Santoro, S.; Meduri, B.; Valentini, V.; Giordano, A.; Bonomo, L. Lung abnormalities at multimodality imaging after radiation therapy for non–small cell lung cancer. *Radiographics* **2011**, *31*, 771–789. [CrossRef] [PubMed]
28. Abravan, A.; Eide, H.A.; Knudtsen, I.S.; Løndalen, A.M.; Helland, Å.; Malinen, E. Assessment of Pulmonary 18F-FDG-PET Uptake and Cytokine Profiles in Non-Small Cell Lung Cancer Patients Treated with Radiotherapy and Erlotinib. *Clin. Transl. Radiat. Oncol.* **2017**, *4*, 57–63. [CrossRef] [PubMed]
29. Zhang, X.; Shin, Y.K.; Zheng, Z.; Zhu, L.; Lee, I.J. Risk of Radiation-Induced Pneumonitis After Helical and Static-Port Tomotherapy in Lung Cancer Patients and Experimental Rats. *Radiat. Oncol.* **2015**, *10*, 195. [CrossRef] [PubMed]
30. Guo, L.; Ding, G.; Xu, W.; Lu, Y.; Ge, H.; Jiang, Y.; Chen, X.; Li, Y. Prognostic Biological Factors of Radiation Pneumonitis after Stereotactic Body Radiation Therapy Combined with Pulmonary Perfusion Imaging. *Exp. Ther. Med.* **2019**, *17*, 244–250. [CrossRef]
31. Wang, J.; Zhou, F.; Li, Z.; Mei, H.; Wang, Y.; Ma, H.; Shi, L.; Huan, A.; Zhang, T.; Lin, Z.; et al. Pharmacological targeting of BET proteins attenuates radiation-induced lung fibrosis. *Sci. Rep.* **2018**, *8*, 998. [CrossRef]
32. Komaki, R.; Travis, E.L.; Cox, J.D. The lung, pleura, and thymus. In *Radiation Oncology: Rationale, Technique, Results*, 9th ed.; Cox, J.D., Ang, K.K., Eds.; Elsevier Health Sciences: Philadelphia, PA, USA, 2009; pp. 424–427.
33. Goldman, L.; Schafer, A.I. *Goldman's Cecil Medicine*, 24th ed.; Elsevier Health Sciences: Philadelphia, PA, USA, 2012; p. 579.
34. Haschek, W.M.; Rousseaux, C.G.; Wallig, M.A. *Haschek and Rousseaux's Handbook of Toxicologic Pathology*, 3rd ed.; Academic Press: Cambridge, MA, USA, 2013; pp. 1462–1464.
35. Belkina, A.C.; Nikolajczyk, B.S.; Denis, G.V. BET protein function is required for inflammation: Brd2 genetic disruption and BET inhibitor JQ1 impair mouse macrophage inflammatory responses. *J. Immunol.* **2013**, *190*, 3670–3678. [CrossRef]
36. Cellini, F.; Morganti, A.G.; Genovesi, D.; Silvestris, N.; Valentini, V. Role of microRNA in response to ionizing radiations: Evidences and potential impact on clinical practice for radiotherapy. *Molecules* **2014**, *19*, 5379–5401. [CrossRef]
37. Metheetrairut, C.; Slack, F.J. MicroRNAs in the ionizing radiation response and in radiotherapy. *Curr. Opin. Genet. Dev.* **2013**, *23*, 12–19. [CrossRef]
38. Wadowska, K.; Bil-Lula, I.; Trembecki, Ł.; Śliwińska-Mossoń, M. Genetic Markers in Lung Cancer Diagnosis: A Review. *Int. J. Mol. Sci.* **2020**, *21*, 4569. [CrossRef]

39. Kramer, E.L.; Clancy, J.P. TGFβ as a therapeutic target in cystic fibrosis. *Expert Opin. Ther. Targets* **2018**, *22*, 177–189. [CrossRef]
40. Stępień-Wyrobiec, O.; Hrycek, A.; Wyrobiec, G. Transforming growth factor beta (TGF-beta): Its structure, function, and role in the pathogenesis of systemic lupus erythematosus. *Postepy Hig. Med. Dosw.* **2008**, *62*, 688–693.
41. Wang, Y.; Wang, X.; Wang, X.; Zhang, D.; Jiang, S. Effect of transforming growth factor-β1 869C/T polymorphism and radiation pneumonitis. *Int. J. Clin. Exp. Pathol.* **2015**, *8*, 2835–2839.
42. Gonzalez-Gonzalez, F.J.; Chandel, N.S.; Jain, M.; Budinger, G.R.S. Reactive oxygen species as signaling molecules in the development of lung fibrosis. *Transl. Res.* **2017**, *190*, 61–68. [CrossRef] [PubMed]
43. Tsoutsou, P.G.; Koukourakis, M.I. Radiation Pneumonitis and Fibrosis: Mechanisms Underlying Its Pathogenesis and Implications for Future Research. *Int. J. Radiat. Oncol.* **2006**, *66*, 1281–1293. [CrossRef]
44. Kong, F.M.; Ao, X.; Wang, L.; Lawrence, T.S. The Use of Blood Biomarkers to Predict Radiation Lung Toxicity: A Potential strategy to individualize thoracic radiation therapy. *Cancer Control* **2008**, *15*, 140–150. [CrossRef]
45. Wang, S.; Campbell, J.; Stenmark, M.H.; Zhao, J.; Stanton, P.; Matuszak, M.M.; Ten Haken, R.K.; Kong, F.S. Plasma Levels of IL-8 and TGF-β1 Predict Radiation-Induced Lung Toxicity in Non-Small Cell Lung Cancer: A Validation Study. *Int. J. Radiat. Oncol. Biol. Phys.* **2017**, *98*, 615–621. [CrossRef] [PubMed]
46. Provatopoulou, X.; Athanasiou, E.; Gounaris, A. Predictive markers of radiation pneumonitis. *Anticancer Res.* **2008**, *28*, 2421–2432. [PubMed]
47. Palmer, J.D.; Zaorsky, N.G.; Witek, M.; Lu, B. Molecular markers to predict clinical outcome and radiation induced toxicity in lung cancer. *J. Thorac. Dis.* **2014**, *6*, 387–398. [PubMed]
48. Crohns, M.; Saarelainen, S.; Laine, S.; Poussa, T.; Alho, H.; Kellokumpu-Lehtinen, P. Cytokines in Bronchoalveolar Lavage Fluid and Serum of Lung Cancer Patients During Radiotherapy—Association of Interleukin-8 and VEGF with Survival. *Cytokine* **2010**, *50*, 30–36. [CrossRef]
49. Gilowska, I. CXCL8 (Interleukina 8)—Główny mediator stanu zapalnego w przewlekłej obturacyjnej chorobie płuc? *Postepy Hig. Med. Dosw.* **2014**, *68*, 842–850. [CrossRef]
50. Arpin, D.; Perol, D.; Blay, J.Y.; Falchero, L.; Line Claude, L.; Vuillermoz-Blas, S.; Martel-Lafay, I.; Ginestet, C.; Alberti, L.; Nosov, D.; et al. Early Variations of Circulating Interleukin-6 and Interleukin-10 Levels During Thoracic Radiotherapy Are Predictive for Radiation Pneumonitis. *J. Clin. Oncol.* **2005**, *23*, 8748–8756. [CrossRef] [PubMed]
51. Verma, S.; Kalita, B.; Bajaj, S.; Prakash, H.; Singh, A.K.; Gupta, M.L. A Combination of Podophyllotoxin and Rutin Alleviates Radiation-Induced Pneumonitis and Fibrosis through Modulation of Lung Inflammation in Mice. *Front. Immunol.* **2017**, *8*, 658. [CrossRef] [PubMed]
52. Chen, C.; Yang, S.; Zhang, M.; Zhang, Z.; Zhang, S.B.; Wu, B.; Hong, J.; Zhang, W.; Lin, J.; Okunieff, P.; et al. Triptolide mitigates radiation-induced pneumonitis via inhibition of alveolar macrophages and related inflammatory molecules. *Oncotarget* **2017**, *8*, 45133–45142. [CrossRef] [PubMed]
53. Li, B.; Chen, S.H.; Lu, H.J.; Tan, Y. Predictive values of TNF-beta1, IL-6, IL-10 for radiation pneumonitis. *Int. J. Radiat. Res.* **2016**, *14*, 173–179.
54. Refahi, S.; Pourissa, M.; Zirak, M.R.; Hadadi, G. Modulation expression of tumor necrosis factor α in the radiation-induced lung injury by glycyrrhizic acid. *J. Med. Phys.* **2015**, *40*, 95–101. [PubMed]
55. Zhang, M.; Qian, J.; Xing, X.; Kong, F.-M.; Zhao, L.; Chen, M.; Theodore, S.; Lawrence, T.D. Inhibition of the Tumor Necrosis Factor-α Pathway is Radioprotective for the Lung. *Clin. Cancer Res.* **2008**, *14*, 1868–1876. [CrossRef]
56. Krishnamurthy, P.M.; Shukla, S.; Ray, P.; Mehra, R.; Nyati, M.K.; Lawrence, T.S.; Ray, D. Involvement of p38-βTrCP-Tristetraprolin-TNFα axis in radiation pneumonitis. *Oncotarget* **2017**, *8*, 47767–47779. [CrossRef]
57. Christofidou-Solomidou, M.; Pietrofesa, R.A.; Arguiri, E.; Koumenis, C.; Segal, R. Radiation Mitigating Properties of Intranasally Administered KL4 Surfactant in a Murine Model of Radiation-Induced Lung Damage. *Radiat. Res.* **2017**, *188*, 491–504. [CrossRef]
58. Yamagishi, T.; Kodaka, N.; Kurose, Y.; Watanabe, K.; Nakano, C.; Kishimoto, K.; Oshio, T.; Niitsuma, K.; Matsuse, H. Analysis of predictive parameters for the development of radiation-induced pneumonitis. *Ann. Thorac. Med.* **2017**, *2*, 252–258.
59. Yamashita, H.; Takahashi, W.; Nakagawa, K. Radiation pneumonitis after stereotactic radiation therapy for lung cancer. *World J. Radiol.* **2014**, *6*, 708–715. [CrossRef]

60. Xu, L.; Jiang, J.; Li, Y.; Zhang, L.; Li, Z.; Xian, J.; Jiang, C.; Diao, Y.; Su, X.; Xu, H.; et al. Genetic variants of SP-D confer susceptibility to radiation pneumonitis in lung cancer patients undergoing thoracic radiation therapy. *Cancer Med.* **2019**, *8*, 2599–2611. [CrossRef] [PubMed]
61. Yamazaki, H.; Aibe, N.; Nakamura, S.; Sasaki, N.; Suzuki, G.; Yoshida, K.; Yamada, K.; Koizumi, M.; Arimoto, T.; Iwasaki, Y.; et al. Measurement of exhaled nitric oxide and serum surfactant protein D levels for monitoring radiation pneumonitis following thoracic radiotherapy. *Oncol. Lett.* **2017**, *14*, 4190–4196. [CrossRef] [PubMed]
62. Sasaki, R.; Soejima, T.; Matsumoto, A.; Maruta, T.; Yamada, K.; Ota, Y.; Kawabe, T.; Nishimura, H.; Sakai, E.; Ejima, Y.; et al. Clinical Significance of Serum Pulmonary Surfactant Proteins A and D for the Early Detection of Radiation Pneumonitis. *Int. J. Radiat. Oncol. Biol. Phys.* **2001**, *50*, 301–307. [CrossRef]
63. Esteves, F.; Calé, S.S.; Badura, R.; De Boer, M.G.; Maltez, F.; Calderón, E.J.; Van der Reijden, T.J.; Márquez-Martín, E.F.; Antunes, F.; Matos, O. Diagnosis of Pneumocystis Pneumonia: Evaluation of Four Serologic Biomarkers. *Clin. Microbiol. Infect.* **2015**, *21*, 379.e1–379.e10. [CrossRef]
64. Sato, S.; Kato, T.; Abe, K.; Hanaoka, T.; Yano, Y.; Kurosaki, A.; Yasuda, M.; Sekino, T.; Fujiwara, K.; Hasegawa, K. Pre-operative evaluation of circulating KL-6 levels as a biomarker for epithelial ovarian carcinoma and its correlation with tumor MUC1 expression. *Oncol. Lett.* **2017**, *14*, 776–786. [CrossRef]
65. Ohyabu, N.; Hinou, H.; Matsushita, T.; Izumi, R.; Shimizu, H.; Kawamoto, K.; Numata, Y.; Togame, H.; Takemoto, H.; Kondo, H.; et al. An Essential Epitope of anti-MUC1 Monoclonal Antibody KL-6 Revealed by Focused Glycopeptide Library. *J. Am. Chem. Soc.* **2009**, *131*, 17102–17109. [CrossRef]
66. Jeremic, B. *Advances in Radiation Oncology in Lung Cancer*; Springer Science & Business Media: Berlin, Germany, 2011; pp. 121–122.
67. Ishikawa, N.; Hattori, N.; Yokoyama, A.; Tanaka, S.; Nishino, R.; Yoshioka, K.; Ohshimo, S.; Fujitaka, K.; Ohnishi, H.; Hamada, H.; et al. Usefulness of monitoring the circulating Krebs von den Lungen-6 levels to predict the clinical outcome of patients with advanced non-small cell lung cancer treated with epidermal growth factor receptor tyrosine kinase inhibitors. *Int. J. Cancer* **2008**, *122*, 2612–2620. [CrossRef]
68. Iwata, H.; Shibamoto, Y.; Baba, F.; Sugie, C.; Ogino, H.; Murata, R.; Yanagi, T.; Otsuka, S.; Kosaki, K.; Murai, T.; et al. Correlation between the serum KL-6 level and the grade of radiation pneumonitis after stereotactic body radiotherapy for stage I lung cancer or small lung metastasis. *Radiother. Oncol.* **2011**, *101*, 267–270. [CrossRef]
69. Ishikawa, N.; Hattori, N.; Yokoyama, A.; Kohno, N. Utility of KL-6/MUC1 in the clinical management of interstitial lung diseases. *Respir. Investig.* **2012**, *50*, 3–13. [CrossRef]
70. Takeda, A.; Tsurugai, Y.; Sanuki, N.; Enomoto, T.; Shinkai, M.; Mizuno, T.; Aoki, Y.; Oku, Y.; Akiba, T.; Hara, Y.; et al. Clarithromycin mitigates radiation pneumonitis in patients with lung cancer treated with stereotactic body radiotherapy. *J. Thorac. Dis.* **2018**, *10*, 247–261. [CrossRef]
71. Hall, J.S.; Taylor, J.; Valentine, H.R.; Irlam, J.; Eustace, A.; Hoskin, P.J.; Miller, C.J.; West, C.M.L. Enhanced stability of microRNA expression facilitates classification of FFPE tumour samples exhibiting near total mRNA degradation. *Br. J. Cancer* **2012**, *107*, 684–694. [CrossRef]
72. Jiang, L.P.; He, C.Y.; Zhu, Z.T. Role of microRNA-21 in radiosensitivity in non-small cell lung cancer cells by targeting PDCD4 gene. *Oncotarget* **2017**, *8*, 23675–23689. [CrossRef]
73. Yin, J.; Zhao, J.; Hu, W.; Yang, G.; Yu, H.; Wang, R.; Wang, L.; Zhang, G.; Fu, W.; Dai, L.; et al. Disturbance of the let-7/LIN28 double-negative feedback loop is associated with radio- and chemo-resistance in non-small cell lung cancer. *PLoS ONE* **2017**, *12*, e0172787. [CrossRef]
74. Weidhaas, J.B.; Babar, I.; Nallur, S.M.; Trang, P.; Roush, S.; Boehm, M.; Gillespie, E.; Slack, F.J. MicroRNAs as Potential Agents to Alter Resistance to Cytotoxic Anticancer Therapy. *Cancer Res.* **2007**, *67*, 11111–11116. [CrossRef]
75. Arora, H.; Qureshi, R.; Jin, S.; Park, A.K.; Park, W.Y. miR-9 and let-7g enhance the sensitivity to ionizing radiation by suppression of NFκB1. *Exp. Mol. Med.* **2011**, *43*, 298–304. [CrossRef]
76. Grosso, S.; Doyen, J.; Parks, S.K.; Bertero, T.; Paye, A.; Cardinaud, B.; Gounon, P.; Lacas-Gervais, S.; Noël, A.; Pouysségur, J.; et al. MiR-210 Promotes a Hypoxic Phenotype and Increases Radioresistance in Human Lung Cancer Cell Lines. *Cell Death Dis.* **2013**, *4*, e544. [CrossRef]
77. Lou, Y.L.; Guo, F.; Liuetal, F. MiR-210 activates notch signaling pathway in angiogenesis induced by cerebral ischemia. *Mol. Cell. Biochem.* **2012**, *370*, 45–51. [CrossRef]

78. Sun, C.; Zeng, X.; Guo, H.; Wang, T.; Wei, L.; Zhang, Y.; Zhao, J.; Ma, X.; Zhang, N. MicroRNA-125a-5p modulates radioresistance in LTEP-a2 non-small cell lung cancer cells by targeting SIRT7. *Cancer Biomark.* **2020**, *27*, 39–49. [CrossRef]
79. Huang, X.; Zhang, T.; Li, G.; Guo, X.; Liu, X. Regulation of miR-125a expression by rs12976445 single-nucleotide polymorphism is associated with radiotherapy-induced pneumonitis in lung carcinoma patients. *J. Cell. Biochem.* **2019**, *120*, 4485–4493. [CrossRef]
80. Liu, Z.L.; Wang, H.; Liu, J.; Wang, Z.X. MicroRNA-21 (miR-21) expression promotes growth, metastasis, and chemo- or radioresistance in non-small cell lung cancer cells by targeting PTEN. *Mol. Cell. Biochem.* **2013**, *372*, 35–45. [CrossRef]
81. Yamada, K.M.; Araki, M. Tumor suppressor PTEN: Modulator of cell signaling, growth, migration and apoptosis. *J. Cell Sci.* **2001**, *114*, 2375–2382. [PubMed]
82. Kwon, O.S.; Kim, K.T.; Lee, E.; Kim, M.; Choi, S.H.; Li, H.; Fornace, A.J., Jr.; Cho, J.H.; Lee, Y.S.; Lee, J.S.; et al. Induction of MiR-21 by Stereotactic Body Radiotherapy Contributes to the Pulmonary Fibrotic Response. *PLoS ONE* **2016**, *11*, e0154942. [CrossRef] [PubMed]
83. Oh, J.S.; Kim, J.J.; Byun, J.Y.; Kim, I.A. Lin28-let7 Modulates Radiosensitivity of Human Cancer Cells with Activation of K-Ras. *Int. J. Radiat. Oncol. Biol. Phys.* **2010**, *76*, 5–8. [CrossRef] [PubMed]
84. Wang, X.C.; Wang, W.; Zhang, Z.B.; Zhao, J.; Tan, X.G.; Luo, J.C. Overexpression of miRNA-21 Promotes Radiation-Resistance of Non-Small Cell Lung Cancer. *Radiat. Oncol.* **2013**, *8*, 146. [PubMed]
85. Balça-Silva, J.; Sousa Neves, S.; Gonçalves, A.C.; Abrantes, A.M.; Casalta-Lopes, J.; Botelho, M.F.; Sarmento-Ribeiro, A.B.; Silva, H.C. Effect of miR-34b overexpression on the radiosensitivity of non-small celllung cancer cell lines. *Anticancer Res.* **2012**, *32*, 1603–1609. [PubMed]
86. Yang, H.; Tang, Y.; Guo, W.; Du, Y.; Wang, Y.; Li, P.; Zang, W.; Yin, X.; Wang, H.; Chu, H.; et al. Up-regulation of microRNA-138 induce radiosensitization in lung cancer cells. *Tumour Biol.* **2014**, *35*, 6557–6565. [CrossRef]
87. Chen, G.; Yu, L.; Dong, H.; Liu, Z.; Sun, Y. MiR-182 Enhances Radioresistance in Non-Small Cell Lung Cancer Cells by Regulating FOXO3. *Clin. Exp. Pharmacol. Physiol.* **2019**, *46*, 137–143. [CrossRef]
88. Chen, S.; Wang, H.; Ng, W.L.; Curran, W.J.; Wang, Y. Radiosensitizing effects of ectopic miR-101 on non-small-cell lung cancer cells depend on the endogenous miR-101 level. *Int. J. Radiat. Oncol. Biol. Phys.* **2011**, *81*, 1524–1529. [CrossRef]

Journal of *Personalized Medicine*

MDPI

Review

Blood-Derived Biomarkers of Diagnosis, Prognosis and Therapy Response in Prostate Cancer Patients

Katalin Balázs, Lilla Antal, Géza Sáfrány and Katalin Lumniczky *

Unit of Radiation Medicine, Department of Radiobiology and Radiohygiene, National Public Health Centre, 1221 Budapest, Hungary; balazs.katalin@osski.hu (K.B.); antal.lilla@osski.hu (L.A.); safrany.geza@osski.hu (G.S.)
* Correspondence: lumniczky.katalin@osski.hu; Tel.: +36-1-482-2011 or +36-30-554-9308

Abstract: Prostate cancer is among the most frequent cancers in men worldwide. Despite the fact that multiple therapeutic alternatives are available for its treatment, it is often discovered in an advanced stage as a metastatic disease. Prostate cancer screening is based on physical examination of prostate size and prostate-specific antigen (PSA) level in the blood as well as biopsy in suspect cases. However, these markers often fail to correctly identify the presence of cancer, or their positivity might lead to overdiagnosis and consequent overtreatment of an otherwise silent non-progressing disease. Moreover, these markers have very limited if any predictive value regarding therapy response or individual risk for therapy-related toxicities. Therefore, novel, optimally liquid biopsy-based (blood-derived) markers or marker panels are needed, which have better prognostic and predictive value than the ones currently used in the everyday routine. In this review the role of circulating tumour cells, extracellular vesicles and their microRNA content, as well as cellular and soluble immunological and inflammation- related blood markers for prostate cancer diagnosis, prognosis and prediction of therapy response is discussed. A special emphasis is placed on markers predicting response to radiotherapy and radiotherapy-related late side effects.

Keywords: prostate cancer; radiotherapy; liquid biopsy; circulating tumour cells; extracellular vesicles; microRNAs; immune system; inflammation

Citation: Balázs, K.; Antal, L.; Sáfrány, G.; Lumniczky, K. Blood-Derived Biomarkers of Diagnosis, Prognosis and Therapy Response in Prostate Cancer Patients. *J. Pers. Med.* **2021**, *11*, 296. https://doi.org/10.3390/jpm11040296

Academic Editors: Christophe Badie and Eric Andreas Rutten

Received: 17 March 2021
Accepted: 3 April 2021
Published: 13 April 2021

1. Introduction

Based on the 2020 cancer statistics of the International Agency for Research on Cancer (IARC) out of 19.3 million newly diagnosed cancers prostate cancer is ranked as the third most common among both sexes (constituting 7.1% of total cases). Regarding mortality rate it is on the eights place with approx. 375,000 deaths per year [1]. There are marked differences in the incidence of prostate cancer among various countries and races. It was reported that Japanese men living in Japan had very low prostate cancer incidence, while the incidence among USA resident Japanese increased and was at an intermediate level between Japanese living in Japan and European American men. Conversely, African American men have the highest incidence and mortality rates from prostate cancer within the United States [2,3]. These observations stress the importance of both genetic susceptibility and lifestyle in disease development and progression.

Among the main reasons for the increased prostate cancer mortality are the lack of reliable and effective prognostic biomarkers and methods which enable to recognise tumours in an early stage, to monitor individual therapy response more effectively, to sensitively detect minimal residual disease and development of distant metastasis as well as predict tumour relapse. These markers would allow patient stratification for optimal response rate to a certain therapy and enable the identification of those patients who are at increased risk for developing therapy-related side effects; thus, they are prerequisites for the development of efficient individualized anticancer treatment protocols.

At present diagnosis of prostate cancer is complex and is based on symptoms such as difficulties in urination, presence of blood in the urine or sperm, physical examination (including rectal digital examination), ultrasound examination, blood test to measure the prostate specific antigen (PSA) and tissue sample testing (biopsy). Due to the rather unspecific symptoms, early diagnosis of prostate cancer is not without problems and often the disease is only diagnosed in an advanced stage, where actually symptoms related to bone metastasis (bone pain and limb weakness caused by spinal marrow compression) are already present. While early detection of prostate cancer is fully curable, the efficiency of anti-cancer treatment in an advanced stage of the disease is very low.

Therefore, regular screening protocols in asymptomatic men with the purpose of identifying early-stage prostate cancer would be very important. Though, regular screening for prostate cancer has certain caveats. One such caveat is that more than 75% of PSA-positive tests (with blood PSA levels above 4 ng/mL, traditionally used as a cut-off value) are followed by a negative biopsy [4]. Biopsy can lead to infections [5], significant drop in quality of life [6] and can cause urinary, bowel and sexual dysfunctions persisting for several months [7,8]. Another caveat is the identification of indolent prostate cancer patients. Based on autopsy material, prostate cancers are identified at a much younger age (31–40 years) than clinically diagnosed in symptomatic patients. It appears that some prostate cancers may pass through a period of latency of up to 15 to 20 years, during which the disease is histologically present but it is completely asymptomatic. PSA-based screening of the population might result in over-diagnosed and therefore over-treated indolent prostate cancers resulting in serious side effects (such as incontinence and impotence), which would have caused no clinical consequences during a man's lifetime if left untreated [9–11].

The issue of regular prostate cancer screening is a dilemma all over the world. Currently, in several European countries the main indications of annual prostate monitoring are age (men over 45 years) and/or family history. Nevertheless, the influence of family history for the risk of developing prostate cancer is recently being under revision due to studies with contradictory conclusions (Selkirk, Wang et al., 2015, Abdel-Rahman 2019). Increasing number of studies are investigating benefits, harms and cost-effectiveness of prostate cancer screening based on experimental and clinical data, clinical trials and model calculations. Two big studies are especially worth mentioning. One such study called the European Randomised Study of Screening for Prostate Cancer (ERSPC) randomized more than 180,000 men from Europe to analyse the longitudinal relationship between PSA values and biopsy (biopsy was carried out if blood PSA level was 3.0 ng/mL or higher) at regular intervals (every 4 years). After 13 years of follow-up the risk of prostate cancer mortality decreased 21% in the surveyed population compared to control group [12]. The other one called the Prostate, Lung, Colorectal and Ovarian (PLCO) carried out in the USA randomised more than 76,000 men using basically similar screening principles to the ERSPC study. Their final, updated conclusion, as a result of an extended follow up was that no significant difference was found in prostate cancer mortality in the screened group compared to control [13]. Thus, regarding the primary endpoint of the two studies, namely, to evaluate the predictive value of PSA screening in reducing prostate cancer mortality the two trials seem to reach contradictory conclusions. However, a recent re-analysis of both trials showed that the discordant results were due to differences in implementation and setting. After correcting them both studies reached the conclusion that screening could significantly reduce prostate cancer death [14]. These clinical trials highlight the overall positive balance of screening even using a marker (PSA) by far not optimal in detecting those patients which indeed should be treated for prostate cancer. More efficient, cost-effective and specific screening methodology is needed to reliably discriminate prostate cancer from benign alterations or other non-cancerous prostate diseases. Screening is especially important in races with an increased incidence of the disease (African American men) in order to reduce racial differences in prostate cancer survival [15].

Over the past decade, liquid biopsy investigations have received more and more attention. This minimal invasive method enables us to study a wide array of blood-based cellular and secreted soluble or vesicular markers, which offer a complex, comprehensive and real-time information on tumour stage, progression, tumour micro- and macro-environment, including the integrity of the anti-tumour immune response. These complex indicators might serve as prognostic and/or predictive markers able to predict patients' outcomes, their response to particular therapies, forecast the formation of late therapy-related side effects (such as secondary tumours after radiotherapy) and ultimately to improve medical decision-making [16]. Blood-based markers of prognosis or therapy responsiveness are especially important in prostate cancer patients because of the high heterogeneity and molecular diversity of prostate cancer and because the prostate gland contains different subclones, which respond differently to treatments [17,18], so prostate gland biopsy can be misleading.

In this review, we summarize the current knowledge on blood-based liquid biopsy analyses in prostate cancer focusing on disease- and therapy-related changes in PSA and related molecules, immune cells and immune- and inflammation-related secreted factors, circulating tumour cells (CTCs) and tumour-derived cell-free circulating nucleic acids as well as extracellular vesicles (EVs) and their micro-RNA (miRNA) content (Figure 1 and Table 1). We also discuss the relevance of these markers in radiotherapy-treated patients, in predicting their therapy-response or their risk for developing radiotherapy-induced late toxicities. Apart of blood-derived markers a large panel of urine and tissue-based potential biomarkers with prognostic and/or predictive value are identified. A few are already in the possession of clinical approval and some are still in an experimental stage. Though, in the present review we do not wish to focus on these. Detailed reviews such as [19–24] are available on these topics. For interested readers we advise consulting these publications.

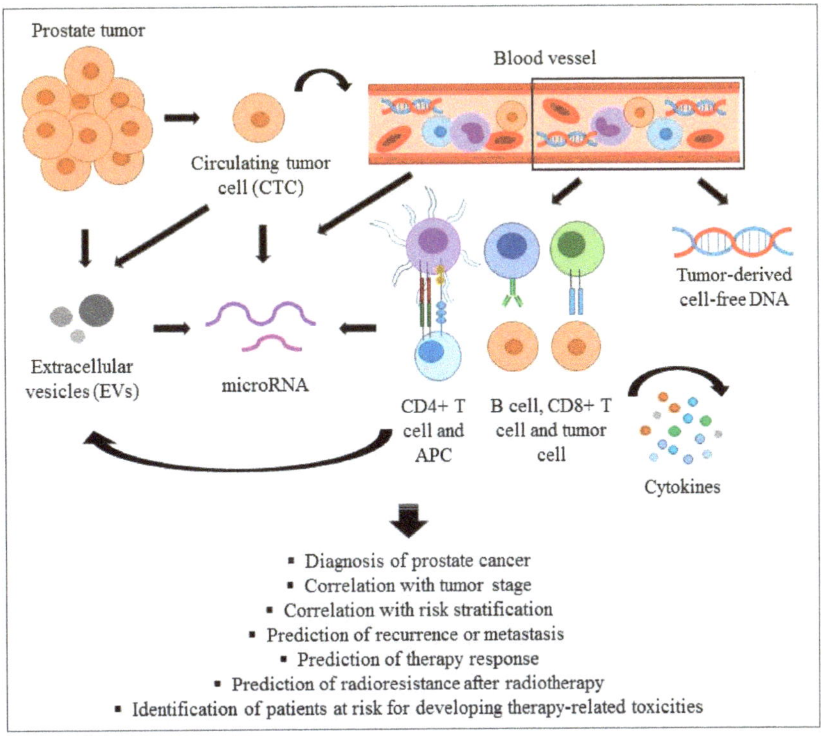

Figure 1. Overview of candidate blood-based liquid biopsy markers in prostate cancer patients.

This schematic picture summarizes the current knowledge on liquid biopsy analyses in prostate cancer focusing on circulating tumour cells (CTCs), immune cells and secreted factors such as tumour-derived cell-free circulating nucleic acids, cytokines and chemokines, as well as EVs released by prostate cancer cells, CTCs or various immune cells and their microRNA (miRNA) content.

2. Blood-Based Liquid Biopsy Marker Candidates

2.1. PSA and Related Molecules

At present, PSA is the most widespread and most accepted biomarker for prostate cancer monitoring; however, it lacks many of the qualities of an ideal tumour marker. PSA is a serine protease secreted physiologically by the prostate gland epithelium [25]. The total PSA (tPSA) is present in the serum in two forms, free (fPSA) and conjugated to serum proteins like alpha1 antichymotripsin, alpha2 macroglobulin and alpha1 protease inhibitor. Free PSA is comprised of pro PSA, benign PSA (BPSA) and intact PSA. Pro PSA is a zymogen precursor of PSA that comes in four different isoforms, as determined by the length of its pro leader peptide sequences [26]. Pro PSA is associated with cancer, BPSA with benign diseases whilst the association of intact PSA is currently unknown [27]. The free component represents about 5%–35% of tPSA [28]. The normal range of tPSA (commonly called as PSA) is 0–4 ng/mL in peripheral blood and levels above 10 ng/mL are considered pathological [29].

Monitoring regular variations in PSA level might serve as rough indicators of cancer progression (and regression after therapy) as well as disease recurrence. Since PSA is a tumour-associated antigen (TAA) and not a tumour-specific one, its specificity in prostate cancer diagnosis is not 100%, since inflammation, benign prostate hyperplasia (BPH) or other non-malignant disorders could also cause increased blood PSA levels, while normal PSA levels do not necessarily exclude the presence of a tumour. Furthermore, the age of cancer patients also influences the risk of cancer-specific death. With 7–10 ng/mL of PSA the risk of death is only 7% for men aged 50–59 but increases to 51% for men aged 80–89, 10 years after diagnosis [30].

As mentioned before, 75% of men with PSA levels above 4 ng/mL are not diagnosed with prostate cancer on biopsy. Only 26% of patients with PSA level within the "grey zone" of 4.1–9.9 ng/mL have cancer [31]. The PSA grey zone needs more accurate non-invasive diagnostic biomarkers to avoid the false-positive results because of benign changes. It was shown that PSA produced by prostate cancer cells escape degradation and occur in complexed form in the serum. When serum PSA is between 4 and 10 ng/mL and free to total PSA ratio (F/T ratio) is less than 25%, one should strongly suspect prostate malignancy, thus avoiding up to 20% of unnecessary prostate biopsies [32].

The so-called 'prostate healthy index' (PHI) reflects the ratio between total PSA, free PSA and pro PSA levels and prostate health index density (PHID) combines PHI parameters with prostate volume. These markers are clear improvement over PSA since they allow a better distinction between benign and malignant prostate gland hypertrophy and improve the prediction of high-grade and clinically aggressive prostatic tumours, especially in cases where PSA levels are in the grey zone [33–38].

The four kallikrein (4K) test measures tPSA, fPSA, intact PSA and human kallikrein-related peptidase 2 (hK2) in serum and is used to get a probability score for prostate cancer [39]. Similar to PHI, it improves the identification of overall and high-grade cancer and helps with reducing unnecessary biopsies [40,41]. Combined with PHI increases their diagnostic value [37]. Both the PHI and 4K test have been approved by the US Food and Drug Administration (FDA) to be used for prostate cancer screening. Recently two novel cancer-related glycoproteins, thrombospondin 1 (THBS1) and cathepsin D (CTSD) were proposed as blood-based biomarkers that outperformed PSA in distinguishing benign disease from prostate cancer in men with enlarged prostate gland [42]. A recently commercialized product—the Proclarix—incorporating THBS1, CTSD, tPSA and % of fPSA, combined with patient age, yielded a significantly better diagnostic accuracy compared to either PSA or % of fPSA alone in discriminating clinically significant from no or insignificant prostate cancer [43,44]. Though we have not found studies comparing the diagnostic efficiency of Proclarix with either PHI or 4K test.

2.2. Circulating Tumour Cells (CTCs) and Cell-Free Circulating Tumour DNA (cfDNA)

Prostate cancer metastasis is initiated by CTCs originating from the primary tumour transported through the blood or lymphatic system [45]. Some CTCs die in the circulation, others proliferate and form metastasis in distant organs [46]. Experimental models indicate that millions of tumour cells continuously circulate through the body, although only few of them can survive by evading the immune response and systemic therapies, reach a distant organ, proliferate and ultimately form metastases [47].

The number of CTCs in peripheral blood is very low, on average one CTC per one million peripheral blood mononuclear cells (PBMCs) [48], so their isolation is challenging. Several approaches have been reported for CTC detection, isolation and characterization in the peripheral blood of cancer patients such as two-stage microfluidic chip technology [49], acoustic separation of CTCs [50] and in situ hybridization (ISH) technology combined with immunomagnetic selection [51]. There are label-free techniques as well, which include size-based and density-based approaches [52] and methods based on Ficoll-Paque centrifugation [53], electrical property-based separation [54] and leukocyte depletion (anti-CD45 immunomagnetic negative selection) [55]. At present, the CellSearch™ method is an FDA-approved technology based on CTC characterisation used to predict the outcome of prostate cancer patients. It enriches CTCs from the peripheral blood using a magnetic ferrofluid containing antibodies against epithelial cell adhesion molecule (EpCAM), which is a common CTC marker. Cells are then stained for expression of cytokeratine (CK) 8, 18, and 19, all of which are intracellular structural proteins found in epithelial cells [56].

CTCs are critical for monitoring anti-cancer therapeutic efficacy such as drug screening [57], since resistance towards various chemotherapeutic agents remains a major clinical challenge [58]. Regular monitoring of CTCs can give a more complex and more realistic view of tumour heterogeneity than conventional biopsy [59]. Furthermore, CTCs are independent prognostic factors of progression-free survival (PFS) and overall survival (OS) in metastatic breast [60], colon [61] and prostate cancers [62] and their presence was implicated in worse cancer prognosis and outcome [63]. Patients with CTC numbers higher than 5 per 7.5 mL whole blood (as compared with the group with CTC numbers lower than 5 per 7.5 mL blood) had shorter median PFS and OS [64]. Quantification of CTCs has been proposed also as a potential surrogate endpoint to promote the selection of treatment algorithms [65] especially in advanced-stage prostate cancer disease, although the small number of cells detectable in the blood of prostate cancer patients and the lack of specific molecular determinants on CTCs indicative of therapy response have limited its clinical utility [66].

Not just CTC numbers can serve as prognostic markers but also the repertoire of their cell surface molecules which could also indicate the efficacy of various therapies such as radiotherapy or immune therapy. The EpCAM glycoprotein was initially described as one of the most commonly used protein CTC markers, however its level was shown to be downregulated during the dissemination of cancer cells from primary tumour [67]. Therefore, using CTCs as biomarkers of therapy response based purely on their immune phenotypical changes might be misleading because of their dynamic evolution during cancer progression [68].

Certain studies suggest that CTCs adopt different strategies to protect themselves from therapy-induced cell death, developing an epithelial to mesenchymal transition (EMT), grouping into clusters or switching between cancer stem cell state and differentiated cancer cell state. Not only individual CTCs, but also CTC clusters, their EMT and the presence of cancer-associated macrophage-like cells (CAMLs) in the blood are indicative for an increased risk of metastatic disease. Compared to single CTCs, CTC clusters may be more aggressive in forming distal metastasis [69]. CTC cluster size and number have been associated with lower overall survival in patients with breast, pancreatic, or prostate cancer [70–72]. These additional features of CTCs apart of their immune phenotypical changes have improved their prognostic value.

The programmed cell death protein (PD-1) and its ligand 1 (PD-L1) are major targets of the immune checkpoint inhibitor therapies in metastatic cancer diseases. PD-L1 expressing circulating epithelial tumour cells (CETCs) are described in 100% of prostate, 94.5% of breast, 95.4% of colorectal and 82% of lung cancer patients. Monitoring the frequency of PD-L1 positive CTCs could reflect individual patient's response to anti-PD-1/PD-L1 therapy [59,73]. Expression of nuclear PD-L1 (nPD-L1) in the CTCs of prostate cancer patients was shown to significantly correlate with short survival rate [74]. In conclusion, the use of CTC-based models for risk assessment can improve standard cancer staging.

The effect of radiotherapy on CTCs is controversial. Martin et al. described that fractionated radiotherapy disrupted the tumour mass in non-small cell lung cancer (NSCLC), thus promoting the passage of tumour cells into the circulation [75]. In contrast, Budna-Tukan et al. analysed the number of CTCs in patients with non-metastatic high-risk prostate cancer with three different innovative CTC enumeration technologies before and after radiotherapy. They did not find any differences and significant therapy-related changes in CTC counts. These latter data do not support the hypothesis that radiotherapy leads to CTC release into the circulation in prostate cancer most probably because radiotherapy efficiently reduces tumour size in patients with prostate cancer, therefore the number of cancer cells in the circulation should also partially or totally decrease. It would be interesting to analyse this CTC number in patients with worse prognosis and metastatic disease as well. Furthermore, the reason for the difference between radiotherapy effects on CTCs in NSCLC and prostate cancer could be that these tumours respond differently to radiotherapy. Less effective radiotherapy leads to a suboptimal tumour response, and possibly an increase in CTC numbers [76].

Some patients undergoing prostate brachytherapy develop distant metastases despite the absence of local recurrence. Although micrometastases were not detected by radiographic images in these patients, cytokeratine positive or PSA positive cells were present in the bone marrow aspirates, which were considered disseminated tumour cells (DTCs) [77]. It has been proposed that in the early phases of radiotherapy, when cancer cells suffer only from sub-lethal damage, the quick increase of CTCs could, in principle, contribute to the development of distant metastases [76]. Another explanation is that surgical manipulation with needles being inserted into the prostate tissue during brachytherapy may pose a potential risk for haematogenous spillage of prostate cancer cells and play a role in distant metastases development [78].

Quantification of cell-free circulating tumour nucleotides in blood samples is another promising new molecular strategy for non-invasive tumour monitoring in prostate cancer [79]. CfDNA may be more suitable than CTCs to estimate therapy efficiency in patients with early-stage disease [80]. CfDNA originates from apoptotic or necrotic cells (including CTCs) or is actively secreted by cancer cells [81] and has been detected in human blood, urine and semen [82].

CTCs carry the complete mutation spectrum of the primary tumours and metastases, [16,83] and therefore genetic and transcriptional analysis of individual CTCs might enable personalized medical decisions for cancer therapy and provide insights into the biological processes involved in metastasis. Somatic mutations are detected in advanced or metastatic tumours, so they are unsuitable for monitoring primary, nonmetastatic disease [84,85]. Conversely chromosomal rearrangements represent an early stage of cancer pathogenesis [86]. The most common chromosomal rearrangement in prostate cancer present in approx. 50% of patients results from the fusion of the androgen-regulated gene, transmembrane protease serine 2 gene (*TMPRSS2*, chr21q22.2), with E-twenty-six (ETS)-related gene (*ERG*, chr21q22.3). This rearrangement is detectable in CTCs or as cfDNA and might be considered as a highly tumour-specific, non-invasive molecular biomarker for therapy assessment, risk stratification and relapse detection [79,87,88]. Furthermore, prostate cancer carrying this rearrangement can regulate the recruitment and infiltration of regulatory T cells (Tregs) in the tumour [89].

Gene expression analysis of CTCs of prostate cancer patients have revealed altered expression levels of eight metastasis-related metabolic genes, such as phosphoglycerate kinase 1 (*PGK1*) and glucose-6-phosphate dehydrogenase (*G6PD*) responsible for optimal glucose metabolism in CTCs. Their increased expression level in CTCs was associated with advanced tumour stage and metastasis proneness [90].

The clonal evolution of cancer cells can be traced at the level of CTC DNA or cfDNA by next generation sequencing or tumour mutation allele frequency analyses. The dynamics and relative abundance of the different clones are suitable to evaluate disease and metastasis heterogeneity, to monitor the emergence of resistance mechanisms as well as therapy resistance [91]. Quantification of cfDNA can reveal treatment ineffectiveness at an early stage of the treatment protocol and also avoid toxicity of ineffective overtreatment. Thus, patients can receive alternative therapies [92]. Since both CTCs and cfDNA can be retrieved basically in a non-invasive manner by blood collection, their regular follow up allows a more precise monitoring of disease progression and a better patient care as well.

2.3. Cellular and Soluble Immunological Markers

Systemic inflammatory conditions as well as the components of adaptive and innate immunity are involved in the initiation and progression of prostate cancer [93–95]. The role of chronic inflammation in this process involves multiple mechanisms such as: (a) mutagenesis caused by oxidative stress, (b) remodelling of the extracellular matrix, (c) recruitment of immune cells including tumour-associated neutrophils (TANs), tumour-infiltrating macrophages (TIMs), myeloid-derived suppressor cells (MDSCs), mast cells, as well as fibroblasts, and endothelial cells, (d) elevated secretion of cytokines and growth factors contributing to a proliferative and angiogenic environment [96–98].

Innate immune cells (macrophages, neutrophils) are triggered by foreign microbial and viral structures, known as pathogen-associated molecular patterns (PAMPs), or normal cellular constituents released upon injury and cell death, known as damage-associated molecular patterns (DAMPs), which are recognized by pattern-recognition receptors (PRRs), like the Toll-like receptor (TLR) family [99]. Innate immune cells are the main players in the early phase of the inflammation and affect tumour progression via intercellular signalling including cytokines and chemokines [100]. Tan et al. found in animal studies that the Cystein-X-Cystein (C-X-C) motif chemokine ligand 9 (CXCL9) regulated the host's response to inflammation by recruiting leukocytes to the inflammatory environment and had important role in promoting prostate tumorigenesis [101]. Activation of the innate immune system implies upregulation of major histocompatibility (MHC) class I and II molecules on the surface of nucleated cells and antigen presenting cells (APCs) like macrophages, dendritic cells (DCs) and B lymphocytes and presentation of tumour associated antigens on their MHC molecules to naive T lymphocytes [102]. These processes induce the production of different inflammatory chemokines and cytokines, which in turn lead to the activation of both the cellular and humoral arm of the adaptive immune response [103].

An important step in prostate cancer development is tumour immune escape manifested among others in defects in antigen presentation (human leukocyte antigen (HLA) class I receptor deficiency on cytotoxic T cells), imbalance in T helper type 1 (Th1) and Th2 cytokine production leading to elevated levels of immunosuppressive cytokines such as interleukine-4 (IL-4), IL-6 and IL-10. Furthermore, induction of T cell death, T cell receptor dysfunction, prostate tumour infiltration with tolerogenic DCs and Tregs are also important indicators of an immune suppressing microenvironment and low tumour immunogenicity [104].

Granulocyte colony-stimulating factor (G-CSF), IL-1β, or tumour necrosis factor (TNF) secreted by tumour cells extend the lifespan of neutrophils and attract them to the tumour microenvironment, where they become immunosuppressive tumour-associated neutrophils, which stimulate proliferation of tumour cells and angiogenesis [105]. Macrophages are important in promoting growth and bone metastasis of prostate cancer [106]. Monocyte chemotactic protein (MCP)-1/C-C motif ligand (CCL)2 secreted by cancer cells recruits tumour-infiltrating macrophages and induces tumour progression [107]. MDSCs are the immature form of myeloid cells and they suppress anti-tumour immune responses in the tumour microenvironment. Tregs are among the most important immune cell populations suppressing antitumour immune responses [108]. Increased Treg infiltration in the tumour microenvironment through C-C chemokine receptor 4 (CCR4) [109] with the high expression level of the cytotoxic T-lymphocyte-associated protein 4 (CTLA-4) and PD-1 markers was linked with a poor prognosis in prostate cancer [110,111]. Several studies published that the number of Tregs showed significant correlation with the number of macrophages with tumour promoting M2 phenotype in the prostate cancer microenvironment and together they were associated with a worse clinical outcome [112,113]. Furthermore, isoforms of cluster of differentiation 44 (CD44) transmembrane glycoprotein receptor serve also as a poor prognostic factor in prostate cancer. This receptor has different isoforms. The standard isoform (CD44std) is expressed in normal epithelial cells [114], while the variant isoforms (CD44v) are highly expressed in several epithelial-type carcinomas [115]. Increased expression of CD44v (also known as CD44 variant 6) was associated with progressive disease and poor prognosis in prostate cancer [116].

Several immune and inflammatory genes harbouring single nucleotide polymorphisms (SNPs) associated with prostate cancer risk were identified, including pattern recognition receptors (macrophage scavenger receptor 1 or *MSR1, TLR1, TLR4, TLR5, TLR6,* and *TLR10*) [117–120]; antiviral genes (ribonuclease L or *RNASEL*) [121,122]; cytokines (macrophage inhibitory cytokine 1 or *MIC1, IL-8, TNF-α,* and IL-1 receptor antagonist or *IL1RN*) [123,124]; and the proinflammatory gene cyclooxygenase 2 (*COX-2*) [125].

Several of the identified gene expression signatures in prostate cancer are also immune-related, highlighting the importance of immune system in disease pathogenesis. Liong et al. developed a blood-based biomarker panel consisting of 7 mRNAs and demonstrated in 739 prostate cancer patients that the panel could identify men with aggressive prostate cancer. It is important to highlight that the majority of the differentially expressed genes were involved in immune processes [126]. Wallace et al. reported differential gene expression signatures in prostate cancer samples from African American and European American men and the majority of the differentially expressed genes was also immune related (immune response, defence response, antigen presentation, B/T cell function, cytokine signalling, chemokines, inflammatory response) [127]. The C-X-C motif chemokine receptor 4 (CXCR4) chemokine, previously linked to tumour metastasis [128] was differentially expressed between tumour and surrounding non-tumour tissue in African American men and the CXCR4 pathway was the highest-ranked pathway showing differential expression pattern among tumour and non-tumour tissue in African American men [127,129]. Clinical application of these gene expression signatures in therapy individualisation holds great promise. Though, we should mention that the so-far tested approaches for molecular characterisation of prostate cancer are based on biopsy tissues. In order to overcome serial biopsies, analysis of CTCs holds great promise in the non-invasive molecular profiling of prostate cancer and in determining both tumour- and patient-derived heterogeneity in disease progression and therapy response. A report on CTC-based liquid biopsy signatures with prognostic relevance and with implications in therapy decision has recently been published [130].

Radiotherapy can influence immune processes by increasing the expression of TAAs and DAMPs, as well as inducing cell death and secondary release of the proinflammatory cytokines and chemokines [131,132]. Radiotherapy-induced DNA, protein and lipid damage was shown to increase free radical levels in the circulation released by directly irradiated cells [133]. Gupta et al. found that IL-6, IL-8, TNF-α and transforming growth factor-beta (TGF-β) were the major mediators of ionizing radiation response in prostate cancer after radiation therapy influencing signalling pathways targeting transcription factors such as nuclear factor kappa B (NF-kB), activator protein-1 (AP-1) and signal transducers and activators of transcription (STATs). These transcription factors further enhanced expression of IL-1β and TNF-α [134]. Furthermore, radiotherapy also upregulated MHC class I on cancer cells, leading to the recognition of TAAs by cytotoxic T cells, enabling them to raise an antitumour response. Thus, prostate radiotherapy could potentially initiate a systemic, or 'abscopal' immune response, resulting in antitumorigenic responses in distant metastases [135]. According to Reits et al., the effect of γ-irradiation on MHC class I molecules could explain immune-mediated abscopal effects [136,137].

It was shown that, in patients responsive to androgen deprivation therapy (ADT), the baseline levels of certain immune markers such as IL-6, IL-10, granulocyte macrophage colony stimulating factor (GM-CSF) was significantly lower, and the level of certain pro-inflammatory cytokines (IL-5, interferon-γ (IFN-γ), TNF-α) during the course of the therapy was significantly higher than in patients resistant to ADT [138]. Both ADT and radiotherapy can damage the endothelium network in prostate cancer and vascular damage is part of radiotherapy-caused late toxicities [139]. It was reported that ADT downregulated vascular endothelial growth factor (VEGF) in normal tissue as well as in malignant prostatic tissue. In the absence of VEGF immature blood vessels underwent selective apoptosis and endothelial dysfunction [140]. Microvascular endothelial cell apoptosis after high dose irradiation constituted a primary lesion, developing into persistent endothelial dysfunction with microvessel collapse, endothelial cell activation and ultimately premature aging and senescence [139]. These effects impact normal tissue homeostasis leading to hypoxia and consequent ischemia, as well as inflammation and fibrosis. The early phases of fibrogenesis after irradiation were characterized by the upregulation of pro-inflammatory cytokines such as TNF-α, IL-1 and IL-6 and many growth factors in the irradiated tissue [141]. It was shown that a complex balance between TGF-β [142] and its downstream effector connective tissue growth factor (CTGF) [143], the antifibrotic proteins such as TNF-α and IFN-γ was important in this process [144].

Prostate cancer is among the more radioresistant malignant tumours [145]; the disease recurs in 30%–40% of prostate cancer patients receiving radiation therapy [146]. A retrospective study investigated the overexpression of 24 genes (DNA damage regulated autophagy modulator 1 or *DRAM1*, keratin 14 or *KRT14*, protein tyrosine phosphatase, non-receptor type 22 or *PTPN22*, zinc finger matrin-type 3 or *ZMAT3*, Rho GTPase activating protein 15 or *ARHGAP1*, *IL-1B*, anillin actin binding protein or *ANLN*, ribosomal protein S27a or *RPS27A*, melanoma associated antigen mutated 1 or *MUM1*, topoisomerase (DNA) II alpha or *TOP2A*, cyclin dependent kinase inhibitor 3 or *CDKN3*, G protein subunit gamma 11 or *GNG11*, haematopoietic cell-specific Lyn substrate 1 or *HCLS1*, denticleless E3 ubiquitin protein ligase homologue or *DTL*, IL-7 receptor or *IL-7R*, ubiquitin like modifier activating enzyme 7 or *UBA7*, NIMA related kinase 1 or *NEK1*, CDKN2A interacting protein or *CDKN2AIP*, apurinic/apyrimidinic endonuclease 2 or *APEX2*, kinesin family member 23 or *KIF23*, sulfatase 2 or *SULF2*, polo like kinase 2 or *PLK2*, essential meiotic structure-specific endonuclease 1 or *EME1*, and bridging integrator 2 or *BIN2*) related to radiotherapy and DNA damage-response and found that their expression signatures predicted response to radiotherapy and radioresistance in prostate cancer patients and helped specifically with selecting patients profiting from radiotherapy [147]. Further predictive markers of radioresistance are oxidative stress markers such as lipid peroxidation 4-hydroxylnonenal (4HNE) or 3-nitrotyrosine (3NT) [148,149]. Preclinical studies showed that hypoxia lead to a radioresistant and metastatic phenotype of prostate tumours [150]. Extracellular vesicles could mediate hypoxia-induced prostate cancer progression, enhanced the invasiveness and stemness of prostate cancer cells and increased the level of signalling molecules such as TGF-β2, TNF-1α, IL-6, tumour susceptibility gene 101 (TSG101), protein kinase B (PKB or Akt), integrin-linked kinase 1 (ILK1), matrix metalloproteinase (MMP), and β-catenin [151]. High level of the IL-8 (CXCL8) chemokine was also associated with increased radioresistance [152]. Sequence variants of several genes such as ataxia-teleangiectasia mutated (*ATM*), breast cancer type 1 susceptibility protein (*BRCA1*), H2A histone family member X (*H2AFX*) and mediator of DNA damage checkpoint protein 1 (*MDC1*) were linked to increased radiosensitivity and could distinguish prostate cancer patients with high radiation toxicity from those with low toxicity [153,154]. Langsenlehner et al. investigated

603 patients treated with three-dimensional conformal radiotherapy and found that single nucleotide polymorphisms in the X-ray repair cross-complementing protein 1 (*XRCC1*) gene was associated with radiation-induced late toxicity in prostate cancer patients [155].

2.4. Extracellular Vesicles

Extracellular vesicles (EVs) received considerable attention in recent years because of their role in intercellular communication. EVs are phospholipid bilayer membrane-coated vesicles released by most cell types in physiological and pathological conditions [156]. Since EVs are highly heterogeneous in size, biogenesis, function, content, membrane markers, and so forth [157], we use "extracellular vesicle" as a generic term to describe any type of membrane-coated vesicles (e.g., exosomes, microvesicles, microparticles, apoptotic bodies, etc.) released into the extracellular matrix. A common feature of all types of EVs is their complex cargo consisting of various bioactive molecules, like proteins, lipids, DNA-fragments, different species of RNAs. These molecules are protected by the lipid membrane of the EVs and thus they are transported in an intact and biologically functional form between cells [156,158,159].

The release of EVs from cells and their journey throughout the body is not random, several regulated mechanisms underlie this process. It was shown that cancer cells produced more EVs compared to normal cells [160]. This might be partly due to the acidic environment characteristic for many cancers. Several studies demonstrated that the extracellular pH was an important modifier of EV traffic, since low pH altered EV membrane fluidity [161] and increased EV release and uptake [162]. Under chronic hypoxia prostate cancer cells secreted more EVs as a survival mechanism to remove metabolic waste [163]. Tumour-derived EVs played a key role in tumour cell growth and in the crosstalk between cancer cells and the tumour microenvironment (TME), contributing to the development of a cancer-supportive microenvironment, angiogenesis [164,165] and metastasis [166,167].

Since tumour derived EVs have specific cargos, which differentiate them from EVs released under physiological conditions, and given the fact that they are released into various human body fluids (e.g., blood, saliva, urine, amniotic fluids, sperm, bile, etc.) [158], EVs represent a source of biomarkers for the early detection of cancer, therapeutic planning and monitoring. EVs can transmit their information to recipient cells in several ways, such as (a) transfer of bioactive molecules which regulate signalling pathways in recipient cells; (b) receptor shuttling to alter cellular activities; (c) delivery of fully functional proteins to accomplish specific functions in target cells; (d) and providing new genetic information with various type of nucleic acids to gain new traits [168]. Accordingly, different types of biomolecules within the EV cargo can serve as prognostic and predictive biomarkers in cancer. Increased plasma EV levels in prostate cancer patients were reported by several studies [169–172] but reports are contradictory whether prostate cancer cell-derived EVs could be distinguished from total plasma EVs based on the presence of prostate-specific membrane antigen (PSMA) on the EV membrane. Plasmatic EVs expressing both CD81 and PSA were significantly higher in prostate cancer patients compared to either healthy controls or patients with BPH, reaching 100% specificity and sensitivity in distinguishing prostate cancer patients from healthy individuals [172]. Biggs et al. reported that prostate-specific plasma EV (identified based on PSMA expression on the EV membrane) numbers were suitable to identify prostate cancer patients with high risk, and those with metastatic disease [169]. On the other hand, Joncas et al. found that PSMA expression on plasma EVs was not a reliable marker for the identification of prostate cancer cell-specific EVs. Their conclusion was based on the proteomic analysis of PSMA-enriched EVs, in which no cancer-specific proteins could be identified [170].

Investigation of plasma EV cargo, mainly their protein and RNA content is receiving much attention as diagnostic and prognostic tools in prostate cancer. EVs isolated from either plasma or urine could be utilized to monitor prostate cancer stages, to discriminate high-grade from low-grade prostate cancer and benign disease, thereby reducing the number of unnecessary biopsies. Although it is not a blood-based marker, it is important to mention that ExoDx Prostate, a commercialized, urine-based test evaluates 3 EV-derived mRNAs, used to identify high-grade prostate cancer in patients with previous negative biopsies or with low initial PSA values [173].

Survivin is an apoptosis inhibitor selectively expressed in different tumours, including prostate cancer, and its main role is to promote cancer cell survival and protect cancer cells from apoptosis. It was shown that survivin was present in EVs secreted by prostate cancer cells and survivin levels in plasma-derived EVs from newly diagnosed prostate cancer patients (both early-stage and advanced cancers) and patients who relapsed after chemotherapy were significantly increased. These findings indicate that plasma EV-derived suvivin might be a promising liquid biopsy marker for the early diagnosis and systemic monitoring of prostate cancer [174].

Lundholm et al. found that NKG2D ligand-expressing prostate tumour-derived EVs selectively induced the downregulation of NKG2D on natural killer (NK) and CD8+ T cells, leading to damaged cytotoxic T cell function in vitro. Consistently with these data, surface NKG2D expression on circulating NK and CD8+ T cells was significantly decreased in patients with castration-resistant prostate cancer (CRPC) compared to healthy individuals [175]. These findings suggest that prostate tumour-derived EVs promote immune suppression and tumour escape by acting as down-regulators of the NKG2D-mediated cytotoxic response in prostate cancer patients.

Androgen receptor splice variant 7 (AR-V7) was associated with resistance to hormonal therapy in castration-resistant prostate cancer and plasma-derived EVs were shown to contain AR-V7 RNA [176]. Validation of AR-V7 as a potential target for treatment of CRPC could make it a clinically predictive biomarker of resistance to hormonal therapy and facilitate the decision-making process and therapy planning in these patients. Additionally, another study suggested that EV AR-V7 RNA was correlated with lower level of sexual steroid hormones in CRPC patients with a poor prognosis [170].

2.5. MicroRNAs

RNA content of EVs is considerably different from their parent cells, suggesting that cells can selectively sort their species of RNA into EVs, including small non-coding RNAs such as miRNAs or miRs with important regulatory functions on protein expression. Each miRNA regulates multiple target messenger RNAs (mRNAs). They control protein expression through the degradation of mRNAs or the inhibition of protein translation of target mRNAs by binding to the 3′-untranslated region (UTR). In view of their complex regulatory ability, it is not surprising that abnormal miRNA expression has been described in the pathogenesis of several diseases including cancer. Incorporation of miRNAs into EVs or binding to RNA-binding protein complexes increases their stability and protects them from degradation by various environmental factors [177]. Therefore, miRNAs are very stable in serum, plasma and other biofluids and are resistant to boiling, pH change, repeated freeze-thaw cycles, and fragmentation by chemical or enzymes [178], making them ideal biomarker candidates for the diagnosis, prognosis, and therapeutic planning in cancer disease, including prostate cancer. So far miRNA research in the prostate cancer field mainly focused on the characterization of differentially expressed miRNAs or miRNA panels involved in tumour progression [179]. Relatively few clinical trials have been conducted to date to explore miRNAs as indicators of prognosis or prediction of therapy response (Table 1).

Recently, plasma-derived EVs have proved to be better sources for miRNAs than unfractionated plasma/serum for certain but not all miRNAs. EV-incorporated miR-200c-3p and miR-21-5p could differentiate between prostate cancer and BPH, similarly EV-incorporated Let-7a-5p level could distinguish prostate cancer patients with Gleason score above 8 from those with Gleason score below 6. Both EV-incorporated and free miR-375 in the blood is an important miRNA biomarker candidate in prostate cancer. Huang et al. found that plasma EV-derived miR-375 and miR-1290 could predict overall survival for CRPC patients [180]. Expression of miR-141 and miR-375 increased in the blood of high risk or metastatic CRPC patients [181,182]. Other groups also confirmed miR-375 as important diagnostic marker but only if tested in the whole plasma [183]. Blood miRNAs were shown to discriminate between prostate cancer and BPH, though studies differ on the type and source of miRNAs. In one study overexpression of plasma-derived EV-containing miR-10a-5p and miR-29b-3p, while in another one downregulation of plasma-derived free hsa-miR-221-5p and hsa-miR-708-3p were indicative of prostate cancer but not BPH [184,185]. Correlated expression levels of miR-20a, miR-21, miR-145, and miR-221 [186], miR-17, miR-20a, miR-20b, miR-106a [187] as well as miR-16, miR-148a and miR-195 [188] in the plasma could significantly distinguish high risk patients from those with low risk and some of these miRNAs were shown to confer an aggressive phenotype upon overexpression in vitro as well as an accelerated biochemical recurrence [187]. Fredsoe et al. validated a blood-based miRNA diagnostic model comprising of 4 miRNAs (miR-375, miR-33a-5p, miR-16-5p and miR-409-3p), called bCaP, in 753 patients with benign prostate lesions and multiple stages of prostate cancer and showed that combined with PSA, digital rectal examination and age bCaP predicted the outcomes of biopsies better than PSA alone [189].

An important miRNA cluster with predictive value towards therapy response is formed by miR-205 and miR-31. These miRNAs regulate apoptosis in prostate cancer cells by targeting antiapoptotic proteins Bcl-w and E2F6 and they are downregulated in prostate cancer cell lines derived from advanced metastatic cancers. It was shown that their decreased expression could contribute to resistance to chemotherapy-induced apoptosis making them key targets to improve prostate cancer response to chemotherapy [190]. In this context, upregulated plasma miR-205 expression in metastatic CRPC was associated with a lower Gleason score and a lower probability of both biochemical recurrence and clinically evident metastatic events after prostatectomy [181].

Several studies highlight the prognostic and predictive value of circulating miRNAs secreted by other than prostate cancer cells, most probably reflecting a systemic response. Bone marrow mesenchymal stem cells EV-derived miR-205 contributed to repress prostate cancer cell proliferation, invasion, migration and enhance apoptosis, which suggests that miR-205 could be a valid prognostic marker and a potential therapeutic target in prostate cancer [191]. It was shown that tumour-associated macrophages (TAM)-derived EVs with increased miR-95 content could mediate prostate cancer progression by promoting proliferation, invasion, and EMT [192].

Ionizing radiation is an important exogenous factor, which modifies miRNA expression in cells, including cancer cells. Altered miRNA expression patterns can influence cancer cell radioresistance and consequently lead to changes in radiation response. There are relatively few studies, which investigate miRNA expression profile changes induced by irradiation in prostate cancer patients, most studies are mainly in vitro investigations. A comprehensive review of miRNA expression alterations after various irradiation schedules in different prostate cancer cell lines was prepared by Labbé et al. The authors also summarize the most important radiotherapy-regulated cellular mechanisms in which miRNAs are involved [193].

MiR-106a and miR-20a overexpression conferred radioresistance to prostate cancer models by increasing clonogenic survival after radiotherapy [187,194]. In another study using prostate cancer cell lines with different intrinsic radiosensitivity miR-200, miR-221, miR-31 and miR-4284 were found to correlate with clonogenic survival of cell lines after irradiation [195]. Increased miR-21 and miR-146a/155 levels were found in radiotherapy-treated prostate cancer patients with acute genitourinary side effects, indicating their potential to predict radiotherapy-related toxicities [196].

Gong et al. showed that circulating miR-145 levels were increased in prostate cancer patients responsive to neoadjuvant radiotherapy indicating that miR-145 might serve both as a predictive marker of therapy response and a novel therapeutic agent able to enhance the efficacy of radiotherapy [197]. MiR-93 and miR-221 plasma levels decreased significantly after either radical prostatectomy or radiotherapy but did not change after ADT and miR-

93 significantly correlated with Gleason score in a cohort of 68 prostate cancer patients compared to the observational cohort (n = 81) [198]. Two studies investigated EV-miRNAs as markers of therapy efficacy. The study by Li et al. identified a panel of 9 serum-derived EV-miRNAs, which could predict therapeutic benefit of carbon ion radiotherapy based on their baseline values. Post-therapy levels of miR-654-3p and miR-379-5p were associated with therapy efficacy [199]. Another study identified hsa-let-7a-5p and hsa-miR-21-5p as increased only in high-risk prostate cancer patients after radiotherapy compared to intermediate-risk patients [200]. It is important to highlight that candidate miRNAs in the two studies did not overlap, which might be due to different patient enrolment criteria, treatment protocol and sampling time after therapy. A further limitation of the cited studies is the low number of enrolled patients (n = 8 and 11, respectively), thus data must be confirmed on larger patient cohorts as well.

Table 1. Summary of representative human studies investigating blood-derived liquid biopsy markers as biomarkers in prostate cancer patients.

Biomarker Types	**Biological Sample**	**Indicative for**	**Patient Numbers and Characteristics**	**References Or Clinical Trials.gov ID**
Clinically Approved or Commercialized Biomarkers				
PHI (total/free/pro PSA)	Plasma	- discrimination of prostate cancer and BPH patients; - prediction of high-grade and clinically aggressive prostatic tumours	892 men with no history of prostate cancer, normal rectal examination, prostate specific antigen between 2 and 10 ng/mL	[34] (Approved by FDA)
4K (Four kallikrein) test	Blood (serum)	- discrimination of prostate cancer and BPH patients	392 prostate cancer patients with PSA $\geq$ 3.0 ng/mL	[39] (Approved by FDA)
Proclarix (THBS1, CTSD)	Blood	- aid in the decision-making process before biopsy	955 prostate cancer patients	[43] (Commercialised)
CellSearch™ CTC isolation	Blood	- prognostic factors of PFS and OS in metastatic prostate cancer	6081 patients with CRPC	[201] (Approved by FDA)
Biomarkers in clinical trial				
MDSCs	Blood	- therapy response indicator	300 patients, age $\geq$ 18, histological diagnosis of prostate cancer	NCT03408964 (Recruiting)
Antioxidant enzymes, oxidative stress markers, DNA damage in leukocytes	Blood	- patients at high risk for developing prostate cancer	40 patients with PSA $\geq$ 4.0 ng/mL; fPSA < 18%; PSA velocity > 0.75 ng/mL within the past year	NCT00898274 (Completed)
NK cells	Blood	- correlation between the level of NKp30 and NKp46 receptor-activators expression on the surface of NK cells	30 patients with metastatic prostate cancer; age $\geq$ 18	NCT02963155 (Active, not recruiting)
CTCs	Blood, plasma, PBMCs	- early markers of prostate cancer relapse and early metastases detected by PSMA-positron emission tomography (PET), who need further assistance in treatment decisions	50 patients in good general health and an expected life expectancy of >10 years diagnosed with prostate cancer relapse and positive lymph nodes as seen on PSMA-PET;	NCT04324983 (Recruiting)

Table 1. *Cont.*

Clinically Approved or Commercialized Biomarkers				
Biomarker Types	**Biological Sample**	**Indicative for**	**Patient Numbers and Characteristics**	**References Or Clinical Trials.gov ID**
Biomarkers in clinical trial				
Androgen receptor (*AR*), Phosphatase, tensin homolog (*PTEN*), *AR-V7* and other gene expression biomarkers in CTCs	Blood, Formalin-fixed paraffin-embedded (FFPE) sample	- predictive of outcome of activity of cabazitaxel treatment in CRPC	94 patients with metastatic CRPC; age $\geq$ 18	NCT03381326 (Active, not recruiting)
Tissue damage, CTCs	Blood, plasma	- prostate cancer patients at highest risk of radiotherapy-related complications	68 patients with prostate adenocarcinoma; age $\geq$ 18	NCT02941029 (Completed)
CTCs	Blood	- decrease the number of unnecessary prostate biopsies	500 patients, age $\geq$ 18; subjects with a PSA 4.00–10.99 ng/mL receiving biopsy within 3 months	NCT03488706 (Recruiting)
Immune checkpoint biomarkers (PD-L1, PD-L2, B7-H3, and CTLA-4) on CTCs	Blood	- metastatic prostate cancer	38 patients with histologically confirmed prostate adenocarcinoma; age $\geq$ 18 years;	NCT02456571 (Completed)
CTCs, cfDNA	Blood, plasma, tissue	- markers of drug resistance	24 patients with histologically confirmed prostate adenocarcinoma; increase PSA value over a baseline measurement	NCT02370355 (Terminated—Sponsor decided not to pursue study)
CTCs, cfDNA, exosomes	Blood	- discrimination of prostate cancer and non-cancer controls, identification of high-risk patients	320 men over 40 suspicious of prostate cancer; with PSA $\geq$ 4 and designated for biopsy	NCT04556916 (Recruiting)
Gamma H2AX Positivity	Blood	- prostate cancer cells response to radiotherapy	10 patients, age $\geq$ 18; histologically confirmed prostate adenocarcinoma	NCT02981797 (Completed)
TNF-α, IL-1β, IL-2, IL-2 CD25 Soluble Receptor, IFN-γ, IL-4, IL-5, IL-6, IL-8, IL-10, IL-12, IL-13	Blood, urine	- different types of cancer treatment can elicit different systemic immune responses from the body's immune system	40 patients with histologically confirmed diagnosis of adenocarcinoma of the prostate	NCT03331367 (Completed)

Table 1. *Cont.*

Clinically Approved or Commercialized Biomarkers				
Biomarker Types	**Biological Sample**	**Indicative for**	**Patient Numbers and Characteristics**	**References Or Clinical Trials.gov ID**
Biomarkers in clinical trial				
170 clinically relevant SNPs	Saliva, blood, urine	- incidence and aggressiveness of prostate cancer	4700 patients, aged 55 to 69; caucasian ethnicity; WHO performance status 0–2	NCT03857477 (Recruiting)
PSA and 40 SNPs	Blood	- risk assessment and early detection of prostate cancer	5000 patients	NCT01739062 (Active, not recruiting)
DNA-repair gene defects	Saliva, Blood, Archival Tumor Tissue	- DNA-repair gene defect status of patients with metastatic prostate cancer	10,000 patients with histologically confirmed prostate adenocarcinoma	NCT03871816 (Recruiting)
miRNA expression of prostate cell-derived exosomes	Blood	- disease progression and relapse	600 patients with elevated PSA or patients with diagnosed prostate cancer; age $\geq$ 18;	NCT03694483 (Recruiting)
miRNA panel	Blood	- predictive value of miRNA and ARV7 status in treatment efficacy	46 CRPC patients with biochemical or clinical progression under hormone therapy; age $\geq$ 18;	NCT04188275 (Recruiting)
five prevalent exosomal miRNAs	Blood	- predicting duration of response to ADT	60 patients with histologically confirmed prostate adenocarcinoma; testosterone level > 30ng/mL; age $\geq$ 18;	NCT02366494 (Active, not recruiting)
miRNA	Not Provided	- predicting prostate cancer outcome	300 patients with clinically localised high risk prostate cancer scheduled for radical prostatectomy	NCT01220427 (Terminated)
Biomarkers in experimental phase				
PD-L1 expressing CTCs/CETCs	Blood	- indicates the efficacy of anti-PD-1/PD-L1 therapy	27 patients	[59]
Nuclear PD-L1 (nPD-L1) in CTCs	Blood	- prognostic indicator (short survival rate)	30 metastatic prostate cancer patients	[74]

Table 1. *Cont.*

Clinically Approved or Commercialized Biomarkers				
Biomarker Types	**Biological Sample**	**Indicative for**	**Patient Numbers and Characteristics**	**References Or Clinical Trials.gov ID**
Biomarkers in experimental phase				
CTLA-4 on Tregs	PBMCs	- immune suppression	32 patients	[202]
IL-4, IL-6, IL-10	Serum	- indicator of hormone refractory prostate cancer	18 hormone sensitive prostate cancer patients	[203]
SAMSN1, CRTAM, CXCR3, FCRL3, KIAA1143, KLF12, TMEM204	Blood mRNA	- indicator of aggressive prostate cancer	739 patients	[126]
SNPs of *TLR1*, *TLR4*, *TLR5*, *TLR6*, *TLR10*	Blood	- prostate cancer risk	18,018 US men (from the ongoing Health Professionals Followup Study)	[117]
SNPs of *MSR1*	Blood	- prostate cancer risk	83 Swedish prostate cancer patients	[118]
SNPs of antiviral genes (*RNASEL*)	Blood	- prostate cancer risk	101 prostate cancer patients with a family history of prostate cancer	[121,122]
SNPs of cytokines (*MIC1*, *IL-8*, *TNF-α*, and *IL1RN*	Blood	- prostate cancer risk	1383 prostate cancer patients, 779 controls	[123,124]
SNP of *COX-2*	Blood	- prostate cancer risk	506 prostate cancer and 506 controls	[125]
ATM, *BRCA1*, genes	Peripheral blood lymphocytes	- discrimination of patients with high and low radiation toxicity	37 prostate cancer patients	[153]
SNP of *XRCC1*	Blood	- radiation-induced late toxicity	603 prostate cancer patients	[155]
miR-141, miR-375	Serum	- high risk; - high Gleason score; - lymph node positivity	7 metastatic, 14 localized prostate cancer + 2 validation studies in different prostate cancer risk groups (n_1 = 45 and n_2 = 71)	[182]

Table 1. *Cont.*

Clinically Approved or Commercialized Biomarkers				
Biomarker Types	**Biological Sample**	**Indicative for**	**Patient Numbers and Characteristics**	**References Or Clinical Trials.gov ID**
Biomarkers in experimental phase				
miR-24, miR-26b, miR-30c, miR-93, miR-106a, miR-223, miR-451, miR-874, miR-1207, miR-5p, miR-1274a	Serum	- diagnosis of prostate cancer; correlation with prognosis	36 prostate cancer, 12 healthy controls	[204]
miR-26a, miR-32, miR-195, miR-let7i	Serum	- discrimination of prostate cancer and BPH patients; - correlation with Gleason score; surgical margin positivity	37 localized, 8 metastatic prostate cancer, 18 BPH, 20 healthy controls	[205]
miR-375, miR-141, miR-378, miR-409-3p	Serum	- correlation with diseases status	26 metastatic CRPC, 28 localized low-risk, 30 high-risk prostate cancer	[206]
miR-141, miR-298, miR-346, miR-375	Serum	- diagnosis of prostate cancer; - prediction of biochemical relapse	25 metastatic CRPC, 25 healthy controls	[207]
miR-16, miR-148a, miR-195	Plasma	- high risk; - high Gleason score; high PSA level;	79 prostate cancer patients, 33 healthy controls	[188]
miR-16, miR-21, miR-126, miR-141, miR-151-3p, miR-152, miR-200c, miR-205, miR-375, miR-423-3p	Plasma	- Gleason score; - lymph node involvement; time to tumour recurrence; - PSA level; - probability of biochemical recurrence in 5 years; - metastasis;	25 metastatic CRPC and 25 localized prostate cancer	[181]
miR-20a, miR-21, miR-145, miR-221	Plasma	- high risk versus intermediate or low risk prostate cancer patients	52 Low risk, 21 intermediate risk, 9 high risk prostate cancer patients	[186]

Table 1. *Cont.*

Clinically Approved or Commercialized Biomarkers				
Biomarker Types	**Biological Sample**	**Indicative for**	**Patient Numbers and Characteristics**	**References Or Clinical Trials.gov ID**
Biomarkers in experimental phase				
let-7c, let-7e, miR-30c, miR-622, miR-1285	Plasma	- diagnosis of prostate cancer; - discrimination from BPH	tested on 25 prostate cancer, 12 BPH, validated on 80 prostate cancer, 44 BPH, 54 healthy control	[208]
miR-375, miR-33a-5p, miR-16-5p, miR-409-3p	Plasma	- discrimination between benign prostate lesions and multiple stages of prostate cancer	753 patients (144 BPH, 464 prostate cancer for training + 145 for test)	[189]
miR-17 miR-20a miR-20b miR-106a	Plasma	- discrimination of high risk versus low risk prostate cancer patients	44 high risk, 31 low risk prostate cancer patients	[187]
miR-93, miR-221	Plasma	- prediction of therapy efficacy (radiotherapy, radical prostatectomy)	149 patients (68—treated, interventional cohort, 81—observational cohort)	[198]
let-7a, miR-141, miR-145, miR-155	Whole blood	- discrimination of prostate cancer versus BPH	75 prostate cancer, 27 BPH	[209]
hsa-miR-221-5p, hsa-miR-708-3p	Whole blood	- discrimination of prostate cancer versus BPH	115 prostate cancer, 39 BHP	[185]
miR-493-5p, miR-323a-3p, miR-411-5p, miR-494-3p, miR-379-5p, miR-654-3p, miR-409-3p, miR-543, miR-200c-3p	Serum EV	- prediction of therapeutic benefit of carbon ion radiotherapy; prediction of therapeutic efficacy	8 patients, localized cancer	[199]
hsa-let-7a-5p, hsa-miR-21-5p	Serum EV	- prediction of radiotherapy efficacy	11 patients (6 high-risk, 5 intermediate risk)	[200]
miR-10a-5p miR-29b-3p miR-99b-5p	Plasma EVs	- discrimination of prostate cancer versus BPH	18 prostate cancer, 7 BPH	[184]
miR-375, miR-1246, miR-1290	Plasma EVs	- correlation with overall survival;	screening in 23 CRPC, validating in 100 CRPC	[180]

Table 1. *Cont.*

Clinically Approved or Commercialized Biomarkers					
Biomarker Types	**Biological Sample**		**Indicative for**	**Patient Numbers and Characteristics**	**References Or Clinical Trials.gov ID**
Biomarkers in experimental phase					
Let7a-5p, miR-21-5p, miR-200c-3p, miR-375	Plasma, EVs	-	discrimination of prostate cancer from BPH	50 prostate cancer, 22 BPH	[183]
miR-107, miR-130b, miR-141, miR-181a-2, miR-301a, miR-326, miR-331-3p, miR-432, miR-484, miR-574-3p, miR-625, miR-2110	Plasma-derived EVs, serum-derived EVs, urine	-	diagnosis and staging of prostate cancer	78 prostate cancer, 28 healthy controls	[210]
miR-21 miR-146a miR-155	Blood PBMCs	-	prediction of radiotherapy-related toxicities	15 prostate cancer, 9 with and 6 without acute gastro-urinary toxicity	[196]

3. Conclusions

Table 1 summarizes the most important liquid biopsy-based biomarkers or biomarker candidates either already approved for clinical use or investigated in ongoing clinical trials or still in experimental phase. The high number of studies focusing on different cellular and secreted blood components as candidate liquid biopsy markers demonstrates the need for validated targets with prognostic and/or predictive value in screening prostate cancer patients.

The following biomarker categories were the most successfully tested in prostate cancer:

(a) Molecular variants of PSA (e.g., f/t PSA ratio) which are markers of malignancy, able to discriminate prostate cancer from BPH and markers of tumour aggressiveness as well. Two diagnostic tests based on quantification of PSA variants (PHI and 4K) have received FDA approval for discriminating benign conditions from prostate cancer and identifying aggressive tumours.

(b) Quantitative and phenotypical analysis of CTCs and their DNA content as well as cfDNA proved to be indicative for tumour aggressiveness and risk of distant metastasis and according to some studies as therapy-response markers. These markers are particularly important in identifying tumour heterogeneity and the clonality of metastases. The CellSearch™ method is an FDA-approved technology based on CTC characterisation used to predict outcome of prostate cancer patients.

(c) Blood miRNAs either free or within EVs. While a high number of miRNAs are proposed as candidate biomarkers there is an increasing consensus across different studies about the following miRNAs: miR-141, miR-145 and miR-375, which are markers of malignancy (discriminating prostate cancer from BPH), risk prediction, metastasis or relapse indicators. Importantly, recently miRNAs have been correlated with response to radiotherapy and prediction of radiotherapy-related toxicities as well. The application of miRNAs as biomarkers in prostate cancer is still in experimental phase despite the very numerous studies published in this topic. A common characteristic of the studies is that they are mostly local initiatives with low patient numbers (see Table 1). While miRNAs are clearly very promising markers, discrepancies in the findings of the different studies do not allow their validation and consequently their transition into the clinic. It is important to mention that assaying miRNA panels for screening from blood (or urine) is a non/minimally invasive and fast method, which is suitable for high-throughput screening and it is cost efficient. Thus, miRNAs could become ideal biomarkers.

(d) Immune and inflammatory markers. A large panel of soluble molecules, mainly cytokines, chemokines or growth factors were correlated in different studies with response to radiotherapy, prediction of tumour radioresistance and patient radiosensitivity as well as predisposition to radiotherapy-related toxicity. These markers are still in experimental phase despite significant efforts invested in better understanding local and systemic immune responses in prostate cancer. Since immunotherapy is rapidly becoming part of the everyday treatment routine, it is extremely important to find suitable markers able to identify patients responsive to immunotherapy.

(e) Gene expression signatures and gene polymorphisms indicative of disease progression and therapy response analysed either in traditional biopsy material or in CTCs from liquid biopsies. Due to differences in gene expression signatures in prostate cancer between European American men and African American men, care must be taken in the interpretation of these genetic traits in African American men. Gene expression panels under development already take into account racial differences, using markers with similar predictive values between European American and African American men [211].

The major requirements and guidelines for biological parameters to be considered as biomarkers and to be clinically approved have been extensively described elsewhere [212,213]. Basically, the procedure of biomarker development should adhere to the REMARK guidelines. Besides their proven clinical relevance, proposed biomarkers should fulfil strict specificity and sensitivity criteria, also they have to be reproducible, easy-to-perform and to interpret and cost-effective. Despite the high number of promising biomarker candidates in prostate cancer very few have actually been approved for clinical use and their spread in the clinical routine is very slow. We believe that the most important reason for this relatively low transition of experimental biomarkers into clinical setting is that most studies stop at the discovery or qualification phase and fail to proceed to biomarker verification and validation. In Table 1 one can see that many of the listed clinical trials recruited very low patient numbers, which were not sufficient for validation purposes. A large-scale validation study of a prioritized biomarker needs substantial financial and collaborative efforts involving multi-institutional and optimally international collaboration, which might take years to be finalized. Within the European Union EU-supported multi-national collaborative projects could be one solution for wide-scale harmonized biomarker validation studies. Additionally, given the wealth of available data on biomarker candidates, a meta-analysis would help in biomarker prioritisation, highlighting the most promising targets for large-scale validation.

Author Contributions: Conceptualisation: K.L., K.B. and L.A. Manuscript drafting: K.B. and L.A. Manuscript editing and reviewing: K.B., G.S. and K.L. All authors have read and agreed to the published version of the manuscript.

Funding: This research was funded by the Hungarian National Research, Development and Innovation Office under grant number NKFI-124879.

Institutional Review Board Statement: Not applicable.

Informed Consent Statement: Not applicable.

Data Availability Statement: Not applicable.

Conflicts of Interest: Authors declare no conflict of interest.

References

1. Sung, H.; Ferlay, J.; Siegel, R.L.; Laversanne, M.; Soerjomataram, I.; Jemal, A.; Bray, F. Global cancer statistics 2020: GLOBOCAN estimates of incidence and mortality worldwide for 36 cancers in 185 countries. *CA A Cancer J. Clin.* **2021**. [CrossRef]
2. Williams, H.; Powell, I.J. Epidemiology, pathology, and genetics of prostate cancer among African Americans compared with other ethnicities. *Methods Mol. Biol.* **2009**, *472*, 439–453.
3. Fukagai, T.; Namiki, T.; Carlile, R.G.; Namiki, M. Racial differences in clinical outcome after prostate cancer treatment. *Methods Mol. Biol.* **2009**, *472*, 455–466.
4. Heijnsdijk, E.A.; Bangma, C.H.; Borràs, J.M.; De Carvalho, T.M.; Castells, X.; Eklund, M.; Espinàs, J.A.; Graefen, M.; Grönberg, H.; Lansdorp-Vogelaar, I.; et al. Summary statement on screening for prostate cancer in Europe. *Int. J. Cancer* **2017**, *142*, 741–746. [CrossRef]
5. Loeb, S.; Heuvel, S.V.D.; Zhu, X.; Bangma, C.H.; Schröder, F.H.; Roobol, M.J. Infectious Complications and Hospital Admissions After Prostate Biopsy in a European Randomized Trial. *Eur. Urol.* **2012**, *61*, 1110–1114. [CrossRef]
6. Korfage, I.J.; De Koning, H.J.; Roobol, M.; Schröder, F.H.; Essink-Bot, M.-L. Prostate cancer diagnosis: The impact on patients' mental health. *Eur. J. Cancer* **2006**, *42*, 165–170. [CrossRef]
7. Resnick, M.J.; Koyama, T.; Fan, K.-H.; Albertsen, P.C.; Goodman, M.; Hamilton, A.S.; Hoffman, R.M.; Potosky, A.L.; Stanford, J.L.; Stroup, A.M.; et al. Long-Term Functional Outcomes after Treatment for Localized Prostate Cancer. *N. Engl. J. Med.* **2013**, *368*, 436–445. [CrossRef] [PubMed]
8. Punnen, S.; Cowan, J.E.; Chan, J.M.; Carroll, P.R.; Cooperberg, M.R. Long-term Health-related Quality of Life After Primary Treatment for Localized Prostate Cancer: Results from the CaPSURE Registry. *Eur. Urol.* **2015**, *68*, 600–608. [CrossRef] [PubMed]
9. Sánchez-Chapado, M.; Olmedilla, G.; Cabeza, M.; Donat, E.; Ruiz, A. Prevalence of prostate cancer and prostatic intraepithelial neoplasia in Caucasian Mediterranean males: An autopsy study. *Prostate* **2002**, *54*, 238–247. [CrossRef]
10. Haas, G.P.; Delongchamps, N.; Brawley, O.W.; Wang, C.Y.; De La Roza, G. The worldwide epidemiology of prostate cancer: Perspectives from autopsy studies. *Can. J. Urol.* **2008**, *15*, 3866–3871. [PubMed]
11. Loeb, S.; Bjurlin, M.A.; Nicholson, J.; Tammela, T.L.; Penson, D.F.; Carter, H.B.; Carroll, P.; Etzioni, R. Overdiagnosis and Overtreatment of Prostate Cancer. *Eur. Urol.* **2014**, *65*, 1046–1055. [CrossRef] [PubMed]
12. Schröder, F.H.; Hugosson, J.; Roobol, M.J.; Tammela, T.L.J.; Zappa, M.; Nelen, V.; Kwiatkowski, M.; Lujan, M.; Määttänen, L.; Lilja, H.; et al. Screening and prostate cancer mortality: Results of the European Randomised Study of Screening for Prostate Cancer (ERSPC) at 13 years of follow-up. *Lancet* **2014**, *384*, 2027–2035. [CrossRef]

13. Pinsky, P.F.; Miller, E.; Prorok, P.; Grubb, R.; Crawford, E.D.; Andriole, G. Extended follow-up for prostate cancer incidence and mortality among participants in the Prostate, Lung, Colorectal and Ovarian randomized cancer screening trial. *BJU Int.* **2019**, *123*, 854–860. [CrossRef] [PubMed]
14. Tsodikov, A.; Gulati, R.; Heijnsdijk, E.A.; Pinsky, P.F.; Moss, S.M.; Qiu, S.; De Carvalho, T.M.; Hugosson, J.; Berg, C.D.; Auvinen, A.; et al. Reconciling the Effects of Screening on Prostate Cancer Mortality in the ERSPC and PLCO Trials. *Ann. Intern. Med.* **2017**, *167*, 449–455. [CrossRef] [PubMed]
15. Powell, I.J.; Vigneau, F.D.; Bock, C.H.; Ruterbusch, J.; Heilbrun, L.K. Reducing Prostate Cancer Racial Disparity: Evidence for Aggressive Early Prostate Cancer PSA Testing of African American Men. *Cancer Epidemiol. Biomark. Prev.* **2014**, *23*, 1505–1511. [CrossRef] [PubMed]
16. Pantel, K.; Hille, C.; Scher, H.I. Circulating Tumor Cells in Prostate Cancer: From Discovery to Clinical Utility. *Clin. Chem.* **2019**, *65*, 87–99. [CrossRef] [PubMed]
17. Tolkach, Y.; Kristiansen, G. The Heterogeneity of Prostate Cancer: A Practical Approach. *Pathobiology* **2018**, *85*, 108–116. [CrossRef]
18. Yadav, S.S.; Stockert, J.A.; Hackert, V.; Yadav, K.K.; Tewari, A.K. Intratumor heterogeneity in prostate cancer. *Urol. Oncol. Semin. Orig. Investig.* **2018**, *36*, 349–360. [CrossRef] [PubMed]
19. Rigau, M.; Olivan, M.; Garcia, M.; Sequeiros, T.; Montes, M.; Colás, E.; Llauradó, M.; Planas, J.; De Torres, I.; Morote, J.; et al. The Present and Future of Prostate Cancer Urine Biomarkers. *Int. J. Mol. Sci.* **2013**, *14*, 12620–12649. [CrossRef]
20. Wu, D.; Ni, J.; Beretov, J.; Cozzi, P.; Willcox, M.; Wasinger, V.; Walsh, B.; Graham, P.; Li, Y. Urinary biomarkers in prostate cancer detection and monitoring progression. *Crit. Rev. Oncol.* **2017**, *118*, 15–26. [CrossRef]
21. Eggener, S.E.; Rumble, R.B.; Armstrong, A.J.; Morgan, T.M.; Crispino, T.; Cornford, P.; Van Der Kwast, T.; Grignon, D.J.; Rai, A.J.; Agarwal, N.; et al. Molecular Biomarkers in Localized Prostate Cancer: ASCO Guideline. *J. Clin. Oncol.* **2020**, *38*, 1474–1494. [CrossRef]
22. Wilkins, A.; Dearnaley, D.; Somaiah, N. Genomic and Histopathological Tissue Biomarkers That Predict Radiotherapy Response in Localised Prostate Cancer. *BioMed Res. Int.* **2015**, *2015*, 1–9. [CrossRef] [PubMed]
23. Zhao, L.; Yu, N.; Guo, T.; Hou, Y.; Zeng, Z.; Yang, X.; Hu, P.; Tang, X.; Wang, J.; Liu, M. Tissue Biomarkers for Prognosis of Prostate Cancer: A Systematic Review and Meta-analysis. *Cancer Epidemiol. Biomark. Prev.* **2014**, *23*, 1047–1054. [CrossRef] [PubMed]
24. Clark, J. Urine-Based Biomarkers for Prostate Cancer. *Mol. Biomark. Urol. Oncol.* **2020**, *1*, 87.
25. Hernández, J.; Thompson, I.M. Prostate-specific antigen: A review of the validation of the most commonly used cancer biomarker. *Cancer* **2004**, *101*, 894–904. [CrossRef] [PubMed]
26. Hori, S.; Blanchet, J.-S.; McLoughlin, J. From prostate-specific antigen (PSA) to precursor PSA (proPSA) isoforms: A review of the emerging role of proPSAs in the detection and management of early prostate cancer. *BJU Int.* **2012**, *112*, 717–728. [CrossRef] [PubMed]
27. Mikolajczyk, S.D.; Marks, L.S.; Partin, A.W.; Rittenhouse, H.G. Free prostate-specific antigen in serum is becoming more complex. *Urology* **2002**, *59*, 797–802. [CrossRef]
28. Tewari, P.C.; Williams, J.S. Analytical Characteristics of Seminal Fluid PSA Differ from Those of Serum PSA. *Clin. Chem.* **1998**, *44*, 191–193. [CrossRef]
29. Tormey, W.P. The complexity of PSA interpretation in clinical practice. *Surgeon* **2014**, *12*, 323–327. [CrossRef]
30. Mackintosh, F.R.; Sprenkle, P.C.; Walter, L.C.; Rawson, L.; Karnes, R.J.; Morrell, C.H.; Kattan, M.W.; Nawaf, C.B.; Neville, T.B. Age and Prostate-Specific Antigen Level Prior to Diagnosis Predict Risk of Death from Prostate Cancer. *Front. Oncol.* **2016**, *6*. [CrossRef]
31. Ross, T.; Ahmed, K.; Raison, N.; Challacombe, B.; Dasgupta, P. Clarifying the PSA grey zone: The management of patients with a borderline PSA. *Int. J. Clin. Pract.* **2016**, *70*, 950–959. [CrossRef] [PubMed]
32. Catalona, W.; Partin, A.; Slawin, K.; Brawer, M.; Flanigan, R.; Patel, A.; Richie, J.; Dekernion, J.; Walsh, P.; Scardino, P.; et al. Use of the Percentage of Free Prostate-Specific Antigen to Enhance Differentiation of Prostate Cancer from Benign Prostatic Disease: A Prospective Multicenter Clinical Trial. *J. Urol.* **1999**, *161*, 353–354. [CrossRef]
33. Yilmaz, S.N.; Yildiz, A.; Ayyıldız, S.N.; Ayyıldız, A. PSA, PSA derivatives, proPSA and prostate health index in the diagnosis of prostate cancer. *Türk Üroloji Dergisi/Turk. J. Urol.* **2014**, *40*, 82–88. [CrossRef]
34. Catalona, W.J.; Partin, A.W.; Sanda, M.G.; Wei, J.T.; Klee, G.G.; Bangma, C.H.; Slawin, K.M.; Marks, L.S.; Loeb, S.; Broyles, D.L.; et al. A Multicenter Study of [-2]Pro-Prostate Specific Antigen Combined With Prostate Specific Antigen and Free Prostate Specific Antigen for Prostate Cancer Detection in the 2.0 to 10.0 ng/mL Prostate Specific Antigen Range. *J. Urol.* **2011**, *185*, 1650–1655. [CrossRef]
35. Stephan, C.; Jung, K.; Lein, M.; Rochow, H.; Friedersdorff, F.; Maxeiner, A. PHI density prospectively improves prostate cancer detection. *World J. Urol.* **2021**, *2021*, 1–7. [CrossRef]
36. Barisiene, M.; Bakavicius, A.; Stanciute, D.; Jurkeviciene, J.; Zelvys, A.; Ulys, A.; Vitkus, D.; Jankevicius, F. Prostate Health Index and Prostate Health Index Density as Diagnostic Tools for Improved Prostate Cancer Detection. *BioMed Res. Int.* **2020**, *2020*, 1–15. [CrossRef] [PubMed]
37. Ferrer-Batallé, M.; Llop, E.; Ramírez, M.; Aleixandre, R.N.; Saez, M.; Comet, J.; De Llorens, R.; Peracaula, R. Comparative Study of Blood-Based Biomarkers, α2,3-Sialic Acid PSA and PHI, for High-Risk Prostate Cancer Detection. *Int. J. Mol. Sci.* **2017**, *18*, 845. [CrossRef]

38. Heidegger, I.; Klocker, H.; Pichler, R.; Pircher, A.; Prokop, W.; Steiner, E.; Ladurner, C.; Comploj, E.; Lunacek, A.; Djordjevic, D.; et al. ProPSA and the Prostate Health Index as predictive markers for aggressiveness in low-risk prostate cancer—Results from an international multicenter study. *Prostate Cancer Prostatic Dis.* **2017**, *20*, 271–275. [CrossRef]
39. Carlsson, S.; Maschino, A.; Schröder, F.; Bangma, C.; Steyerberg, E.W.; van der Kwast, T.; van Leenders, G.; Vickers, A.; Lilja, H.; Roobol, M.J. Predictive Value of Four Kallikrein Markers for Pathologically Insignificant Compared with Aggressive Prostate Cancer in Radical Prostatectomy Specimens: Results From the European Randomized Study of Screening for Prostate Cancer Section Rotterdam. *Eur. Urol.* **2013**, *64*, 693–699. [CrossRef]
40. Darst, B.F.; Chou, A.; Wan, P.; Pooler, L.; Sheng, X.; Vertosick, E.A.; Conti, D.V.; Wilkens, L.R.; Le Marchand, L.; Vickers, A.J.; et al. The Four-Kallikrein Panel Is Effective in Identifying Aggressive Prostate Cancer in a Multiethnic Population. *Cancer Epidemiol. Biomark. Prev.* **2020**, *29*, 1381–1388. [CrossRef]
41. Lin, D.W.; Newcomb, L.F.; Brown, M.D.; Sjoberg, D.D.; Dong, Y.; Brooks, J.D.; Carroll, P.R.; Cooperberg, M.; Dash, A.; Ellis, W.J.; et al. Evaluating the Four Kallikrein Panel of the 4Kscore for Prediction of High-grade Prostate Cancer in Men in the Canary Prostate Active Surveillance Study. *Eur. Urol.* **2017**, *72*, 448–454. [CrossRef]
42. Steuber, T.; Tennstedt, P.; Macagno, A.; Athanasiou, A.; Wittig, A.; Huber, R.; Golding, B.; Schiess, R.; Gillessen, S. Thrombospondin 1 and cathepsin D improve prostate cancer diagnosis by avoiding potentially unnecessary prostate biopsies. *BJU Int.* **2018**, *123*, 826–833. [CrossRef] [PubMed]
43. Klocker, H.; Golding, B.; Weber, S.; Steiner, E.; Tennstedt, P.; Keller, T.; Schiess, R.; Gillessen, S.; Horninger, W.; Steuber, T. Development and validation of a novel multivariate risk score to guide biopsy decision for the diagnosis of clinically significant prostate cancer. *BJUI Compass* **2020**, *1*, 15–20. [CrossRef]
44. Steuber, T.; Heidegger, I.; Kafka, M.; Roeder, M.A.; Chun, F.; Preisser, F.; Palisaar, R.-J.; Hanske, J.; Budaeus, L.; Schiess, R.; et al. PROPOSe: A Real-life Prospective Study of Proclarix, a Novel Blood-based Test to Support Challenging Biopsy Decision-making in Prostate Cancer. *Eur. Urol. Oncol.* **2021**. [CrossRef]
45. Yu, M.; Stott, S.; Toner, M.; Maheswaran, S.; Haber, D.A. Circulating tumor cells: Approaches to isolation and characterization. *J. Cell Biol.* **2011**, *192*, 373–382. [CrossRef] [PubMed]
46. Nakagawa, T.; Martinez, S.R.; Goto, Y.; Koyanagi, K.; Kitago, M.; Shingai, T.; Elashoff, D.A.; Ye, X.; Singer, F.R.; Giuliano, A.E.; et al. Detection of Circulating Tumor Cells in Early-Stage Breast Cancer Metastasis to Axillary Lymph Nodes. *Clin. Cancer Res.* **2007**, *13*, 4105–4110. [CrossRef]
47. Kang, Y.; Pantel, K. Tumor Cell Dissemination: Emerging Biological Insights from Animal Models and Cancer Patients. *Cancer Cell* **2013**, *23*, 573–581. [CrossRef]
48. Awe, J.A.; Xu, M.C.; Wechsler, J.; Benali-Furet, N.; Cayre, Y.E.; Saranchuk, J.; Drachenberg, D.; Mai, S. Three-Dimensional Telomeric Analysis of Isolated Circulating Tumor Cells (CTCs) Defines CTC Subpopulations. *Transl. Oncol.* **2013**, *6*, 51-IN4. [CrossRef]
49. Hyun, K.-A.; Lee, T.Y.; Lee, S.H.; Jung, H.-I. Two-stage microfluidic chip for selective isolation of circulating tumor cells (CTCs). *Biosens. Bioelectron.* **2015**, *67*, 86–92. [CrossRef]
50. Li, P.; Mao, Z.; Peng, Z.; Zhou, L.; Chen, Y.; Huang, P.-H.; Truica, C.I.; Drabick, J.J.; El-Deiry, W.S.; Dao, M.; et al. Acoustic separation of circulating tumor cells. *Proc. Natl. Acad. Sci. USA* **2015**, *112*, 4970–4975. [CrossRef]
51. Ortega, F.G.; Lorente, J.A.; Puche, J.L.G.; Ruiz, M.P.; Sanchez-Martin, R.M.; De Miguel-Pérez, D.; Diaz-Mochon, J.J.; Serrano, M.J. miRNA in situ hybridization in circulating tumor cells—MishCTC. *Sci. Rep.* **2015**, *5*, 9207. [CrossRef]
52. A Joosse, S.; Gorges, T.M.; Pantel, K. Biology, detection, and clinical implications of circulating tumor cells. *EMBO Mol. Med.* **2015**, *7*, 1–11. [CrossRef] [PubMed]
53. Fizazi, K.; Morat, L.; Chauveinc, L.; Prapotnich, D.; De Crevoisier, R.; Escudier, B.; Cathelineau, X.; Rozet, F.; Vallancien, G.; Sabatier, L.; et al. High detection rate of circulating tumor cells in blood of patients with prostate cancer using telomerase activity. *Ann. Oncol.* **2007**, *18*, 518–521. [CrossRef]
54. Huang, S.-B.; Wu, M.-H.; Lin, Y.-H.; Hsieh, C.-H.; Yang, C.-L.; Lin, H.-C.; Tseng, C.-P.; Lee, G.-B. High-purity and label-free isolation of circulating tumor cells (CTCs) in a microfluidic platform by using optically-induced-dielectrophoretic (ODEP) force. *Lab Chip* **2013**, *13*, 1371–1383. [CrossRef]
55. He, W.; Kularatne, S.A.; Kalli, K.R.; Prendergast, F.G.; Amato, R.J.; Klee, G.G.; Hartmann, L.C.; Low, P.S. Quantitation of circulating tumor cells in blood samples from ovarian and prostate cancer patients using tumor-specific fluorescent ligands. *Int. J. Cancer* **2008**, *123*, 1968–1973. [CrossRef]
56. Folkersma, L.R.; Gómez, C.O.; Manso, L.S.J.; De Castro, S.V.; Romo, I.G.; Lázaro, M.V.; De La Orden, G.V.; Fernández, M.A.; Rubio, E.D.; Moyano, A.S.; et al. Immunomagnetic quantification of circulating tumoral cells in patients with prostate cancer: Clinical and pathological correlation. *Arch. Esp. Urol.* **2010**, *63*, 23–31.
57. Ruan, D.; So, S.; King, B.; Wang, R. Novel method to detect, isolate, and culture prostate culturing circulating tumor cells. *Transl. Androl. Urol.* **2019**, *8*, 686–695. [CrossRef] [PubMed]
58. Galletti, G.; Worroll, D.; Nanus, D.M.; Giannakakou, P. Using circulating tumor cells to advance precision medicine in prostate cancer. *J. Cancer Metastasis Treat.* **2017**, *3*, 190–205. [CrossRef] [PubMed]
59. Schott, D.S.; Pizon, M.; Pachmann, U.; Pachmann, K. Sensitive detection of PD-L1 expression on circulating epithelial tumor cells (CETCs) could be a potential biomarker to select patients for treatment with PD-1/PD-L1 inhibitors in early and metastatic solid tumors. *Oncotarget* **2017**, *8*, 72755–72772. [CrossRef]

60. Giordano, A.; Cristofanilli, M. CTCs in metastatic breast cancer. *Recent Results Cancer Res.* **2012**, *195*, 193–201.
61. Cohen, S.J.; Punt, C.J.A.; Iannotti, N.; Saidman, B.H.; Sabbath, K.D.; Gabrail, N.Y.; Picus, J.; Morse, M.A.; Mitchell, E.; Miller, M.C.; et al. Prognostic significance of circulating tumor cells in patients with metastatic colorectal cancer. *Ann. Oncol.* **2009**, *20*, 1223–1229. [CrossRef]
62. Moreno, J.G.; Miller, M.C.; Gross, S.; Allard, W.J.; Gomella, L.G.; Terstappen, L.W. Circulating tumor cells predict survival in patients with metastatic prostate cancer. *Urology* **2005**, *65*, 713–718. [CrossRef] [PubMed]
63. Cristofanilli, M.; Budd, G.T.; Ellis, M.J.; Stopeck, A.; Matera, J.; Miller, M.C.; Reuben, J.M.; Doyle, G.V.; Allard, W.J.; Terstappen, L.W.; et al. Circulating Tumor Cells, Disease Progression, and Survival in Metastatic Breast Cancer. *N. Engl. J. Med.* **2004**, *351*, 781–791. [CrossRef] [PubMed]
64. Millner, L.M.; Linder, M.W.; Valdes, R. Circulating Tumor Cells: A Review of Present Methods and the Need to Identify Heterogeneous Phenotypes. *Ann. Clin. Lab. Sci.* **2013**, *43*, 295–304. [PubMed]
65. Scher, H.I.; Heller, G.; Molina, A.; Attard, G.; Danila, D.C.; Jia, X.; Peng, W.; Sandhu, S.K.; Olmos, D.; Riisnaes, R.; et al. Circulating Tumor Cell Biomarker Panel as an Individual-Level Surrogate for Survival in Metastatic Castration-Resistant Prostate Cancer. *J. Clin. Oncol.* **2015**, *33*, 1348–1355. [CrossRef] [PubMed]
66. Miyamoto, D.T.; Sequist, L.V.; Lee, R.J. Circulating tumour cells—Monitoring treatment response in prostate cancer. *Nat. Rev. Clin. Oncol.* **2014**, *11*, 401–412. [CrossRef] [PubMed]
67. Gires, O.; Stoecklein, N.H. Dynamic EpCAM expression on circulating and disseminating tumor cells: Causes and consequences. *Cell. Mol. Life Sci.* **2014**, *71*, 4393–4402. [CrossRef]
68. Alix-Panabières, C.; Pantel, K. Challenges in circulating tumour cell research. *Nat. Rev. Cancer* **2014**, *14*, 623–631. [CrossRef]
69. Gkountela, S.; Castro-Giner, F.; Szczerba, B.M.; Vetter, M.; Landin, J.; Scherrer, R.; Krol, I.; Scheidmann, M.C.; Beisel, C.; Stirnimann, C.U.; et al. Circulating Tumor Cell Clustering Shapes DNA Methylation to Enable Metastasis Seeding. *Cell* **2019**, *176*, 98–112.e14. [CrossRef]
70. Wang, C.; Mu, Z.; Chervoneva, I.; Austin, L.; Ye, Z.; Rossi, G.; Palazzo, J.P.; Sun, C.; Abu-Khalaf, M.; Myers, R.E.; et al. Longitudinally collected CTCs and CTC-clusters and clinical outcomes of metastatic breast cancer. *Breast Cancer Res. Treat.* **2017**, *161*, 83–94. [CrossRef]
71. Fabisiewicz, A.; Grzybowska, E. CTC clusters in cancer progression and metastasis. *Med. Oncol.* **2016**, *34*, 12. [CrossRef]
72. Aceto, N.; Bardia, A.; Miyamoto, D.T.; Donaldson, M.C.; Wittner, B.S.; Spencer, J.A.; Yu, M.; Pely, A.; Engstrom, A.; Zhu, H.; et al. Circulating Tumor Cell Clusters Are Oligoclonal Precursors of Breast Cancer Metastasis. *Cell* **2014**, *158*, 1110–1122. [CrossRef]
73. Kloten, V.; Lampignano, R.; Krahn, T.; Schlange, T. Circulating Tumor Cell PD-L1 Expression as Biomarker for Therapeutic Efficacy of Immune Checkpoint Inhibition in NSCLC. *Cells* **2019**, *8*, 809. [CrossRef]
74. Satelli, A.; Batth, I.S.; Brownlee, Z.; Rojas, C.; Meng, Q.H.; Kopetz, S.; Li, S. Potential role of nuclear PD-L1 expression in cell-surface vimentin positive circulating tumor cells as a prognostic marker in cancer patients. *Sci. Rep.* **2016**, *6*, 28910. [CrossRef]
75. Martin, O.A.; Anderson, R.L.; Russell, P.A.; Cox, R.A.; Ivashkevich, A.; Swierczak, A.; Doherty, J.P.; Jacobs, D.H.; Smith, J.; Siva, S.; et al. Mobilization of Viable Tumor Cells Into the Circulation During Radiation Therapy. *Int. J. Radiat. Oncol.* **2014**, *88*, 395–403. [CrossRef]
76. Budna-Tukan, J.; Świerczewska, M.; Mazel, M.; Cieślikowski, W.A.; Ida, A.; Jankowiak, A.; Antczak, A.; Nowicki, M.; Pantel, K.; Azria, D.; et al. Analysis of Circulating Tumor Cells in Patients with Non-Metastatic High-Risk Prostate Cancer before and after Radiotherapy Using Three Different Enumeration Assays. *Cancers* **2019**, *11*, 802. [CrossRef] [PubMed]
77. Murray, N.; Reyes, E.; Tapia, P.; Badínez, L.; Orellana, N.; Fuentealba, C.; Olivares, R.; Porcell, J.; Dueñas, R. Redefining micrometastasis in prostate cancer—A comparison of circulating prostate cells, bone marrow disseminated tumor cells and micrometastasis: Implications in determining local or systemic treatment for biochemical failure after radical prostatectomy. *Int. J. Mol. Med.* **2012**, *30*, 896–904. [CrossRef]
78. Levine, E.S.; Cisek, V.J.; Mulvihill, M.N.; Cohen, E.L. Role of transurethral resection in dissemination of cancer of prostate. *Urology* **1986**, *28*, 179–183. [CrossRef]
79. Krumbholz, M.; Agaimy, A.; Stoehr, R.; Burger, M.; Wach, S.; Taubert, H.; Wullich, B.; Hartmann, A.; Metzler, M. Molecular Composition of Genomic TMPRSS2-ERG Rearrangements in Prostate Cancer. *Dis. Markers* **2019**, *2019*, 1–8. [CrossRef] [PubMed]
80. Wu, A.; Attard, G. Plasma DNA Analysis in Prostate Cancer: Opportunities for Improving Clinical Management. *Clin. Chem.* **2019**, *65*, 100–107. [CrossRef] [PubMed]
81. Stroun, M.; Lyautey, J.; Lederrey, C.; Olson-Sand, A.; Anker, P. About the possible origin and mechanism of circulating DNA apoptosis and active DNA release. *Clin. Chim. Acta* **2001**, *313*, 139–142. [CrossRef]
82. Li, H.-G.; Huang, S.-Y.; Zhou, H.; Liao, A.-H.; Xiong, C.-L. Quick recovery and characterization of cell-free DNA in seminal plasma of normozoospermia and azoospermia: Implications for non-invasive genetic utilities. *Asian J. Androl.* **2009**, *11*, 703–709. [CrossRef] [PubMed]
83. Schwarzenbach, H.; Alix-Panabières, C.; Müller, I.; Letang, N.; Vendrell, J.-P.; Rebillard, X.; Pantel, K. Cell-free Tumor DNA in Blood Plasma as a Marker for Circulating Tumor Cells in Prostate Cancer. *Clin. Cancer Res.* **2009**, *15*, 1032–1038. [CrossRef]
84. Baca, S.C.; Garraway, L.A. The genomic landscape of prostate cancer. *Front. Endocrinol.* **2012**, *3*, 69. [CrossRef] [PubMed]
85. Grasso, C.S.; Wu, Y.-M.; Robinson, D.R.; Cao, X.; Dhanasekaran, S.M.; Khan, A.P.; Quist, M.J.; Jing, X.; Lonigro, R.J.; Brenner, J.C.; et al. The mutational landscape of lethal castration-resistant prostate cancer. *Nature* **2012**, *487*, 239–243. [CrossRef] [PubMed]

86. Guo, C.C.; Wang, Y.; Xiao, L.; Troncoso, P.; Czerniak, B.A. The relationship of TMPRSS2-ERG gene fusion between primary and metastatic prostate cancers. *Hum. Pathol.* **2012**, *43*, 644–649. [CrossRef]
87. Tomlins, S.A.; Bjartell, A.; Chinnaiyan, A.M.; Jenster, G.; Nam, R.K.; Rubin, M.A.; Schalken, J.A. ETS Gene Fusions in Prostate Cancer: From Discovery to Daily Clinical Practice. *Eur. Urol.* **2009**, *56*, 275–286. [CrossRef]
88. Stott, S.L.; Lee, R.J.; Nagrath, S.; Yu, M.; Miyamoto, D.T.; Ulkus, L.; Inserra, E.J.; Ulman, M.; Springer, S.; Nakamura, Z.; et al. Isolation and Characterization of Circulating Tumor Cells from Patients with Localized and Metastatic Prostate Cancer. *Sci. Transl. Med.* **2010**, *2*, 25ra23. [CrossRef]
89. Shan, L.; Ji, T.; Su, X.; Shao, Q.; Du, T.; Zhang, S. TMPRSS2-ERG Fusion Promotes Recruitment of Regulatory T cells and Tumor Growth in Prostate Cancer. *Am. J. Med Sci.* **2018**, *356*, 72–78. [CrossRef]
90. Chen, J.; Cao, S.; Situ, B.; Zhong, J.; Hu, Y.; Li, S.; Huang, J.; Xu, J.; Wu, S.; Lin, J.; et al. Metabolic reprogramming-based characterization of circulating tumor cells in prostate cancer. *J. Exp. Clin. Cancer Res.* **2018**, *37*, 127. [CrossRef]
91. Carreira, S.; Romanel, A.; Goodall, J.; Grist, E.; Ferraldeschi, R.; Miranda, S.; Prandi, D.; Lorente, D.; Frenel, J.-S.; Pezaro, C.; et al. Tumor clone dynamics in lethal prostate cancer. *Sci. Transl. Med.* **2014**, *6*, 254ra125. [CrossRef] [PubMed]
92. Goodall, J.; Mateo, J.; Yuan, W.; Mossop, H.; Porta, N.; Miranda, S.; Perez-Lopez, R.; Dolling, D.; Robinson, D.R.; Sandhu, S.; et al. Circulating Cell-Free DNA to Guide Prostate Cancer Treatment with PARP Inhibition. *Cancer Discov.* **2017**, *7*, 1006–1017. [CrossRef] [PubMed]
93. Kazma, R.; Mefford, J.A.; Cheng, I.; Plummer, S.J.; Levin, A.M.; Rybicki, B.A.; Casey, G.; Witte, J.S. Association of the Innate Immunity and Inflammation Pathway with Advanced Prostate Cancer Risk. *PLoS ONE* **2012**, *7*, e51680. [CrossRef]
94. Nakai, Y.; Nonomura, N. Inflammation and prostate carcinogenesis. *Int. J. Urol.* **2013**, *20*, 150–160. [CrossRef]
95. Veeranki, S. Role of inflammasomes and their regulators in prostate cancer initiation, progression and metastasis. *Cell. Mol. Biol. Lett.* **2013**, *18*, 355–367. [CrossRef]
96. Coussens, L.M.; Werb, Z. Inflammation and cancer. *Nature* **2002**, *420*, 860–867. [CrossRef]
97. De Visser, K.E.; Coussens, L.M. The interplay between innate and adaptive immunity regulates cancer development. *Cancer Immunol. Immunother.* **2005**, *54*, 1143–1152. [CrossRef] [PubMed]
98. Hanahan, D.; Weinberg, R.A. The Hallmarks of Cancer. *Cell* **2000**, *100*, 57–70. [CrossRef]
99. Brubaker, S.W.; Bonham, K.S.; Zanoni, I.; Kagan, J.C. Innate Immune Pattern Recognition: A Cell Biological Perspective. *Annu. Rev. Immunol.* **2015**, *33*, 257–290. [CrossRef] [PubMed]
100. Shalapour, S.; Karin, M. Immunity, inflammation, and cancer: An eternal fight between good and evil. *J. Clin. Investig.* **2015**, *125*, 3347–3355. [CrossRef] [PubMed]
101. Tan, S.; Wang, K.; Sun, F.; Li, Y.; Gao, Y. CXCL9 promotes prostate cancer progression through inhibition of cytokines from T cells. *Mol. Med. Rep.* **2018**, *18*, 1305–1310. [CrossRef]
102. Wieczorek, M.; Abualrous, E.T.; Sticht, J.; Álvaro-Benito, M.; Stolzenberg, S.; Noé, F.; Freund, C. Major Histocompatibility Complex (MHC) Class I and MHC Class II Proteins: Conformational Plasticity in Antigen Presentation. *Front. Immunol.* **2017**, *8*, 292. [CrossRef]
103. Sokol, C.L.; Luster, A.D. The Chemokine System in Innate Immunity. *Cold Spring Harb. Perspect. Biol.* **2015**, *7*, a016303. [CrossRef]
104. Miller, A.M.; Pisa, P. Tumor escape mechanisms in prostate cancer. *Cancer Immunol. Immunother.* **2005**, *56*, 81–87. [CrossRef] [PubMed]
105. Shaul, M.E.; Fridlender, Z.G. Tumour-associated neutrophils in patients with cancer. *Nat. Rev. Clin. Oncol.* **2019**, *16*, 601–620. [CrossRef] [PubMed]
106. Lo, C.H.; Lynch, C.C. Multifaceted Roles for Macrophages in Prostate Cancer Skeletal Metastasis. *Front. Endocrinol.* **2018**, *9*, 247. [CrossRef]
107. Zhang, J.; Lu, Y.; Pienta, K.J. Multiple Roles of Chemokine (C-C Motif) Ligand 2 in Promoting Prostate Cancer Growth. *J. Natl. Cancer Inst.* **2010**, *102*, 522–528. [CrossRef] [PubMed]
108. Yano, H.; Andrews, L.P.; Workman, C.J.; Vignali, D.A.A. Intratumoral regulatory T cells: Markers, subsets and their impact on anti-tumor immunity. *Immunology* **2019**, *157*, 232–247. [CrossRef] [PubMed]
109. Watanabe, M.; Kanao, K.; Suzuki, S.; Muramatsu, H.; Morinaga, S.; Kajikawa, K.; Kobayashi, I.; Nishikawa, G.; Kato, Y.; Zennami, K.; et al. Increased infiltration of CCR4-positive regulatory T cells in prostate cancer tissue is associated with a poor prognosis. *Prostate* **2019**, *79*, 1658–1665. [CrossRef]
110. Pfannenstiel, L.W.; Diaz-Montero, C.M.; Tian, Y.F.; Scharpf, J.; Ko, J.S.; Gastman, B.R.; Diaz-Montero, M. Immune-Checkpoint Blockade Opposes CD8+ T-cell Suppression in Human and Murine Cancer. *Cancer Immunol. Res.* **2019**, *7*, 510–525. [CrossRef]
111. Matoba, T.; Imai, M.; Ohkura, N.; Kawakita, D.; Ijichi, K.; Toyama, T.; Morita, A.; Murakami, S.; Sakaguchi, S.; Yamazaki, S. Regulatory T cells expressing abundant CTLA-4 on the cell surface with a proliferative gene profile are key features of human head and neck cancer. *Int. J. Cancer* **2019**, *144*, 2811–2822. [CrossRef]
112. Erlandsson, A.; Carlsson, J.; Lundholm, M.; Fält, A.; Andersson, S.-O.; Andrén, O.; Davidsson, S. M2 macrophages and regulatory T cells in lethal prostate cancer. *Prostate* **2019**, *79*, 363–369. [CrossRef] [PubMed]
113. Liu, Z.; Zhong, J.; Cai, C.; Lu, J.; Wu, W.; Zeng, G. Immune-related biomarker risk score predicts prognosis in prostate cancer. *Aging* **2020**, *12*, 22776–22793. [CrossRef]
114. Naor, D.; Sionov, R.V.; Ish-Shalom, D. CD44: Structure, Function and Association with the Malignant Process. *Adv. Cancer Res.* **1997**, *71*, 241–319. [CrossRef] [PubMed]

115. Nagano, O.; Okazaki, S.; Saya, H. Redox regulation in stem-like cancer cells by CD44 variant isoforms. *Oncogene* **2013**, *32*, 5191–5198. [CrossRef]
116. Ni, J.; Cozzi, P.J.; Hao, J.L.; Beretov, J.; Chang, L.; Duan, W.; Shigdar, S.; Delprado, W.J.; Graham, P.H.; Bucci, J.; et al. CD44 variant 6 is associated with prostate cancer metastasis and chemo-/radioresistance. *Prostate* **2014**, *74*, 602–617. [CrossRef]
117. Chen, Y.-C.; Giovannucci, E.; Lazarus, R.; Kraft, P.; Ketkar, S.; Hunter, D.J. Sequence Variants of Toll-Like Receptor 4 and Susceptibility to Prostate Cancer. *Cancer Res.* **2005**, *65*, 11771–11778. [CrossRef]
118. Lindmark, F.; Jonsson, B.-A.; Bergh, A.; Stattin, P.; Zheng, S.L.; Meyers, D.A.; Xu, J.; Grönberg, H. Analysis of the macrophage scavenger receptor 1 gene in Swedish hereditary and sporadic prostate cancer. *Prostate* **2003**, *59*, 132–140. [CrossRef] [PubMed]
119. Rennert, H.; Zeigler-Johnson, C.M.; Addya, K.; Finley, M.J.; Walker, A.H.; Spangler, E.; Leonard, D.G.; Wein, A.; Malkowicz, S.B.; Rebbeck, T.R. Association of Susceptibility Alleles in ELAC2/HPC2, RNASEL/HPC1, and MSR1 with Prostate Cancer Severity in European American and African American Men. *Cancer Epidemiol. Biomark. Prev.* **2005**, *14*, 949–957. [CrossRef] [PubMed]
120. Xu, J.; Lowey, J.; Wiklund, F.; Sun, J.; Lindmark, F.; Hsu, F.-C.; Dimitrov, L.; Chang, B.; Turner, A.R.; Liu, W.; et al. The Interaction of Four Genes in the Inflammation Pathway Significantly Predicts Prostate Cancer Risk. *Cancer Epidemiol. Biomark. Prev.* **2005**, *14*, 2563–2568. [CrossRef]
121. Casey, G.; Neville, P.J.; Plummer, S.J.; Xiang, Y.; Krumroy, L.M.; Klein, E.A.; Catalona, W.J.; Nupponen, N.; Carpten, J.D.; Trent, J.M.; et al. RNASEL Arg462Gln variant is implicated in up to 13% of prostate cancer cases. *Nat. Genet.* **2002**, *32*, 581–583. [CrossRef]
122. Nakazato, H.; Suzuki, K.; Matsui, H.; Ohtake, N.; Nakata, S.; Yamanaka, H. Role of genetic polymorphisms of the RNASEL gene on familial prostate cancer risk in a Japanese population. *Br. J. Cancer* **2003**, *89*, 691–696. [CrossRef]
123. Lindmark, F.; Zheng, S.L.; Wiklund, F.; Balter, K.; Sun, J.; Chang, B.; Hedelin, M.; Clark, J.S.; Johansson, J.-E.; A Meyers, D.; et al. Interleukin-1 receptor antagonist haplotype associated with prostate cancer risk. *Br. J. Cancer* **2005**, *93*, 493–497. [CrossRef]
124. Lindmark, F.; Zheng, S.L.; Wiklund, F.; Bensen, J.; Bälter, K.A.; Chang, B.; Hedelin, M.; Clark, J.; Stattin, P.; Meyers, D.A.; et al. H6D Polymorphism in Macrophage-Inhibitory Cytokine-1 Gene Associated with Prostate Cancer. *J. Natl. Cancer Inst.* **2004**, *96*, 1248–1254. [CrossRef]
125. Cheng, I.; Liu, X.; Plummer, S.J.; Krumroy, L.M.; Casey, G.; Witte, J.S. COX2 genetic variation, NSAIDs, and advanced prostate cancer risk. *Br. J. Cancer* **2007**, *97*, 557–561. [CrossRef]
126. Liong, M.L.; Lim, C.R.; Yang, H.; Chao, S.; Bong, C.W.; Leong, W.S.; Das, P.K.; Loh, C.S.; Lau, B.E.; Yu, C.G.; et al. Blood-Based Biomarkers of Aggressive Prostate Cancer. *PLoS ONE* **2012**, *7*, e45802. [CrossRef] [PubMed]
127. Wallace, T.A.; Prueitt, R.L.; Yi, M.; Howe, T.M.; Gillespie, J.W.; Yfantis, H.G.; Stephens, R.M.; Caporaso, N.E.; Loffredo, C.A.; Ambs, S. Tumor Immunobiological Differences in Prostate Cancer between African-American and European-American Men. *Cancer Res.* **2008**, *68*, 927–936. [CrossRef] [PubMed]
128. Taichman, R.S.; Cooper, C.; Keller, E.T.; Pienta, K.J.; Taichman, N.S.; McCauley, L.K. Use of the stromal cell-derived fac-tor-1/CXCR4 pathway in prostate cancer metastasis to bone. *Cancer Res.* **2002**, *62*, 1832–1837.
129. Powell, I.J.; Dyson, G.; Land, S.; Ruterbusch, J.; Bock, C.H.; Lenk, S.; Herawi, M.; Everson, R.; Giroux, C.N.; Schwartz, A.G.; et al. Genes Associated with Prostate Cancer Are Differentially Expressed in African American and European American Men. *Cancer Epidemiol. Biomark. Prev.* **2013**, *22*, 891–897. [CrossRef] [PubMed]
130. Singhal, U.; Wang, Y.; Henderson, J.; Niknafs, Y.S.; Qiao, Y.; Gursky, A.; Zaslavsky, A.; Chung, J.-S.; Smith, D.C.; Karnes, R.J.; et al. Multigene Profiling of CTCs in mCRPC Identifies a Clinically Relevant Prognostic Signature. *Mol. Cancer Res.* **2018**, *16*, 643–654. [CrossRef]
131. Golden, E.B.; Apetoh, L. Radiotherapy and Immunogenic Cell Death. *Semin. Radiat. Oncol.* **2015**, *25*, 11–17. [CrossRef]
132. Garg, A.D.; Nowis, D.; Golab, J.; Vandenabeele, P.; Krysko, D.V.; Agostinis, P. Immunogenic cell death, DAMPs and anticancer therapeutics: An emerging amalgamation. *Biochim. Biophys. Acta (BBA) Bioenerg.* **2010**, *1805*, 53–71. [CrossRef]
133. Barcellos-Hoff, M.H.; Park, C.; Wright, E.G. Radiation and the microenvironment—Tumorigenesis and therapy. *Nat. Rev. Cancer* **2005**, *5*, 867–875. [CrossRef] [PubMed]
134. Gupta, S.C.; Hevia, D.; Patchva, S.; Park, B.; Koh, W.; Aggarwal, B.B. Upsides and Downsides of Reactive Oxygen Species for Cancer: The Roles of Reactive Oxygen Species in Tumorigenesis, Prevention, and Therapy. *Antioxid. Redox Signal.* **2012**, *16*, 1295–1322. [CrossRef] [PubMed]
135. Frey, B.; Mika, J.; Jelonek, K.; Cruz-Garcia, L.; Roelants, C.; Testard, I.; Cherradi, N.; Lumniczky, K.; Polozov, S.; Napieralska, A.; et al. Systemic modulation of stress and immune parameters in patients treated for prostate adenocarcinoma by intensity-modulated radiation therapy or stereotactic ablative body radiotherapy. *Strahlenther. Onkol.* **2020**, *196*, 1018–1033. [CrossRef] [PubMed]
136. Reits, E.A.; Hodge, J.W.; Herberts, C.A.; Groothuis, T.A.; Chakraborty, M.; Wansley, E.K.; Camphausen, K.; Luiten, R.M.; De Ru, A.H.; Neijssen, J.; et al. Radiation modulates the peptide repertoire, enhances MHC class I expression, and induces successful antitumor immunotherapy. *J. Exp. Med.* **2006**, *203*, 1259–1271. [CrossRef] [PubMed]
137. Harris, T.J.; Hipkiss, E.L.; Borzillary, S.; Wada, S.; Grosso, J.F.; Yen, H.-R.; Getnet, D.; Bruno, T.C.; Goldberg, M.V.; Pardoll, D.M.; et al. Radiotherapy augments the immune response to prostate cancer in a time-dependent manner. *Prostate* **2008**, *68*, 1319–1329. [CrossRef]

138. Pal, S.K.; Moreira, D.; Won, H.; White, S.W.; Duttagupta, P.; Lucia, M.; Jones, J.; Hsu, J.; Kortylewski, M. Reduced T-cell Numbers and Elevated Levels of Immunomodulatory Cytokines in Metastatic Prostate Cancer Patients De Novo Resistant to Abiraterone and/or Enzalutamide Therapy. *Int. J. Mol. Sci.* **2019**, *20*, 1831. [CrossRef]
139. Corre, I.; Guillonneau, M.; Paris, F. Membrane Signaling Induced by High Doses of Ionizing Radiation in the Endothelial Compartment. Relevance in Radiation Toxicity. *Int. J. Mol. Sci.* **2013**, *14*, 22678–22696. [CrossRef] [PubMed]
140. A Woodward, W.; Wachsberger, P.; Burd, R.; Dicker, A.P. Effects of androgen suppression and radiation on prostate cancer suggest a role for angiogenesis blockade. *Prostate Cancer Prostatic Dis.* **2005**, *8*, 127–132. [CrossRef] [PubMed]
141. Bentzen, S.M. Preventing or reducing late side effects of radiation therapy: Radiobiology meets molecular pathology. *Nat. Rev. Cancer* **2006**, *6*, 702–713. [CrossRef]
142. Border, W.A.; Noble, N.A. Transforming growth factor beta in tissue fibrosis. *N. Engl. J. Med.* **1994**, *331*, 1286–1292.
143. Moussad, E.E.-D.A.; Brigstock, D.R. Connective Tissue Growth Factor: What's in a Name? *Mol. Genet. Metab.* **2000**, *71*, 276–292. [CrossRef] [PubMed]
144. Leask, A.; Abraham, D.J. TGF-beta signaling and the fibrotic response. *FASEB J.* **2004**, *18*, 816–827. [CrossRef]
145. Leith, J.T. In vitro radiation sensitivity of the lncap prostatic tumor cell line. *Prostate* **1994**, *24*, 119–124. [CrossRef] [PubMed]
146. Thompson, I.; Thrasher, J.B.; Aus, G.; Burnett, A.L.; Canby-Hagino, E.D.; Cookson, M.S.; D'Amico, A.V.; Dmochowski, R.R.; Eton, D.T.; Forman, J.D.; et al. Guideline for the Management of Clinically Localized Prostate Cancer: 2007 Update. *J. Urol.* **2007**, *177*, 2106–2131. [CrossRef] [PubMed]
147. Zhao, S.G.; Chang, S.L.; E Spratt, D.; Erho, N.; Yu, M.; Ashab, H.A.-D.; Alshalalfa, M.; Speers, C.; A Tomlins, S.; Davicioni, E.; et al. Development and validation of a 24-gene predictor of response to postoperative radiotherapy in prostate cancer: A matched, retrospective analysis. *Lancet Oncol.* **2016**, *17*, 1612–1620. [CrossRef]
148. Bostwick, D.G.; Alexander, E.E.; Singh, R.; Shan, A.; Qian, J.; Santella, R.M.; Oberley, L.W.; Yan, T.; Zhong, W.; Jiang, X.; et al. Antioxidant enzyme expression and reactive oxygen species damage in prostatic intraepithelial neoplasia and cancer. *Cancer* **2000**, *89*, 123–134. [CrossRef]
149. Chaiswing, L.; Weiss, H.L.; Jayswal, R.D.; Clair, D.K.S.; Kyprianou, N. Profiles of Radioresistance Mechanisms in Prostate Cancer. *Crit. Rev. Oncog.* **2018**, *23*, 39–67. [CrossRef]
150. Bristow, R.G.; Hill, R.P. Hypoxia, DNA repair and genetic instability. *Nat. Rev. Cancer* **2008**, *8*, 180–192. [CrossRef]
151. Ramteke, A.; Ting, H.; Agarwal, C.; Mateen, S.; Somasagara, R.; Hussain, A.; Graner, M.; Frederick, B.; Agarwal, R.; Deep, G. Exosomes secreted under hypoxia enhance invasiveness and stemness of prostate cancer cells by targeting adherens junction molecules. *Mol. Carcinog.* **2015**, *54*, 554–565. [CrossRef] [PubMed]
152. Caruso, D.J.; Carmack, A.J.; Lokeshwar, V.B.; Duncan, R.C.; Soloway, M.S.; Lokeshwar, B.L. Osteopontin and Interleukin-8 Expression is Independently Associated with Prostate Cancer Recurrence. *Clin. Cancer Res.* **2008**, *14*, 4111–4118. [CrossRef] [PubMed]
153. Cesaretti, J.A.; Stock, R.G.; Lehrer, S.; Atencio, D.A.; Bernstein, J.L.; Stone, N.N.; Wallenstein, S.; Green, S.; Loeb, K.; Kollmeier, M.; et al. ATM sequence variants are predictive of adverse radiotherapy response among patients treated for prostate cancer. *Int. J. Radiat. Oncol.* **2005**, *61*, 196–202. [CrossRef] [PubMed]
154. Pugh, T.J.; Keyes, M.; Barclay, L.; Delaney, A.; Krzywinski, M.; Thomas, D.; Novik, K.; Yang, C.; Agranovich, A.; McKenzie, M.; et al. Sequence Variant Discovery in DNA Repair Genes from Radiosensitive and Radiotolerant Prostate Brachytherapy Patients. *Clin. Cancer Res.* **2009**, *15*, 5008–5016. [CrossRef]
155. Langsenlehner, T.; Renner, W.; Gerger, A.; Hofmann, G.; Thurner, E.-M.; Kapp, K.S.; Langsenlehner, U. Association between single nucleotide polymorphisms in the gene for XRCC1 and radiation-induced late toxicity in prostate cancer patients. *Radiother. Oncol.* **2011**, *98*, 387–393. [CrossRef]
156. Yáñez-Mó, M.; Siljander, P.R.M.; Andreu, Z.; Zavec, A.B.; Borràs, F.E.; Buzas, E.I.; Buzas, K.; Casal, E.; Cappello, F.; Carvalho, J.; et al. Biological Properties of Extracellular Vesicles and their Physiological Functions. *J. Extracell. Vesicles* **2015**, *4*, 27066. [CrossRef]
157. Gould, S.J.; Raposo, G. As we wait: Coping with an imperfect nomenclature for extracellular vesicles. *J. Extracell. Vesicles* **2013**, *2*. [CrossRef]
158. Fais, S.; O'Driscoll, L.; Borras, F.E.; Buzas, E.; Camussi, G.; Cappello, F.; Carvalho, J.; Da Silva, A.C.; Del Portillo, H.; El Andaloussi, S.; et al. Evidence-Based Clinical Use of Nanoscale Extracellular Vesicles in Nanomedicine. *ACS Nano* **2016**, *10*, 3886–3899. [CrossRef]
159. Skog, J.; Würdinger, T.; Van Rijn, S.; Meijer, D.H.; Gainche, L.; Curry, W.T., Jr.; Carter, B.S.; Krichevsky, A.M.; Breakefield, X.O. Glioblastoma microvesicles transport RNA and proteins that promote tumour growth and provide diagnostic biomarkers. *Nat. Cell Biol.* **2008**, *10*, 1470–1476. [CrossRef]
160. Taylor, D.D.; Gerceltaylor, C. Tumour-derived exosomes and their role in cancer-associated T-cell signalling defects. *Br. J. Cancer* **2005**, *92*, 305–311. [CrossRef]
161. Parolini, I.; Federici, C.; Raggi, C.; Lugini, L.; Palleschi, S.; De Milito, A.; Coscia, C.; Iessi, E.; Logozzi, M.; Molinari, A.; et al. Microenvironmental pH Is a Key Factor for Exosome Traffic in Tumor Cells. *J. Biol. Chem.* **2009**, *284*, 34211–34222. [CrossRef] [PubMed]

162. Boussadia, Z.; Lamberti, J.; Mattei, F.; Pizzi, E.; Puglisi, R.; Zanetti, C.; Pasquini, L.; Fratini, F.; Fantozzi, L.; Felicetti, F.; et al. Acidic microenvironment plays a key role in human melanoma progression through a sustained exosome mediated transfer of clinically relevant metastatic molecules. *J. Exp. Clin. Cancer Res.* **2018**, *37*, 245. [CrossRef] [PubMed]
163. Panigrahi, G.K.; Praharaj, P.P.; Peak, T.C.; Long, J.; Singh, R.; Rhim, J.S.; Abd Elmageed, Z.Y.; Deep, G. Hypoxia-induced exosome secretion promotes survival of African-American and Caucasian prostate cancer cells. *Sci. Rep.* **2018**, *8*, 3853. [CrossRef]
164. Krishn, S.R.; Salem, I.; Quaglia, F.; Naranjo, N.M.; Agarwal, E.; Liu, Q.; Sarker, S.; Kopenhaver, J.; McCue, P.A.; Weinreb, P.H.; et al. The alphavbeta6 integrin in cancer cell-derived small extracellular vesicles enhances angiogenesis. *J. Extracell. Vesicles* **2020**, *9*, 1763594. [CrossRef] [PubMed]
165. Franzen, C.A.; Blackwell, R.H.; Foreman, K.E.; Kuo, P.C.; Flanigan, R.C.; Gupta, G.N. Urinary Exosomes: The Potential for Biomarker Utility, Intercellular Signaling and Therapeutics in Urological Malignancy. *J. Urol.* **2016**, *195*, 1331–1339. [CrossRef]
166. Bijnsdorp, I.V.; Geldof, A.A.; Lavaei, M.; Piersma, S.R.; Van Moorselaar, R.J.A.; Jimenez, C.R. Exosomal ITGA3 interferes with non-cancerous prostate cell functions and is increased in urine exosomes of metastatic prostate cancer patients. *J. Extracell. Vesicles* **2013**, *2*. [CrossRef] [PubMed]
167. Probert, C.; Dottorini, T.; Speakman, A.; Hunt, S.; Nafee, T.; Fazeli, A.; Wood, S.; Brown, J.E.; James, V. Communication of prostate cancer cells with bone cells via extracellular vesicle RNA; a potential mechanism of metastasis. *Oncogene* **2019**, *38*, 1751–1763. [CrossRef]
168. Saber, S.H.; Ali, H.E.A.; Gaballa, R.; Gaballah, M.; Ali, H.I.; Zerfaoui, M.; Elmageed, Z.Y.A. Exosomes are the Driving Force in Preparing the Soil for the Metastatic Seeds: Lessons from the Prostate Cancer. *Cells* **2020**, *9*, 564. [CrossRef]
169. Biggs, C.N.; Siddiqui, K.M.; Al-Zahrani, A.A.; Pardhan, S.; Brett, S.I.; Guo, Q.Q.; Yang, J.; Wolf, P.; Power, N.E.; Durfee, P.N.; et al. Prostate extracellular vesicles in patient plasma as a liquid biopsy platform for prostate cancer using nanoscale flow cytometry. *Oncotarget* **2016**, *7*, 8839–8849. [CrossRef]
170. Joncas, F.; Lucien, F.; Rouleau, M.; Morin, F.; Leong, H.S.; Pouliot, F.; Fradet, Y.; Gilbert, C.; Toren, P. Plasma extracellular vesicles as phenotypic biomarkers in prostate cancer patients. *Prostate* **2019**, *79*, 1767–1776. [CrossRef]
171. Logozzi, M.; Angelini, D.F.; Iessi, E.; Mizzoni, D.; Di Raimo, R.; Federici, C.; Lugini, L.; Borsellino, G.; Gentilucci, A.; Pierella, F.; et al. Increased PSA expression on prostate cancer exosomes in in vitro condition and in cancer patients. *Cancer Lett.* **2017**, *403*, 318–329. [CrossRef]
172. Logozzi, M.; Angelini, D.F.; Giuliani, A.; Mizzoni, D.; Di Raimo, R.; Maggi, M.; Gentilucci, A.; Marzio, V.; Salciccia, S.; Borsellino, G.; et al. Increased Plasmatic Levels of PSA-Expressing Exosomes Distinguish Prostate Cancer Patients from Benign Prostatic Hyperplasia: A Prospective Study. *Cancers* **2019**, *11*, 1449. [CrossRef]
173. McKiernan, J.; Donovan, M.J.; O'Neill, V.; Bentink, S.; Noerholm, M.; Belzer, S.; Skog, J.; Kattan, M.W.; Partin, A.; Andriole, G.; et al. A Novel Urine Exosome Gene Expression Assay to Predict High-grade Prostate Cancer at Initial Biopsy. *JAMA Oncol.* **2016**, *2*, 882–889. [CrossRef]
174. Khan, S.; Jutzy, J.M.S.; Valenzuela, M.M.A.; Turay, D.; Aspe, J.R.; Ashok, A.; Mirshahidi, S.; Mercola, D.; Lilly, M.B.; Wall, N.R. Plasma-Derived Exosomal Survivin, a Plausible Biomarker for Early Detection of Prostate Cancer. *PLoS ONE* **2012**, *7*, e46737. [CrossRef] [PubMed]
175. Lundholm, M.; Schröder, M.; Nagaeva, O.; Baranov, V.; Widmark, A.; Mincheva-Nilsson, L.; Wikström, P. Prostate Tumor-Derived Exosomes Down-Regulate NKG2D Expression on Natural Killer Cells and CD8+ T Cells: Mechanism of Immune Evasion. *PLoS ONE* **2014**, *9*, e108925. [CrossRef]
176. Del Re, M.; Biasco, E.; Crucitta, S.; DeRosa, L.; Rofi, E.; Orlandini, C.; Miccoli, M.; Galli, L.; Falcone, A.; Jenster, G.W.; et al. The Detection of Androgen Receptor Splice Variant 7 in Plasma-derived Exosomal RNA Strongly Predicts Resistance to Hormonal Therapy in Metastatic Prostate Cancer Patients. *Eur. Urol.* **2017**, *71*, 680–687. [CrossRef] [PubMed]
177. Etheridge, A.; Lee, I.; Hood, L.; Galas, D.; Wang, K. Extracellular microRNA: A new source of biomarkers. *Mutat. Res. Mol. Mech. Mutagen.* **2011**, *717*, 85–90. [CrossRef] [PubMed]
178. Mitchell, P.S.; Parkin, R.K.; Kroh, E.M.; Fritz, B.R.; Wyman, S.K.; Pogosova-Agadjanyan, E.L.; Peterson, A.; Noteboom, J.; O'Briant, K.C.; Allen, A.; et al. Circulating microRNAs as stable blood-based markers for cancer detection. *Proc. Natl. Acad. Sci. USA* **2008**, *105*, 10513–10518. [CrossRef]
179. Zenner, M.L.; Baumann, B.; Nonn, L. Oncogenic and tumor-suppressive microRNAs in prostate cancer. *Curr. Opin. Endocr. Metab. Res.* **2020**, *10*, 50–59. [CrossRef]
180. Huang, X.; Yuan, T.; Liang, M.; Du, M.; Xia, S.; Dittmar, R.; Wang, D.; See, W.; Costello, B.A.; Quevedo, F.; et al. Exosomal miR-1290 and miR-375 as Prognostic Markers in Castration-resistant Prostate Cancer. *Eur. Urol.* **2015**, *67*, 33–41. [CrossRef]
181. Watahiki, A.; Macfarlane, R.J.; Gleave, M.E.; Crea, F.; Wang, Y.; Helgason, C.D.; Chi, K.N. Plasma miRNAs as Biomarkers to Identify Patients with Castration-Resistant Metastatic Prostate Cancer. *Int. J. Mol. Sci.* **2013**, *14*, 7757–7770. [CrossRef]
182. Brase, J.C.; Johannes, M.; Schlomm, T.; Fälth, M.; Haese, A.; Steuber, T.; Beissbarth, T.; Kuner, R.; Sültmann, H. Circulating miRNAs are correlated with tumor progression in prostate cancer. *Int. J. Cancer* **2010**, *128*, 608–616. [CrossRef] [PubMed]
183. Endzeliņš, E.; Berger, A.; Melne, V.; Bajo-Santos, C.; Soboļevska, K.; Ābols, A.; Rodriguez, M.; Šantare, D.; Rudņickiha, A.; Lietuvietis, V.; et al. Detection of circulating miRNAs: Comparative analysis of extracellular vesicle-incorporated miRNAs and cell-free miRNAs in whole plasma of prostate cancer patients. *BMC Cancer* **2017**, *17*, 1–13. [CrossRef] [PubMed]

184. Worst, T.S.; Previti, C.; Nitschke, K.; Diessl, N.; Gross, J.C.; Hoffmann, L.; Frey, L.; Thomas, V.; Kahlert, C.; Bieback, K.; et al. miR-10a-5p and miR-29b-3p as Extracellular Vesicle-Associated Prostate Cancer Detection Markers. *Cancers* **2019**, *12*, 43. [CrossRef] [PubMed]
185. Leidinger, P.; Hart, M.; Backes, C.; Rheinheimer, S.; Keck, B.; Wullich, B.; Keller, A.; Meese, E. Differential blood-based diagnosis between benign prostatic hyperplasia and prostate cancer: miRNA as source for biomarkers independent of PSA level, Gleason score, or TNM status. *Tumor Biol.* **2016**, *37*, 10177–10185. [CrossRef]
186. Shen, J.; Hruby, G.W.; McKiernan, J.M.; Gurvich, I.; Lipsky, M.J.; Benson, M.C.; Santella, R.M. Dysregulation of circulating microRNAs and prediction of aggressive prostate cancer. *Prostate* **2012**, *72*, 1469–1477. [CrossRef]
187. Hoey, C.; Ahmed, M.; Ghiam, A.F.; Vesprini, D.; Huang, X.; Commisso, K.; Ray, J.; Fokas, E.; Loblaw, D.A.; He, H.H.; et al. Circulating miRNAs as non-invasive biomarkers to predict aggressive prostate cancer after radical prostatectomy. *J. Transl. Med.* **2019**, *17*, 173. [CrossRef]
188. Al-Qatati, A.; Akrong, C.; Stevic, I.; Pantel, K.; Awe, J.; Saranchuk, J.; Drachenberg, D.; Mai, S.; Schwarzenbach, H. Plasma microRNA signature is associated with risk stratification in prostate cancer patients. *Int. J. Cancer* **2017**, *141*, 1231–1239. [CrossRef]
189. Fredsøe, J.; Rasmussen, A.K.I.; Mouritzen, P.; Bjerre, M.T.; Østergren, P.; Fode, M.; Borre, M.; Sørensen, K.D. Profiling of Circulating microRNAs in Prostate Cancer Reveals Diagnostic Biomarker Potential. *Diagnostics* **2020**, *10*, 188. [CrossRef] [PubMed]
190. Bhatnagar, N.; Li, X.; Padi, S.K.R.; Zhang, Q.; Tang, M.-S.; Guo, B. Downregulation of miR-205 and miR-31 confers resistance to chemotherapy-induced apoptosis in prostate cancer cells. *Cell Death Dis.* **2010**, *1*, e105. [CrossRef]
191. Jiang, S.; Mo, C.; Guo, S.; Zhuang, J.; Huang, B.; Mao, X. Human bone marrow mesenchymal stem cells-derived microRNA-205-containing exosomes impede the progression of prostate cancer through suppression of RHPN2. *J. Exp. Clin. Cancer Res.* **2019**, *38*, 1–16. [CrossRef] [PubMed]
192. Guan, H.; Peng, R.; Fang, F.; Mao, L.; Chen, Z.; Yang, S.; Dai, C.; Wu, H.; Wang, C.; Feng, N.; et al. Tumor-associated macrophages promote prostate cancer progression via exosome-mediated miR-95 transfer. *J. Cell. Physiol.* **2020**, *235*, 9729–9742. [CrossRef] [PubMed]
193. Labbé, M.; Hoey, C.; Ray, J.; Potiron, V.; Supiot, S.; Liu, S.K.; Fradin, D. microRNAs identified in prostate cancer: Correlative studies on response to ionizing radiation. *Mol. Cancer* **2020**, *19*, 1–18. [CrossRef]
194. Hoey, C.; Ray, J.; Jeon, J.; Huang, X.; Taeb, S.; Ylanko, J.; Andrews, D.W.; Boutros, P.C.; Liu, S.K. miRNA-106a and pros-tate cancer radioresistance: A novel role for LITAF in ATM regulation. *Mol. Oncol.* **2018**, *12*, 1324–1341. [CrossRef]
195. McDermott, N.; Meunier, A.; Wong, S.; Buchete, V.; Marignol, L. Profiling of a panel of radioresistant prostate cancer cells identifies deregulation of key miRNAs. *Clin. Transl. Radiat. Oncol.* **2017**, *2*, 63–68. [CrossRef]
196. Kopcalic, K.; Petrovic, N.; Stanojkovic, T.P.; Stankovic, V.; Bukumiric, Z.; Roganovic, J.; Malisic, E.; Nikitovic, M. Associ-ation between miR-21/146a/155 level changes and acute genitourinary radiotoxicity in prostate cancer patients: A pilot study. *Pathol. Res. Pract.* **2019**, *215*, 626–631. [CrossRef]
197. Gong, P.; Zhang, T.; He, D.; Hsieh, J.-T. MicroRNA-145 Modulates Tumor Sensitivity to Radiation in Prostate Cancer. *Radiat. Res.* **2015**, *184*, 630–638. [CrossRef]
198. Zedan, A.H.; Hansen, T.F.; Assenholt, J.; Madsen, J.S.; Osther, P.J.S. Circulating miRNAs in localized/locally advanced prostate cancer patients after radical prostatectomy and radiotherapy. *Prostate* **2018**, *79*, 425–432. [CrossRef]
199. Yu, Q.; Li, P.; Weng, M.; Wu, S.; Zhang, Y.; Chen, X.; Zhang, Q.; Shen, G.; Ding, X.; Fu, S. Nano-Vesicles are a Potential Tool to Monitor Therapeutic Efficacy of Carbon Ion Radiotherapy in Prostate Cancer. *J. Biomed. Nanotechnol.* **2018**, *14*, 168–178. [CrossRef] [PubMed]
200. Malla, B.; Aebersold, D.M.; Pra, A.D. Protocol for serum exosomal miRNAs analysis in prostate cancer patients treated with radiotherapy. *J. Transl. Med.* **2018**, *16*, 223. [CrossRef]
201. Heller, G.; McCormack, R.; Kheoh, T.; Molina, A.; Smith, M.R.; Dreicer, R.; Saad, F.; De Wit, R.; Aftab, D.T.; Hirmand, M.; et al. Circulating Tumor Cell Number as a Response Measure of Prolonged Survival for Metastatic Castration-Resistant Prostate Cancer: A Comparison with Prostate-Specific Antigen Across Five Randomized Phase III Clinical Trials. *J. Clin. Oncol.* **2018**, *36*, 572–580. [CrossRef]
202. Vergati, M.; Cereda, V.; Madan, R.A.; Gulley, J.L.; Huen, N.-Y.; Rogers, C.J.; Hance, K.W.; Arlen, P.M.; Schlom, J.; Tsangsa, K.Y. Analysis of circulating regulatory T cells in patients with metastatic prostate cancer pre- versus post-vaccination. *Cancer Immunol. Immunother.* **2011**, *60*, 197–206. [CrossRef] [PubMed]
203. Wise, G.J.; Marella, V.K.; Talluri, G.; Shirazian, D. Cytokine variations in patients with hormone treated prostate cancer. *J. Urol.* **2000**, *164*, 722–725. [CrossRef]
204. Moltzahn, F.; Olshen, A.B.; Baehner, L.; Peek, A.; Fong, L.; Stöppler, H.; Simko, J.; Hilton, J.F.; Carroll, P.; Blelloch, R. Microfluidic-based multiplex qRT-PCR identifies diagnostic and prognostic microRNA signatures in the sera of prostate cancer patients. *Cancer Res.* **2011**, *71*, 550–560. [CrossRef]
205. Mahn, R.; Heukamp, L.C.; Rogenhofer, S.; von Ruecker, A.; Müller, S.C.; Ellinger, J. Circulating microRNAs (miRNA) in serum of patients with prostate cancer. *Urology* **2011**, *77*, 1265.e9–1265.e16. [CrossRef] [PubMed]
206. Nguyen, H.C.N.; Xie, W.; Yang, M.; Hsieh, C.-L.; Drouin, S.; Lee, G.-S.M.; Kantoff, P.W. Expression differences of circulating microRNAs in metastatic castration resistant prostate cancer and low-risk, localized prostate cancer. *Prostate* **2013**, *73*, 346–354. [CrossRef] [PubMed]

207. Selth, L.A.; Townley, S.; Gillis, J.L.; Ochnik, A.M.; Murti, K.; Macfarlane, R.J.; Chi, K.N.; Marshall, V.R.; Tilley, W.D.; Butler, L.M. Discovery of circulating microRNAs associated with human prostate cancer using a mouse model of disease. *Int. J. Cancer* **2011**, *131*, 652–661. [CrossRef] [PubMed]
208. Chen, Z.-H.; Zhang, G.-L.; Li, H.-R.; Luo, J.-D.; Li, Z.-X.; Chen, G.-M.; Yang, J. A panel of five circulating microRNAs as potential biomarkers for prostate cancer. *Prostate* **2012**, *72*, 1443–1452. [CrossRef]
209. Kelly, B.D.; Miller, N.; Sweeney, K.J.; Durkan, G.C.; Rogers, E.; Walsh, K.; Kerin, M.J. A Circulating MicroRNA Signature as a Biomarker for Prostate Cancer in a High Risk Group. *J. Clin. Med.* **2015**, *4*, 1369–1379. [CrossRef] [PubMed]
210. Bryant, R.J.; Pawlowski, T.; Catto, J.W.F.; Marsden, G.; Vessella, R.L.; Rhees, B.; Kuslich, C.; Visakorpi, T.; Hamdy, F.C. Changes in circulating microRNA levels associated with prostate cancer. *Br. J. Cancer* **2012**, *106*, 768–774. [CrossRef] [PubMed]
211. Murphy, A.B.; Carbunaru, S.; Nettey, O.S.; Gornbein, C.; Dixon, M.A.; Macias, V.; Sharifi, R.; Kittles, R.A.; Yang, X.; Kajdacsy-Balla, A.; et al. A 17-Gene Panel Genomic Prostate Score Has Similar Predictive Accuracy for Adverse Pathology at Radical Prostatectomy in African American and European American Men. *Urology* **2020**, *142*, 166–173. [CrossRef] [PubMed]
212. Reis, L.O. Basics of Biomarker Development and Interpretation. In *Molecular Biomarkers in Urologic Oncology*; World Urologic Oncology Federation (WUOF), 2020; pp. 5–21.
213. Sauerbrei, W.; Taube, S.E.; McShane, L.M.; Cavenagh, M.M.; Altman, D.G. Reporting Recommendations for Tumor Marker Prognostic Studies (REMARK): An Abridged Explanation and Elaboration. *J. Natl. Cancer Inst.* **2018**, *110*, 803–811. [CrossRef] [PubMed]

Journal of
Personalized Medicine

MDPI

Review

Radiation Response in the Tumour Microenvironment: Predictive Biomarkers and Future Perspectives

Niall M. Byrne , Prajakta Tambe and Jonathan A. Coulter *

School of Pharmacy, Queens University Belfast, Lisburn Road, Belfast BT9 7BL, UK; n.byrne@qub.ac.uk (N.M.B.); tprajakta05@gmail.com (P.T.)
* Correspondence: j.coulter@qub.ac.uk; Tel.: +44-0-28-9097-2253

Abstract: Radiotherapy (RT) is a primary treatment modality for a number of cancers, offering potentially curative outcomes. Despite its success, tumour *cells* can become resistant to RT, leading to disease recurrence. Components of the tumour microenvironment (TME) likely play an integral role in managing RT success or failure including infiltrating immune *cells*, the tumour vasculature and stroma. Furthermore, genomic profiling of the TME could identify predictive biomarkers or gene signatures indicative of RT response. In this review, we will discuss proposed mechanisms of radioresistance within the TME, biomarkers that may predict RT outcomes, and future perspectives on radiation treatment in the era of personalised medicine.

Keywords: biomarkers; immune infiltrate; radiotherapy; stroma; tumour microenvironment

check for updates

Citation: Byrne, N.M.; Tambe, P.; Coulter, J.A. Radiation Response in the Tumour Microenvironment: Predictive Biomarkers and Future Perspectives. *J. Pers. Med.* **2021**, *11*, 53. https://doi.org/10.3390/jpm11010053

Received: 9 December 2020
Accepted: 13 January 2021
Published: 16 January 2021

Publisher's Note: MDPI stays neutral with regard to jurisdictional claims in published maps and institutional affiliations.

1. Introduction

Radiotherapy (RT) is a primary treatment modality for a number of cancers, offering potentially curative outcomes [1]. Radiation treatment modalities have significantly improved over the last two decades with the introduction of advanced techniques including stereotactic radiotherapy (SRT) and enhanced imaging methodologies to improve the precision of RT delivery, thus limiting damage to healthy tissue. However, despite these advancements, resistance to radiotherapy still occurs, resulting in disease recurrence. Characterisation of radioresistance has traditionally focused on the effects of RT on tumour *cells*, overlooking the impact on supporting stromal and immune *cells* that make up the tumour microenvironment (TME) [2]. Although components of the TME have been shown to regulate angiogenesis [3] and promote malignant progression and metastasis [4], their role in the response to RT and their contribution to radioresistance is less well characterised [5]. As such, a greater understanding of the TME response could identify predictive biomarkers indicative of RT success or failure.

Predictive biomarkers offer an approach for stratifying patients who will respond favourably to a particular treatment, in turn sparing those for whom the modality may be less effective. While radiotherapy is intrinsically a precision treatment, directed to the specific architecture of the patient's tumour, it has so far lacked a personalised approach, taking into consideration patient-specific genomic alterations or TME composition, factors that could predict the outcome of radiotherapy [6,7]. In this review, we summarise some of the recent advances in understanding the TME response to ionising radiation. In particular, we discuss the effect of radiotherapy on the tumour stroma and immune response, and how this may contribute to radioresistance. This review will also consider the biomarkers or gene expression signatures that have been developed to predict radiation outcomes. Lastly, we conclude by exploring how these approaches could be used to develop personalised radiotherapy treatment plans to improve patient outcomes.

2. Radiation Response in the Tumour Microenvironment

RT can be a cure for many; however, for some patients, the treatment fails or resistance occurs. Though ionizing radiation can induce DNA damage in tumour *cells*, a potential barrier to the success of RT may be its effects on the other components of the local TME, including the vasculature, stroma and the immune infiltrate (Figure 1). These components can influence tumour progression and response to treatment. Understanding how they are influenced by RT may be critical in predicting disease outcomes. Extracellular vesicles (EVs) including exosomes have also been shown to play a role in cancer progression, immunomodulation and importantly, in modifying the response to radiation; key examples of which are below. However, recent detailed articles focusing on the role of EV-modulated radiation response exist; as such, EVs will not form a primary focus of this review [8,9].

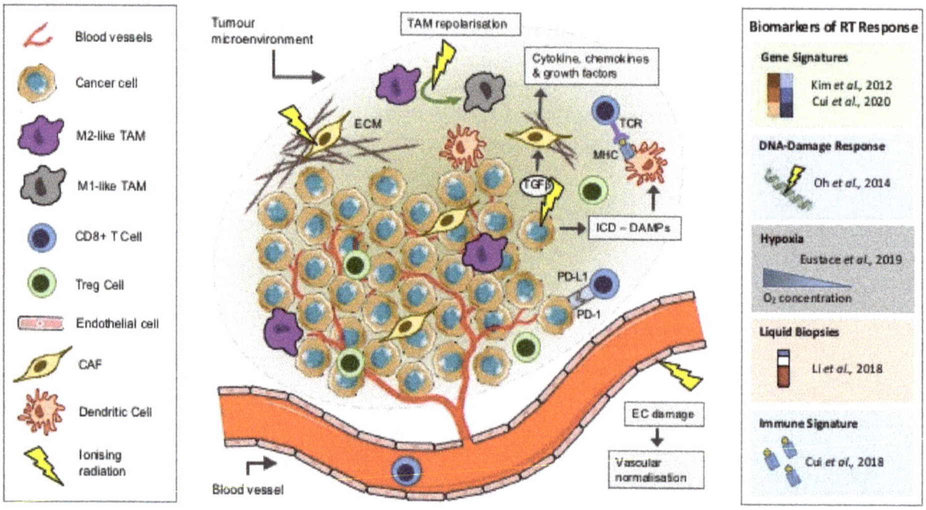

Figure 1. The effect of radiation on the TME. Schematic showing the role of ionizing radiation on components of the TME and predictive biomarkers of radiation response. DAMPs, damage-associated molecular patterns; EC, endothelial cell; ECM, extracellular matrix; ICD, immunogenic cell death; MHC, major histocompatibility complex; PD-1, programmed cell death protein 1; PD-L1, programmed death ligand-1; RT, radiotherapy; TAM, tumour-associated macrophage; TCR, T-cell receptor; TGFβ, transforming growth factor beta; TME, tumour microenvironment.

2.1. Tumour Immune Microenvironment

Immune evasion, the process by which tumour *cells* can avoid immune recognition and destruction, has become one of the hallmarks of cancer [10]. Subsequently, more recent therapeutic developments have focused on shifting the TME from an immunosuppressive environment to an immune-activated one through the use of immunotherapeutics: treatments that can effectively remove the brakes on immune signals mounting an anti-tumour response. RT has been shown to have contradictory immunomodulatory effects, influencing both proinflammatory and immunosuppressive responses, which likely influence response to treatment [5]. The inflammatory milieu of the TME, or the tumour immune microenvironment (TIME), is composed of T *cells*, natural killer (NK) *cells*, dendritic *cells* (DCs) and tumour-infiltrating myeloid *cells* (TIMs) including tumour-associated macrophages (TAMs), myeloid-derived suppressor *cells* (MDSCs) and dendritic *cells* (DCs), all of which are recruited into the TME through altered chemokine and cytokine signalling [11]. The extent and relative proportion of immune infiltration can also influence the response to treatment and progression. Tumours can be broadly separated into two categories based on their TIME: those that are immune "hot", being infiltrated with T lymphocytes; and those that are immune "cold", with poor infiltration [12]. In immune "hot" tumours, regulatory

T *cells* (Tregs) and TAMs cooperate to support the immunosuppressive TME and may be more susceptible to the immunomodulatory effects of radiotherapy [13]. Furthermore, these immune-inflamed tumours, including non-small cell lung cancer and melanoma, are more likely to respond favourably to immune checkpoint inhibitors in comparison to immune "cold" tumours, including pancreatic and prostate tumours [14]. Lack of tumour antigens, defects in antigen presentation and poor T-cell homing to the TME by the stroma may all contribute to a "cold" tumour immune phenotype; mechanisms to modulate immune infiltration and turn these tumours "hot" could improve response to therapy [14–16].

The ability of radiotherapy to modulate systemic immune responses may contribute towards the observations of tumour regression at non-irradiated sites, an effect described as an abscopal response. Abscopal effects are particularly relevant when RT is combined with immune checkpoint blockade. In preclinical syngeneic models of prostate cancer, a combination of radiotherapy (20 Gy in two fractions) with antibodies against programmed death-1 (anti-PD-1) or programmed death ligand-1 (anti-PD-L1) (iRT) significantly increased median survival (70–130%) in comparison to anti-PD-1 monotherapy, contributing to an abscopal response in which the unirradiated tumours responded similarly to the irradiated tumours. Importantly, this effect was shown to be mediated through antitumour CD8+ (cytotoxic) T *cells* [17]. Clinical observations of the abscopal effect have been rare in radiation oncology; however, with the development and advancement of immunotherapeutics, these observations are becoming more frequent across a variety of tumour types [18]. Clinically, in patients with unresectable melanoma combining anti-PD-1 therapy with hypofractionated RT (typically 26 Gy in 3–5 fractions) resulted in abscopal treatment responses in 36% of patients [19,20]. Targeting of another immune checkpoint, cytotoxic T-lymphocyte antigen 4 (CTLA-4), with the monoclonal antibody ipilimumab in combination with RT has also been shown to result in abscopal responses both preclinically in models of breast cancer and clinically in melanoma and lung cancer patients [21–24]. Interestingly, EVs isolated from irradiated tumour *cells* (H22 cells and 4T1 *cells*; 8 Gy) in vitro were shown to have immunomodulatory effects when mice were inoculated in vivo, enhancing CD8+ and CD4+ T-cell infiltration in lung metastasis in comparison to nonirradiated EVs [25]. Dose and fractionation are likely to play a critical role in the immunological responses to RT; however, the molecular and cellular mechanisms underpinning this immune-priming effect are still poorly understood [26].

RT-induced cell death is typically thought to occur through DNA damage, particularly in the form of double-strand breaks (DSB). Subsequently, the tumour cell response to radiation-induced DNA damage (RIDD) is dependent on its DNA damage response (DDR), which can activate downstream signalling to repair damage, thus contributing to radioresistance [27]. While the immune cell compartment, including lymphocyte and myeloid populations, may be more resistant to RIDD, RT can modulate immune signalling within the TME, promoting immune cell recruitment and activation and triggering immunogenic cell death [28]. RT-induced immunogenic cell death results in a cascade of events, starting with the release of damage-associated molecular patterns (DAMPs) (Figure 1) [29]. These "danger" signals released by tumour *cells* include high-mobility group box 1 (HMGB1) and ATP, triggering innate and adaptive immune responses through the expression of major histocompatibility complex (MHC) class I and MHC-II molecules. These antigen-presenting *cells* (APCs) can in turn can prime CD8+ T *cells* to induce an antitumour response [28]. In fact, RT has been shown to upregulate MHC-I expression preclinically in tumour cell lines in vivo, an observation that has been recapitulated in ex vivo-irradiated tumour biopsies [30]. Cytosolic double-stranded DNA (dsDNA) released as a result of RIDD can also promote dendritic cell activation through guanosine monophosphate–adenosine monophosphate synthase (cGAS)/stimulator of IFN *genes* (STING)/interferon (IFN) signalling, leading to CD8+ T-cell activation [31].

TIM populations, including TAMs, form another important component of the TIME and although they have a complex plasticity, they are usually organised as classically activated (M1) or alternatively activated (M2) *cells*. Numerous stimuli including chemokines can influence TAM polarisation from a proinflammatory (antitumour) M1 to an anti-inflammatory (protumour) M2 phenotype, which promotes tumour angiogenesis, tissue remodelling and tumour progression [32]. Interestingly, the frequency of TAMs has also been associated with clinical treatment response and disease progression [33,34]. In murine tumour models, low-dose gamma irradiation (LDI; 2 Gy) has been shown to promote repolarisation of M2-like TAMs towards M1-like inducible nitric oxide synthase (iNOS)-expressing TAMs, contributing to T-cell recruitment and tumour regression (Figure 1) [35]. TAMs and MDSCs are dependent on colony-stimulating factor (CSF1) signalling for recruitment into the TME. In murine models of breast cancer, blocking CSF1/CSF1R signalling inhibited TAM recruitment and delayed tumour regrowth following RT (5 Gy), an effect associated with an increase in CD8+ T *cells* and a reduction in CD4+ (helper) T *cells* [36]. Similar effects were observed following CSF1R signalling blockade in combination with RT (3 Gy, five fractions) in syngeneic models of prostate cancer in vivo. Furthermore, serum levels of CSF1 were also shown to be elevated in prostate cancer patients following RT [37]. Clinically, in patients with T3 rectal cancer, a short course of radiotherapy (neoadjuvant hyperfractionated 25 Gy in 10 fractions; surgery performed on day 2–5) promoted TAM repolarisation towards an M1-like proinflammatory phenotype. Interestingly, ex vivo modelling of this response suggested that HMGB1 in EVs from irradiated tumour *cells* could be responsible for this effect on TAM polarisation [38].

2.2. Cancer-Associated Fibroblasts

The stromal compartment of the TME plays an integral role in the response to treatment, including RT (Figure 1). Radiotherapy-induced tissue fibrosis is a late side effect where myofibroblast transformation leads to the excess production of collagen and deposition of components of the extracellular matrix (ECM) [39]. RT can also lead to the release of the pleotropic cytokine transforming growth factor beta (TGFβ), which can modulate fibroblast phenotype and function [40]. Fibroblasts recruited into the TME are transformed into cancer-associated fibroblasts (CAFs), where they play a role in regulating the extracellular matrix [41]. Furthermore, CAFs are responsible for the secretion of a number of cytokines (including interleukin 6 (IL6) and IL8), chemokines (including C-X-C motif ligand 12 (CXCL12)) and growth factors (including TGF-β and platelet-derived growth factor (PDGF)) that can influence immune cell fate and tumour progression, often contributing to the immunosuppressive TIME [42]. However, the effects of RT on the stromal compartment of the TME including CAFs are less well understood and they appear to have contradictory roles, contributing to both tumour growth and suppression [43]. Coimplantation of A549 lung tumour xenografts with preirradiated CAFs (at both 18 Gy $\times$ 1 fraction or 6 Gy $\times$ 3 fractions) abrogated the protumour growth effect observed in tumours coimplanted with nonirradiated CAFs [44]. In contrast, irradiated fibroblasts (1, 6 or 12 Gy) have been shown to express high levels of TGF-β1 and promote human T3M-1 squamous cell carcinoma (SCC) invasion and growth [45]. Furthermore, EVs derived from CAFs were shown to contribute to colorectal cancer cell stemness and radioresistance (6 Gy) in vitro, through the activation of the TGF-β signalling pathway [46]. It is therefore clear that more work is needed to understand the complex role of CAFs in the tumour response to RT.

2.3. Tumour Vasculature

The integrity of the tumour vasculature differs significantly from that of physiologically normal vessels, characterised by abnormal recruitment of pericytes, leading to increased tortuosity and porosity. This, in part, contributes to treatment failure through poor drug penetration into the TME, establishing local hypoxia gradients and increasing the yield of reactive oxygen species [47]. The effect of RT on the tumour vasculature has been well studied, with tumour blood vessels and their endothelial *cells* proven to exhibit increased sensitivity to radiation, a response likely dependent on total radiation dose and fractionation schedule [5,48,49]. Vascular damage is mainly witnessed at radiation doses exceeding 5 Gy. Conversely, individual, low-dose fractions have been shown to temporarily stimulate blood flow, while at higher or cumulative doses, the vascular network is disrupted, promoting hypoxic stress that can trigger tumour cell death [50,51]. In a recent dose-escalation study, single administration of 2, 4 or 8 Gy doses were shown to compromise the tumour vasculature in a dose-dependent manner, prolonging the survival of mice bearing CT-2A (high-grade glioma) tumours. Interestingly, this was also associated with changes in the TIME, promoting an increase in CD8+ T *cells* and a reduction in M2-like TAMs [52]. Potiron et al. [53] reported that RT (at both 10×2 Gy and 2×12 Gy) induces tumour vasculature normalisation and remodelling, thus improving the distribution and efficacy of the anticancer drug doxorubicin (DOX) [53]. Further evidence of the effects of RT effects on endothelial cell permeability has been demonstrated in vitro. Monotherapy radiation doses to primary human umbilical vein endothelial *cells* (HUVECs) increased permeability and transmigration of tumour *cells*, owing to altered metalloprotease ADAM10 expression and degradation of VE-cadherin, both of which play an integral role in maintaining intercellular junctions and vascular integrity [54]. High radiation doses (>20 Gy) were also found to cause transient endothelial dysfunction, platelet leukocyte adhesion and increased expression of hypoxia-inducible factor-1α (HIF-1α) in pancreatic tumours [55]. However, a recent study indicated that high-dose RT (>8 Gy) induced expression of Notch1 signalling in HUVEC monolayers. Consequently, in vivo high-dose RT, in combination with inhibition of Notch1 signalling, resulted in a significant reduction in tumour vessel endothelial cell coverage in comparison to high-dose RT alone, suggesting Notch1 signalling may protect tumour vessels from radiation-induced damage [56]. Furthermore, it is also well understood that oxygenated tumour *cells* are preferentially killed by RT, due to oxygen-induced fixation of radiation-induced DNA damage. However, this effect has been proven to accelerate the production of proangiogenic cytokines, inhibiting treatment-induced apoptosis, stimulating a postradiotherapy angiogenic burst that can contribute to eventual tumour regrowth [57].

3. Predictive Biomarkers of Radiation Response

Precision medicine based on common tumour-specific alterations, emerging from high-throughput molecular profiling, has become a reality in recent years. This approach underpins the discovery of clinically validated prognostic and/or predictive biomarkers, allowing for stratification of patients based either on those most likely to derive benefit or have treatment-related harm limited. This strategy gained significant momentum in the chemotherapy field with the development of various commercially produced kits such as Prosigna (NanoString Technologies, Inc., Seattle, USA) and MammaPrint (Agendia, Amsterdam, The Netherlands), designed to aid clinical decision-making [58,59]. However, equivalence in radiotherapy has not yet been achieved due to the variability in radiation response, an effect attributed to tumour heterogeneity. Heterogeneity is an umbrella term used to describe both intra- and intertumour variability at the morphological, physiological and more recently, genetic levels. Divergence of these features exerts a profound influence on localised factors such as vascular integrity, tumour oxygenation and immune infiltrate, ultimately influencing treatment outcome (detailed in Section 2 [5,13,48]). In an effort to address the issue of heterogeneity, research efforts have shifted from focusing on macroscopic phenotypic or environmental variation to the identification of commonality at the molecular level. Table 1 provides an outline of biomarkers for radiotherapy response in a number of tumour types (summarised in Figure 1); these are discussed further in the sections below.

Table 1. Biomarkers of radiotherapy response.

	Year	Cancer Type	Biomarker	Results	Ref
Gene signatures	2012	NCI-60 human tumor cell lines screen	A 31-*gene* signature developed from meta-analysis of microarray data correlated with clonogenic assay data to identify radiosensitive or radioresistant *cells*	*Genes* involved in cell cycle progression (*CCNA2, CDK6, CCND1*) and DNA damage repair were associated with increased radiosensitivity	[60]
	2014	Breast cancer	A 7-gene signature applied to the Danish Breast Cancer Cooperative Group (DBCG82bc) cohort to stratify patients into either high-risk locoregional recurrence (LRR) or low-risk LRR	Identified that post-mastectomy RT would benefit only those identified as high risk, providing no benefit to low-risk patients	[61]
	2015	Breast cancer	Radiation sensitivity gene signature developed from correlating radiation sensitivity (SF2) of a panel of breast cancer models against gene expression changes	Gene signature significantly predicted loco-regional recurrence; beating all clinicopathologic features used in clinical practice	[62]
	2016	Prostate cancer	A 24-gene signature applied to prostate cancer patients who had undergone radical prostatectomy to identify those most likely to benefit from postoperative radiotherapy	Retrospective analysis identified that those patients with a high PROTOS (post-operative radiation therapy outcomes score), indicative of radiation sensitive tumours, were less likely to develop metastasis at 10 years post-RT. In the low PROTOS score group, radiotherapy proved detrimental	[63]
	2020	HNSCC	A 12-gene signature	Classified patients with a higher radiosensitivity for whom RT would be beneficial and could predict overall survival.	[64]
DNA-damage response	2010	Breast cancer	*Gene* expression signature associated with DDR, correlated against publicly available breast cancer microarray data	DDR-associated *genes* induced by radiation correlated positively with those who responded favourably to radiation treatment	[65]
	2014	Breast cancer	Radiation-induced 30-gene DDR signature	Gene signature was capable of discriminating between breast cancer patients likely to achieve a pathological complete response (pCR) to neoadjuvant chemotherapy and poor-responding patients	[66]
Hypoxia	2013	Laryngeal cancer	A 26-hypoxia gene signature	Could predict those patients receiving RT for whom hypoxia-modifying ARCON (accelerated radiotherapy with carbogen and nicotinamide) therapy would be of benefit	[67]
	2012	HNSCC	A 15-gene hypoxia signature	Classified patients who would benefit from combining RT with hypoxia modification (nimorazole)	[68]

Table 1. *Cont.*

	Year	Cancer Type	Biomarker	Results	Ref
Liquid biopsies	2011	Prostate cancer	Altered miRNA expression: developed through screening of miRNAs in prostate cancer *cells* (LNCaP) in response to RT	Suppressed miR-221 expression linked with increased radiation sensitivity: data subsequently correlated in clinical datasets where low serum levels of miR-221 are indicative of low-risk prostate cancer	[69]
	2018	Nonmetastatic rectal cancer and head and neck cancers	miRNA expression rations: prediction classifier	The expressions of three miRNAs—miR-374a-5p, miR-342-5p and miR-519d-3p—were significantly different between responsive and poor-responsive RT groups. miRNA classifier successfully predicted radiotherapy outcomes	[70]
Immune signature	2018	Breast cancer	Combined radiation sensitivity (RS) gene signature with an antigen-presentation (AP) immune signature	Both RS and AP signatures capable of predicting increased disease specific survival (DSS) in patients identified with either radio-sensitive or immune-effective tumours	[71]

3.1. Gene Signatures of Radiation Sensitivity

An early example of this approach used the clonogenic assay to profile radiation sensitivity, based on survival fraction data at 2 Gy (SF2), of the NCI-60 cancer cell line panel [60]. This was then correlated against gene expression data from four published microarray platforms, identifying significant alterations in expression profiles for 31 *genes*, common to each microarray dataset. Unsurprisingly, significant suppression of *genes* which regulate cell cycle progression (*CCNA2, CDK6, CCND1)* and DNA damage repair were associated with increased radiosensitivity. *CCND1*, the gene encoding for cyclin D_1, stalls cell cycle progression, providing time for DNA damage repair, ultimately suppressing radiation-induced apoptosis [72]. Therefore, suppressed *CCND1* and other cell cycle regulatory *genes* may contribute, in part, towards a genetic signature for identifying radiosensitive tumours. A second set of *genes* common to the top 10% most radiosensitive (SF2 < 0.2) *cells*, and totally absent from the most radioresistant (SF2 > 0.8), were those involved in integrin signalling, cell adhesion and cytoskeletal remodelling. Cell-adhesion complexes and integrin signalling act both directly and indirectly to influence radiation response [73]. Cell-to-cell contact and adhesion with the extracellular matrix are central features of the protumour phenotypes of migration and invasion. Along with integrin β1, the 31-gene profile identified downregulation of *ITGB5*, the gene encoding integrin β5, as a highly significant indicator of radiosensitivity [60]. Indeed, radiosensitisation achieved through the antagonism of αvβ5 integrin using a cyclic-RGD (arginine-glycine-aspartate) containing peptide was the focus of a large phase III clinical trial for the treatment of glioblastoma multiforme [74]. This was based on the rationale that αvβ5 antagonism suppresses tumour angiogenesis and metastasis, an effect in part attributed to the dampening of major cancer-related signalling pathways, including *Wnt* and *PI3K* [75]. Developed as a universal predicator of radiation sensitivity, independent of tumour type, many of the 31 *genes* identified likely hold predictive value in relation to radiation response. However, stringent application using only the most radiosensitive or radioresistant *cells* again highlights the problem of heterogeneity, where 80% tumour models analysed exhibited intermediary gene expression alterations, diluting the predictive power of the signature.

Recent approaches adopting a similar strategy tend to focus on a specific disease type. Breast cancer radiotherapy is most commonly used in the adjuvant setting to improve treatment outcomes, forming a core strategy of breast conservation surgery and mastectomy. However, not all patients benefit from adjuvant radiotherapy and some experience significant debilitating late effects [76]. The importance of identifying those who will benefit most from adjuvant radiotherapy was neatly demonstrated in a study using FFPE tumour tissue from the Danish Breast Cancer Cooperative Group (DBCG82bc) cohort. Applying a seven-gene signature to stratify patients into either high-risk loco regional recurrence (LRR) or low-risk LRR, the authors were able to establish that postmastectomy radiotherapy would benefit only those identified as high risk, providing no benefit to low-risk patients [61]. Adopting a similar strategy to the 31-gene signature, Speers et al. [62] correlated the radiation sensitivity (SF2) of a panel of breast cancer models against gene expression changes, developing a radiation sensitivity signature (RSS), which was subsequently shown to be the most significant factor in prediction of loco-regional recurrence, beating all clinicopathologic features used in clinical practice [62]. While a clear step forward, RRS remains a prognostic signature for loco-regional control, and not predictive of radiation response. Similar predictive gene signatures have been developed, including a six-gene signature (including *genes* such as HOXB13 and NKX2-2) that was also shown to predict radiotherapy sensitivity in breast cancer [77]. Applying a 24-gene signature to prostate cancer patients who had undergone radical prostatectomy to identify those most likely to benefit from postoperative radiotherapy similarly found that those with a high PROTOS (postoperative radiation therapy outcomes score), indicative of radiation-sensitive tumours, significantly benefited from radiotherapy, with a 10-year metastasis rate of 4% (95% CI 0–10) versus 35% (CI 7–54) for those not receiving radiotherapy. However, in the low PROTOS score group, radiotherapy proved detrimental (HR 2.5 (CI 1.6–4.1); $p < 0.0001$) in the 157-patient cohort training group and of no benefit in the 248-patient validation cohort [63]. Liu et al. [64] recently used multiple omics data to develop a prediction model of sensitivity to radiation in head and neck squamous cell carcinoma (HNSCC) tumours. A 12-gene signature was established from differentially expressed *genes* in patients treated with or without RT and used to develop a scoring system. Those HNSCC patients with a low score had a higher radiosensitivity and were shown to benefit from RT [64].

3.2. DNA Damage Response Biomarkers

The antitumour effects of radiotherapy are directly proportional to the degree to which potentially lethal DNA DSBs are both induced by radiation and are sustained by the cell following activation of DDR processes. Continual refinements to the delivery of radiotherapy have ensured that the DNA-damaging properties of the most commonly utilised radiation sources, such as X-rays and γ-rays, minimise dose to surrounding healthy tissue, while focusing dose on the target volume. In parallel, intensive research efforts have led to the development of numerous small-molecule inhibitors targeting key DNA damage repair proteins, thus sustaining radiation-induced damage, resulting in increased tumour cell death. This is the fundamental basis of many radiosensitising strategies. Key targets of the DNA damage response pathways for which clinically utilised inhibitors have been developed include the ATM/ATR (ataxia–telangiectasia mutated and Rad3-related) signalling pathways, PARP (poly (ADP-ribose) polymerase), DNA-PKcs (DNA-dependent protein kinase, catalytic subunit), BRAC1 (breast cancer1 C terminal) and HIF-1, amongst others. While reviewing the full therapeutic potential of these inhibitors is beyond the scope of the current article, several recent publications provide comprehensive details of this field [27,78,79]. Herein, we aim to focus on the utility of gene expression alterations in DDR *genes* as prognostic/predictive indicators of radiation response. Piening et al. [65] developed an early radiation-derived gene signature, evaluated for prognostic utility in breast cancer. The signature was derived from gene expression alterations following a 5 Gy dose across a panel of nontumour lymphoblast *cells*, a relevant point given that genomic instability in tumours support aberrant DDR activity. Expression levels of 219 *genes* were altered with 160 being induced and 59 repressed by radiation. Using a gene set enrichment algorithm [80], the prognostic utility of the signature was evaluated against publicly available breast cancer microarray data. With respect to the repressed *genes*, tumour samples neatly clustered into two groups, aligning with gene repression or not, where the former strongly correlated with increased proliferation and poor overall treatment outcomes. Similarly, *genes* induced by radiation correlated positively with those who responded favourably to radiation treatment, promoting the expression of *genes* involved in negative regulation of the cell cycle, apoptosis (e.g., caspases) and DNA damage repair proteins. Importantly, applying the same approach but using the NCI-60 cancer cell line panel to derive the radiation signature failed to discriminate between favourable and poor outcomes, with no overlap between the altered gene set signature [65]. This clearly illustrates the impact of genomic instability in influencing the DDR response and an important point for consideration in the development of radiation biomarkers.

Another study exploited the overlapping DNA damage responses activated by both chemotherapy and radiotherapy, producing a radiation-induced 30-gene signature. This signature was proven capable of discriminating between breast cancer patients likely to achieve a pathological complete response (pCR) to neoadjuvant chemotherapy and poor-responding patients. Importantly, pCR represents the most relevant clinical end point for predicting improved overall and disease-free survival [81]. In addition to *genes* clearly linked to DNA damage pathways, such as the extracellular signal-regulated kinase (*ERK*) pathway, *AKT*, *mTOR* and *NF-kB*, radiation significantly elevated the expression of metabolism processing *genes*, in particular *PDHA1* and *LDHB*. These genes encode for key proteins driving pyruvate metabolism and energy production, along with the catalytic conversion of pyruvate to lactate, thus indicating that tumours with a high metabolic demand are more likely to prove sensitive to the effects of chemo- and radiotherapy [66].

3.3. Hypoxia Biomarkers

As outlined previously, hypoxia resulting from aberrant tumour vasculature can influence RT resistance. As such, there is a strong rationale for identifying robust biomarkers of tumour hypoxia that predict response to RT [82]. Traditionally, tumour hypoxia was measured using oxygen electrode probes, endogenous HIF-1α levels, physiological markers such as pimonidazole staining or other imaging methodologies (MRI). However, gene signatures may better represent the nuances of hypoxia within the TME that might predict response to RT. To this end, Eustace et al. [67] developed a 26-hypoxia gene signature (informed by a 121-gene hypoxia meta-signature derived from datasets of head and neck, breast and lung cancers [83]) predicting treatment response in laryngeal cancer. This hypoxia signature, composed of *genes* involved in glucose metabolism (*ALDOA*, *ENO1*, *LDHA*), cell proliferation (*CDKN3*, *FOSL1*) and angiogenesis (*VEGFA*), could predict those patients receiving RT for whom hypoxia-modifying ARCON (accelerated radiotherapy with carbogen and nicotinamide) therapy would be of benefit in laryngeal carcinomas [67]. The approach of stratifying patients for hypoxic modification of RT has also been performed by Troustrup et al. [68] to classify HNSCC tumours as "more" or "less" hypoxic [84]. A 15-gene hypoxic signature including *genes* for stress response (ADM, HIG2), cell proliferation (FOSL2, IGFBP3) and glucose metabolism (ALDOA, FKBP3) was developed from HNSCC cell lines under hypoxic conditions, and subsequently validated in patients that had previously been hypoxia-evaluated [85,86]. The predictive power of this gene signature was validated in a clinical cohort of HPV-negative HNSCC tumours, with those classified as having "more" hypoxic tumours having more favourable outcomes (loco-regional tumour control and disease-specific survival) after combining RT with hypoxia modification using nimorazole [68].

3.4. Liquid Biopsies

Minimally invasive liquid biopsies represent an area of intense research interest. While the field is in relative infancy, with no commercially validated tests, the identification of circulating biomarkers predicative of radiation response holds tremendous potential. MicroRNAs (miRNAs) are differentially regulated in a number of disease types and following exposure to ionizing radiation; they therefore offer a potential biomarker to predict treatment response in cancer [87–89]. A radiotherapeutic response predication was developed for patients with lower-grade glioma (LGG), based on the expression of five miRNAs. The signature was capable of classifying those as low-risk or high-risk in terms of survival and radiation response, based on the analysis of miRNA expression profiles in 624 patients. This signature was found to be superior to isocitrate dehydrogenase (IDH) mutational status in predicting survival in LGG [90]. Of particular interest is free plasma or exosome secretion of miRNAs predictive of radiation response: Li et al. [69] linked low-level miR-221 expression with increased radiation sensitivity, a finding subsequently correlated with several patient studies reporting that low serum levels of miR-221 and miR-125b are indicative of low-risk prostate cancer [69,91,92]. Furthermore, Li et al. [70] associated the levels of three miRNAs (miR-374a-5p, miR-342-5p and miR-519d-3p) with radiation responses in the plasma of patients with nonmetastatic rectal cancer and head and neck cancers. Prediction classifiers were developed from miRNA signatures in pre- and postradiotherapy samples and could significantly distinguish between radiation responders and poor responders 6 months postradiotherapy [70]. The importance of effective biomarkers, particularly in the prostate cancer setting, is evident considering that prostate-specific antigen (PSA) screening has formed the bedrock of prostate cancer diagnosis for over 25 years—a test lacking in specificity—resulting in significant treatment related morbidities from overdiagnosis and overtreatment [93]. Given the role of the TIME in influencing tumour fate postradiotherapy (detailed in Section 2), immune infiltrate composition in the TME may predict radiotherapy response and prognosis in cancer patients [5,94]. Cui et al. [71] pioneered a combined radiation sensitivity (RS) gene signature with an antigen-presentation (AP) immune signature, establishing a dual-modality approach with predictive capabilities of radiation response. Independently, both RS and AP signatures were proven capable of predicting increased disease-specific survival (DSS) in patients identified with either radiosensitive or immune-effective tumours, with the reverse observed in radioresistant and immune defective individuals. Importantly, integration of both signatures further strengthened the predictive capabilities of either signature used independently [71].

4. Conclusions and Future Perspectives

RT is the treatment of choice for a number of cancer, designed to target and kill tumour *cells*; however, it triggers a myriad of effects on other components of the TME, including the vasculature, stroma and the immune compartment [5]. The immunomodulatory effects of RT are complex, with reported changes to the proportions and functionality of T *cells* and antigen-presenting dendritic *cells*, and effects on TAM polarisation within the TME. This effect is further complicated by clinical observations of an increase in the abscopal effect reported in patients receiving RT in combination with immunotherapeutics. RT has also been shown to affect tumour vascular architecture, inducing tissue fibrosis. It is important to note that the majority of responses to RT in the TME reported above are in the context of conventional X-ray or photon radiation therapy. Recent advances in the clinical delivery of RT, including high-energy proton beam therapy and heavy ion therapy, have the improvement of delivering more dose in the Bragg peak with a lower dependence on tissue oxygenation and improved biological effectiveness [95]. While these newer treatment modalities are likely to have biological effects on the components of the TME outlined in this review, their response has been less well characterised [96,97]. Therefore it is of critical importance to take into consideration the role of the TME when considering radiobiological responses and disease recurrence. As RT techniques have evolved over the last two decades, so too have their physical precision, aided by improved imaging guidance and technological advancements. However, genomic precision has lagged, as most RT treatment planning is designed around the tumour and local tissue architecture, with the aim to deliver the maximum dose to the tumour while sparing healthy tissue. However as highlighted above, genomic signatures could allow for a greater prediction of those patients for whom RT would be of benefit as a single therapy or in combination with radiation sensitizers or hypoxia modifiers [6]. Yet, of critical importance, these findings further stress the necessity for a precision medicine approach, in that not only do patients with radioresistant tumours fail to experience radiotherapy benefit, but that treatment is actually detrimental both in terms of DSS and toxicities associated with radiation-induced late effects [71]. Taking a more "personalised" approach to RT could ensure patients receive the most benefit from their treatment.

Author Contributions: Conceptualization, N.M.B. and J.A.C.; writing—original draft preparation, review and editing, N.M.B., P.T. and J.A.C. All authors have read and agreed to the published version of the manuscript.

Funding: This research received no external funding.

Institutional Review Board Statement: Not applicable.

Informed Consent Statement: Not applicable.

Data Availability Statement: Data sharing not applicable.

Acknowledgments: Figures created using MedART (creative commons license): https://smart.servier.com/.

Conflicts of Interest: The authors declare no conflict of interest.

References

1. Bernier, J.; Hall, E.J.; Giaccia, A. Radiation oncology: A century of achievements. *Nat. Rev. Cancer* **2004**, *4*, 737–747. [CrossRef] [PubMed]
2. Barcellos-Hoff, M.H.; Park, C.; Wright, E.G. Radiation and the microenvironment—tumorigenesis and therapy. *Nat. Rev. Cancer* **2005**, *5*, 867–875. [CrossRef] [PubMed]
3. De Palma, M.; Biziato, D.; Petrova, T.V. Microenvironmental regulation of tumour angiogenesis. *Nat. Rev. Cancer* **2017**, *17*, 457–474. [CrossRef] [PubMed]
4. Quail, D.F.; Joyce, J.A. Microenvironmental regulation of tumor progression and metastasis. *Nat. Med.* **2013**, *19*, 1423–1437. [CrossRef]
5. Barker, H.E.; Paget, J.T.; Khan, A.A.; Harrington, K.J. The tumour microenvironment after radiotherapy: Mechanisms of resistance and recurrence. *Nat. Rev. Cancer* **2015**, *15*, 409–425. [CrossRef]
6. Bratman, S.V.; Milosevic, M.F.; Liu, F.F.; Haibe-Kains, B. Genomic biomarkers for precision radiation medicine. *Lancet Oncol.* **2017**, *18*, e238. [CrossRef]
7. Scott, J.G.; Berglund, A.; Schell, M.J.; Mihaylov, I.; Fulp, W.J.; Yue, B.; Welsh, E.; Caudell, J.J.; Ahmed, K.; Strom, T.S.; et al. A genome-based model for adjusting radiotherapy dose (GARD): A retrospective, cohort-based study. *Lancet Oncol.* **2017**, *18*, 202–211. [CrossRef]
8. Ni, J.; Bucci, J.; Malouf, D.; Knox, M.; Graham, P.; Li, Y. Exosomes in Cancer Radioresistance. *Front. Oncol.* **2019**, *9*, 869. [CrossRef]
9. Szatmári, T.; Hargitai, R.; Sáfrány, G.; Lumniczky, K. Extracellular Vesicles in Modifying the Effects of Ionizing Radiation. *Int. J. Mol. Sci.* **2019**, *20*, 5527. [CrossRef]
10. Hanahan, D.; Weinberg, R.A. Hallmarks of cancer: The next generation. *Cell* **2011**, *144*, 646–674. [CrossRef]
11. Binnewies, M.; Roberts, E.W.; Kersten, K.; Chan, V.; Fearon, D.F.; Merad, M.; Coussens, L.M.; Gabrilovich, D.I.; Ostrand-Rosenberg, S.; Hedrick, C.C.; et al. Understanding the tumor immune microenvironment (TIME) for effective therapy. *Nat. Med.* **2018**, *24*, 541–550. [CrossRef] [PubMed]
12. Gajewski, T.F. The Next Hurdle in Cancer Immunotherapy: Overcoming the Non-T-Cell-Inflamed Tumor Microenvironment. *Semin. Oncol.* **2015**, *42*, 663–671. [CrossRef] [PubMed]
13. Fridman, W.H.; Pagès, F.; Sautès-Fridman, C.; Galon, J. The immune contexture in human tumours: Impact on clinical outcome. *Nat. Rev. Cancer* **2012**, *12*, 298–306. [CrossRef] [PubMed]
14. Bonaventura, P.; Shekarian, T.; Alcazer, V.; Valladeau-Guilemond, J.; Valsesia-Wittmann, S.; Amigorena, S.; Caux, C.; Depil, S. Cold Tumors: A Therapeutic Challenge for Immunotherapy. *Front. Immunol.* **2019**, *10*, 168. [CrossRef] [PubMed]
15. Duan, Q.; Zhang, H.; Zheng, J.; Zhang, L. Turning Cold into Hot: Firing up the Tumor Microenvironment. *Trends Cancer* **2020**, *6*, 605–618. [CrossRef] [PubMed]
16. Galon, J.; Bruni, D. Approaches to treat immune hot, altered and cold tumours with combination immunotherapies. *Nat. Rev. Drug Discov.* **2019**, *18*, 197–218. [CrossRef]
17. Dudzinski, S.O.; Cameron, B.D.; Wang, J.; Rathmell, J.C.; Giorgio, T.D.; Kirschner, A.N. Combination immunotherapy and radiotherapy causes an abscopal treatment response in a mouse model of castration resistant prostate cancer. *J. Immunother. Cancer* **2019**, *7*, 218. [CrossRef]

18. Reynders, K.; Illidge, T.; Siva, S.; Chang, J.Y.; De Ruysscher, D. The abscopal effect of local radiotherapy: Using immunotherapy to make a rare event clinically relevant. *Cancer Treat. Rev.* **2015**, *41*, 503–510. [CrossRef]
19. Gong, J.; Le, T.Q.; Massarelli, E.; Hendifar, A.E.; Tuli, R. Radiation therapy and PD-1/PD-L1 blockade: The clinical development of an evolving anticancer combination. *J. Immunother. Cancer* **2018**, *6*, 46. [CrossRef]
20. Roger, A.; Finet, A.; Boru, B.; Beauchet, A.; Mazeron, J.J.; Otzmeguine, Y.; Blom, A.; Longvert, C.; de Maleissye, M.F.; Fort, M.; et al. Efficacy of combined hypo-fractionated radiotherapy and anti-PD-1 monotherapy in difficult-to-treat advanced melanoma patients. *Oncoimmunology* **2018**, *7*, e1442166. [CrossRef]
21. Demaria, S.; Kawashima, N.; Yang, A.M.; Devitt, M.L.; Babb, J.S.; Allison, J.P.; Formenti, S.C. Immune-mediated inhibition of metastases after treatment with local radiation and CTLA-4 blockade in a mouse model of breast cancer. *Clin. Cancer Res.* **2005**, *11*, 728–734. [PubMed]
22. Postow, M.A.; Callahan, M.K.; Barker, C.A.; Yamada, Y.; Yuan, J.; Kitano, S.; Mu, Z.; Rasalan, T.; Adamow, M.; Ritter, E.; et al. Immunologic correlates of the abscopal effect in a patient with melanoma. *N. Engl. J. Med.* **2012**, *366*, 925–931. [CrossRef] [PubMed]
23. Chandra, R.A.; Wilhite, T.J.; Balboni, T.A.; Alexander, B.M.; Spektor, A.; Ott, P.A.; Ng, A.K.; Hodi, F.S.; Schoenfeld, J.D. A systematic evaluation of abscopal responses following radiotherapy in patients with metastatic melanoma treated with ipilimumab. *Oncoimmunology* **2015**, *4*, e1046028. [CrossRef] [PubMed]
24. Garelli, E.; Rittmeyer, A.; Putora, P.M.; Glatzer, M.; Dressel, R.; Andreas, S. Abscopal effect in lung cancer: Three case reports and a concise review. *Immunotherapy* **2019**, *11*, 1445–1461. [CrossRef] [PubMed]
25. Lin, W.; Xu, Y.; Chen, X.; Liu, J.; Weng, Y.; Zhuang, Q.; Lin, F.; Huang, Z.; Wu, S.; Ding, J.; et al. Radiation-induced small extracellular vesicles as "carriages" promote tumor antigen release and trigger antitumor immunity. *Theranostics* **2020**, *10*, 4871–4884. [CrossRef] [PubMed]
26. Rodríguez-Ruiz, M.E.; Vanpouille-Box, C.; Melero, I.; Formenti, S.C.; Demaria, S. Immunological Mechanisms Responsible for Radiation-Induced Abscopal Effect. *Trends Immunol.* **2018**, *39*, 644–655. [CrossRef]
27. Huang, R.X.; Zhou, P.K. DNA damage response signaling pathways and targets for radiotherapy sensitization in cancer. *Signal Transduct. Target. Ther.* **2020**, *5*, 60. [CrossRef]
28. Golden, E.B.; Apetoh, L. Radiotherapy and immunogenic cell death. *Semin. Radiat. Oncol.* **2015**, *25*, 11–17. [CrossRef]
29. Golden, E.B.; Frances, D.; Pellicciotta, I.; Demaria, S.; Helen Barcellos-Hoff, M.; Formenti, S.C. Radiation fosters dose-dependent and chemotherapy-induced immunogenic cell death. *Oncoimmunology* **2014**, *3*, e28518. [CrossRef]
30. Sharma, A.; Bode, B.; Wenger, R.H.; Lehmann, K.; Sartori, A.A.; Moch, H.; Knuth, A.; Boehmer, L.; Broek, M. γ-Radiation promotes immunological recognition of cancer *cells* through increased expression of cancer-testis antigens in vitro and in vivo. *PLoS ONE* **2011**, *6*, e28217. [CrossRef]
31. Deng, L.; Liang, H.; Xu, M.; Yang, X.; Burnette, B.; Arina, A.; Li, X.D.; Mauceri, H.; Beckett, M.; Darga, T.; et al. STING-Dependent Cytosolic DNA Sensing Promotes Radiation-Induced Type I Interferon-Dependent Antitumor Immunity in Immunogenic Tumors. *Immunity* **2014**, *41*, 843–852. [CrossRef] [PubMed]
32. Mantovani, A.; Marchesi, F.; Malesci, A.; Laghi, L.; Allavena, P. Tumour-associated macrophages as treatment targets in oncology. *Nat. Rev. Clin. Oncol.* **2017**, *14*, 399–416. [CrossRef] [PubMed]
33. Zhao, X.; Qu, J.; Sun, Y.; Wang, J.; Liu, X.; Wang, F.; Zhang, H.; Wang, W.; Ma, X.; Gao, X.; et al. Prognostic significance of tumor-associated macrophages in breast cancer: A meta-analysis of the literature. *Oncotarget* **2017**, *8*, 30576–30586. [CrossRef] [PubMed]
34. Yuri, P.; Shigemura, K.; Kitagawa, K.; Hadibrata, E.; Risan, M.; Zulfiqqar, A.; Soeroharjo, I.; Hendri, A.Z.; Danarto, R.; Ishii, A.; et al. Increased tumor-associated macrophages in the prostate cancer microenvironment predicted patients' survival and responses to androgen deprivation therapies in Indonesian patients cohort. *Prostate Int.* **2020**, *8*, 62–69. [CrossRef] [PubMed]
35. Klug, F.; Prakash, H.; Huber, P.E.; Seibel, T.; Bender, N.; Halama, N.; Pfirschke, C.; Voss, R.H.; Timke, C.; Umansky, L.; et al. Low-dose irradiation programs macrophage differentiation to an $iNOS^+$/M1 phenotype that orchestrates effective T cell immunotherapy. *Cancer Cell* **2013**, *24*, 589–602. [CrossRef] [PubMed]
36. Shiao, S.L.; Ruffell, B.; DeNardo, D.G.; Faddegon, B.A.; Park, C.C.; Coussens, L.M. TH2-Polarized CD4(+) T *Cells* and Macrophages Limit Efficacy of Radiotherapy. *Cancer Immunol. Res.* **2015**, *3*, 518–525. [CrossRef] [PubMed]
37. Xu, J.; Escamilla, J.; Mok, S.; David, J.; Priceman, S.; West, B.; Bollag, G.; McBride, W.; Wu, L. CSF1R signaling blockade stanches tumor-infiltrating myeloid *cells* and improves the efficacy of radiotherapy in prostate cancer. *Cancer Res.* **2013**, *73*, 2782–2794. [CrossRef] [PubMed]
38. Stary, V.; Wolf, B.; Unterleuthner, D.; List, J.; Talic, M.; Laengle, J.; Beer, A.; Strobl, J.; Stary, G.; Dolznig, H.; et al. Short-course radiotherapy promotes pro-inflammatory macrophages via extracellular vesicles in human rectal cancer. *J. Immunother. Cancer* **2020**, *8*. [CrossRef]
39. Straub, J.M.; New, J.; Hamilton, C.D.; Lominska, C.; Shnayder, Y.; Thomas, S.M. Radiation-induced fibrosis: Mechanisms and implications for therapy. *J. Cancer Res. Clin. Oncol.* **2015**, *141*, 1985–1994. [CrossRef]
40. Dancea, H.C.; Shareef, M.M.; Ahmed, M.M. Role of Radiation-induced TGF-beta Signaling in Cancer Therapy. *Mol. Cell. Pharmacol.* **2009**, *1*, 44–56. [CrossRef]

41. Sahai, E.; Astsaturov, I.; Cukierman, E.; DeNardo, D.G.; Egeblad, M.; Evans, R.M.; Fearon, D.; Greten, F.R.; Hingorani, S.R.; Hunter, T.; et al. A framework for advancing our understanding of cancer-associated fibroblasts. *Nat. Rev. Cancer* **2020**, *20*, 174–186. [CrossRef] [PubMed]
42. Ganguly, D.; Chandra, R.; Karalis, J.; Teke, M.; Aguilera, T.; Maddipati, R.; Wachsmann, M.B.; Ghersi, D.; Siravegna, G.; Zeh, H.J., 3rd; et al. Cancer-Associated Fibroblasts: Versatile Players in the Tumor Microenvironment. *Cancers (Basel)* **2020**, *12*, 2652. [CrossRef] [PubMed]
43. Wang, Z.; Tang, Y.; Tan, Y.; Wei, Q.; Yu, W. Cancer-associated fibroblasts in radiotherapy: Challenges and new opportunities. *Cell Commun. Signal.* **2019**, *17*, 47. [CrossRef] [PubMed]
44. Grinde, M.T.; Vik, J.; Camilio, K.A.; Martinez-Zubiaurre, I.; Hellevik, T. Ionizing radiation abrogates the pro-tumorigenic capacity of cancer-associated fibroblasts co-implanted in xenografts. *Sci. Rep.* **2017**, *7*, 46714. [CrossRef] [PubMed]
45. Kamochi, N.; Nakashima, M.; Aoki, S.; Uchihashi, K.; Sugihara, H.; Toda, S.; Kudo, S. Irradiated fibroblast-induced bystander effects on invasive growth of squamous cell carcinoma under cancer-stromal cell interaction. *Cancer Sci.* **2008**, *99*, 2417–2427. [CrossRef] [PubMed]
46. Liu, L.; Zhang, Z.; Zhou, L.; Hu, L.; Yin, C.; Qing, D.; Huang, S.; Cai, X.; Chen, Y. Cancer associated fibroblasts-derived exosomes contribute to radioresistance through promoting colorectal cancer stem *cells* phenotype. *Exp. Cell Res.* **2020**, *391*, 111956. [CrossRef]
47. Colton, M.; Cheadle, E.J.; Honeychurch, J.; Illidge, T.M. Reprogramming the tumour microenvironment by radiotherapy: Implications for radiotherapy and immunotherapy combinations. *Radiat. Oncol.* **2020**, *15*, 254. [CrossRef] [PubMed]
48. Brown, J.M. Radiation Damage to Tumor Vasculature Initiates a Program That Promotes Tumor Recurrences. *Int. J. Radiat. Oncol. Biol. Phys.* **2020**, *108*, 734–744. [CrossRef]
49. Castle, K.D.; Kirsch, D.G. Establishing the Impact of Vascular Damage on Tumor Response to High-Dose Radiation Therapy. *Cancer Res.* **2019**, *79*, 5685–5692. [CrossRef]
50. Arnold, K.M.; Flynn, N.J.; Raben, A.; Romak, L.; Yu, Y.; Dicker, A.P.; Mourtada, F.; Sims-Mourtada, J. The Impact of Radiation on the Tumor Microenvironment: Effect of Dose and Fractionation Schedules. *Cancer Growth Metastasis* **2018**, *11*, 1179064418761639. [CrossRef]
51. Park, H.J.; Griffin, R.J.; Hui, S.; Levitt, S.H.; Song, C.W. Radiation-induced vascular damage in tumors: Implications of vascular damage in ablative hypofractionated radiotherapy (SBRT and SRS). *Radiat. Res.* **2012**, *177*, 311–327. [CrossRef] [PubMed]
52. Riva, M.; Wouters, R.; Nittner, D.; Ceuster, J.; Sterpin, E.; Giovannoni, R.; Himmelreich, U.; Gsell, W.; Van Ranst, M.; Coosemans, A. Radiation dose-escalation and dose-fractionation modulate the immune microenvironment, cancer stem *cells* and vasculature in experimental high-grade gliomas. *J. Neurosurg. Sci.* **2020**. [CrossRef] [PubMed]
53. Potiron, V.; Clément-Colmou, K.; Jouglar, E.; Pietri, M.; Chiavassa, S.; Delpon, G.; Paris, F.; Supiot, S. Tumor vasculature remodeling by radiation therapy increases doxorubicin distribution and efficacy. *Cancer Lett.* **2019**, *457*, 1–9. [CrossRef] [PubMed]
54. Kouam, P.N.; Rezniczek, G.A.; Adamietz, I.A.; Bühler, H. Ionizing radiation increases the endothelial permeability and the transendothelial migration of tumor *cells* through ADAM10-activation and subsequent degradation of VE-cadherin. *BMC Cancer* **2019**, *19*, 958. [CrossRef] [PubMed]
55. Maeda, A.; Chen, Y.; Bu, J.; Mujcic, H.; Wouters, B.G.; DaCosta, R.S. In Vivo Imaging Reveals Significant Tumor Vascular Dysfunction and Increased Tumor Hypoxia-Inducible Factor-1α Expression Induced by High Single-Dose Irradiation in a Pancreatic Tumor Model. *Int. J. Radiat. Oncol. Biol. Phys.* **2017**, *97*, 184–194. [CrossRef]
56. Banerjee, D.; Barton, S.M.; Grabham, P.W.; Rumeld, A.L.; Okochi, S.; Street, C.; Kadenhe-Chiweshe, A.; Boboila, S.; Yamashiro, D.J.; Connolly, E.P. High-Dose Radiation Increases Notch1 in Tumor Vasculature. *Int. J. Radiat. Oncol. Biol. Phys.* **2020**, *106*, 857–866. [CrossRef] [PubMed]
57. Stapleton, S.; Jaffray, D.; Milosevic, M. Radiation effects on the tumor microenvironment: Implications for nanomedicine delivery. *Adv. Drug Deliv. Rev.* **2017**, *109*, 119–130. [CrossRef]
58. Jensen, M.B.; Lænkholm, A.V.; Balslev, E.; Buckingham, W.; Ferree, S.; Glavicic, V.; Dupont Jensen, J.; Søegaard Knoop, A.; Mouridsen, H.T.; Nielsen, D.; et al. The Prosigna 50-gene profile and responsiveness to adjuvant anthracycline-based chemotherapy in high-risk breast cancer patients. *NPJ Breast Cancer* **2020**, *6*, 7. [CrossRef]
59. Cardoso, F.; van't Veer, L.J.; Bogaerts, J.; Slaets, L.; Viale, G.; Delaloge, S.; Pierga, J.Y.; Brain, E.; Causeret, S.; DeLorenzi, M.; et al. 70-Gene Signature as an Aid to Treatment Decisions in Early-Stage Breast Cancer. *N. Engl. J. Med.* **2016**, *375*, 717–729. [CrossRef]
60. Kim, H.S.; Kim, S.C.; Kim, S.J.; Park, C.H.; Jeung, H.C.; Kim, Y.B.; Ahn, J.B.; Chung, H.C.; Rha, S.Y. Identification of a radiosensitivity signature using integrative metaanalysis of published microarray data for NCI-60 cancer *cells*. *BMC Genom.* **2012**, *13*, 348. [CrossRef]
61. Tramm, T.; Mohammed, H.; Myhre, S.; Kyndi, M.; Alsner, J.; Børresen-Dale, A.L.; Sørlie, T.; Frigessi, A.; Overgaard, J. Development and validation of a gene profile predicting benefit of postmastectomy radiotherapy in patients with high-risk breast cancer: A study of gene expression in the DBCG82bc cohort. *Clin. Cancer Res.* **2014**, *20*, 5272–5280. [CrossRef] [PubMed]
62. Speers, C.; Zhao, S.; Liu, M.; Bartelink, H.; Pierce, L.J.; Feng, F.Y. Development and Validation of a Novel Radiosensitivity Signature in Human Breast Cancer. *Clin. Cancer Res.* **2015**, *21*, 3667–3677. [CrossRef] [PubMed]
63. Zhao, S.G.; Chang, S.L.; Spratt, D.E.; Erho, N.; Yu, M.; Ashab, H.A.; Alshalalfa, M.; Speers, C.; Tomlins, S.A.; Davicioni, E.; et al. Development and validation of a 24-gene predictor of response to postoperative radiotherapy in prostate cancer: A matched, retrospective analysis. *Lancet Oncol.* **2016**, *17*, 1612–1620. [CrossRef]

64. Liu, J.; Han, M.; Yue, Z.; Dong, C.; Wen, P.; Zhao, G.; Wu, L.; Xia, J.; Bin, Y. Prediction of Radiosensitivity in Head and Neck Squamous Cell Carcinoma Based on Multiple Omics Data. *Front. Genet.* **2020**, *11*, 960. [CrossRef] [PubMed]
65. Piening, B.D.; Wang, P.; Subramanian, A.; Paulovich, A.G. A radiation-derived gene expression signature predicts clinical outcome for breast cancer patients. *Radiat. Res.* **2009**, *171*, 141–154. [CrossRef]
66. Oh, D.S.; Cheang, M.C.; Fan, C.; Perou, C.M. Radiation-induced gene signature predicts pathologic complete response to neoadjuvant chemotherapy in breast cancer patients. *Radiat. Res.* **2014**, *181*, 193–207. [CrossRef]
67. Eustace, A.; Mani, N.; Span, P.N.; Irlam, J.J.; Taylor, J.; Betts, G.N.; Denley, H.; Miller, C.J.; Homer, J.J.; Rojas, A.M.; et al. A 26-gene hypoxia signature predicts benefit from hypoxia-modifying therapy in laryngeal cancer but not bladder cancer. *Clin. Cancer Res.* **2013**, *19*, 4879–4888. [CrossRef]
68. Toustrup, K.; Sørensen, B.S.; Lassen, P.; Wiuf, C.; Alsner, J.; Overgaard, J. Gene expression classifier predicts for hypoxic modification of radiotherapy with nimorazole in squamous cell carcinomas of the head and neck. *Radiother. Oncol.* **2012**, *102*, 122–129. [CrossRef]
69. Li, B.; Shi, X.B.; Nori, D.; Chao, C.K.; Chen, A.M.; Valicenti, R.; White Rde, V. Down-regulation of microRNA 106b is involved in p21-mediated cell cycle arrest in response to radiation in prostate cancer *cells. Prostate* **2011**, *71*, 567–574. [CrossRef]
70. Li, A.L.; Chung, T.S.; Chan, Y.N.; Chen, C.L.; Lin, S.C.; Chiang, Y.R.; Lin, C.H.; Chen, C.C.; Ma, N. microRNA expression pattern as an ancillary prognostic signature for radiotherapy. *J. Transl. Med.* **2018**, *16*, 341. [CrossRef]
71. Cui, Y.; Li, B.; Pollom, E.L.; Horst, K.C.; Li, R. Integrating Radiosensitivity and Immune Gene Signatures for Predicting Benefit of Radiotherapy in Breast Cancer. *Clin. Cancer Res.* **2018**, *24*, 4754–4762. [CrossRef] [PubMed]
72. Wang, Q.; He, G.; Hou, M.; Chen, L.; Chen, S.; Xu, A.; Fu, Y. Cell Cycle Regulation by Alternative Polyadenylation of CCND1. *Sci. Rep.* **2018**, *8*, 6824. [CrossRef] [PubMed]
73. Goel, H.L.; Mercurio, A.M. VEGF targets the tumour cell. *Nat. Rev. Cancer* **2013**, *13*, 871–882. [CrossRef] [PubMed]
74. Stupp, R.; Hegi, M.E.; Gorlia, T.; Erridge, S.C.; Perry, J.; Hong, Y.K.; Aldape, K.D.; Lhermitte, B.; Pietsch, T.; Grujicic, D.; et al. Cilengitide combined with standard treatment for patients with newly diagnosed glioblastoma with methylated MGMT promoter (CENTRIC EORTC 26071-22072 study): A multicentre, randomised, open-label, phase 3 trial. *Lancet Oncol.* **2014**, *15*, 1100–1108. [CrossRef]
75. Gvozdenovic, A.; Boro, A.; Meier, D.; Bode-Lesniewska, B.; Born, W.; Muff, R.; Fuchs, B. Targeting αvβ3 and αvβ5 integrins inhibits pulmonary metastasis in an intratibial xenograft osteosarcoma mouse model. *Oncotarget* **2016**, *7*, 55141–55154. [CrossRef] [PubMed]
76. Noal, S.; Levy, C.; Hardouin, A.; Rieux, C.; Heutte, N.; Ségura, C.; Collet, F.; Allouache, D.; Switsers, O.; Delcambre, C.; et al. One-year longitudinal study of fatigue, cognitive functions, and quality of life after adjuvant radiotherapy for breast cancer. *Int J. Radiat. Oncol. Biol. Phys.* **2011**, *81*, 795–803. [CrossRef]
77. Chen, X.; Zheng, J.; Zhuo, M.L.; Zhang, A.; You, Z. A six-gene-based signature for breast cancer radiotherapy sensitivity estimation. *Biosci. Rep.* **2020**, *40*. [CrossRef]
78. Hu, Y.; Guo, M. Synthetic lethality strategies: Beyond BRCA1/2 mutations in pancreatic cancer. *Cancer Sci.* **2020**, *111*, 3111–3121. [CrossRef]
79. Reichert, Z.R.; Wahl, D.R.; Morgan, M.A. Translation of Targeted Radiation Sensitizers into Clinical Trials. *Semin. Radiat. Oncol.* **2016**, *26*, 261–270. [CrossRef]
80. Subramanian, A.; Tamayo, P.; Mootha, V.K.; Mukherjee, S.; Ebert, B.L.; Gillette, M.A.; Paulovich, A.; Pomeroy, S.L.; Golub, T.R.; Lander, E.S.; et al. Gene set enrichment analysis: A knowledge-based approach for interpreting genome-wide expression profiles. *Proc. Natl. Acad. Sci. USA* **2005**, *102*, 15545–15550. [CrossRef]
81. Rastogi, P.; Anderson, S.J.; Bear, H.D.; Geyer, C.E.; Kahlenberg, M.S.; Robidoux, A.; Margolese, R.G.; Hoehn, J.L.; Vogel, V.G.; Dakhil, S.R.; et al. Preoperative chemotherapy: Updates of National Surgical Adjuvant Breast and Bowel Project Protocols B-18 and B-27. *J. Clin. Oncol.* **2008**, *26*, 778–785. [CrossRef] [PubMed]
82. Yang, L.; West, C.M. Hypoxia gene expression signatures as predictive biomarkers for personalising radiotherapy. *Br. J. Radiol.* **2019**, *92*, 20180036. [CrossRef] [PubMed]
83. Buffa, F.M.; Harris, A.L.; West, C.M.; Miller, C.J. Large meta-analysis of multiple cancers reveals a common, compact and highly prognostic hypoxia metagene. *Br. J. Cancer* **2010**, *102*, 428–435. [CrossRef] [PubMed]
84. Toustrup, K.; Sørensen, B.S.; Nordsmark, M.; Busk, M.; Wiuf, C.; Alsner, J.; Overgaard, J. Development of a hypoxia gene expression classifier with predictive impact for hypoxic modification of radiotherapy in head and neck cancer. *Cancer Res.* **2011**, *71*, 5923–5931. [CrossRef] [PubMed]
85. Nordsmark, M.; Overgaard, M.; Overgaard, J. Pretreatment oxygenation predicts radiation response in advanced squamous cell carcinoma of the head and neck. *Radiother. Oncol.* **1996**, *41*, 31–39. [CrossRef]
86. Nordsmark, M.; Overgaard, J. A confirmatory prognostic study on oxygenation status and loco-regional control in advanced head and neck squamous cell carcinoma treated by radiation therapy. *Radiother. Oncol.* **2000**, *57*, 39–43. [CrossRef]
87. Małachowska, B.; Tomasik, B.; Stawiski, K.; Kulkarni, S.; Guha, C.; Chowdhury, D.; Fendler, W. Circulating microRNAs as Biomarkers of Radiation Exposure: A Systematic Review and Meta-Analysis. *Int. J. Radiat. Oncol. Biol. Phys.* **2020**, *106*, 390–402. [CrossRef]

88. Asakura, K.; Kadota, T.; Matsuzaki, J.; Yoshida, Y.; Yamamoto, Y.; Nakagawa, K.; Takizawa, S.; Aoki, Y.; Nakamura, E.; Miura, J.; et al. A miRNA-based diagnostic model predicts resectable lung cancer in humans with high accuracy. *Commun. Biol.* **2020**, *3*, 134. [CrossRef]
89. Hamam, R.; Hamam, D.; Alsaleh, K.A.; Kassem, M.; Zaher, W.; Alfayez, M.; Aldahmash, A.; Alajez, N.M. Circulating microRNAs in breast cancer: Novel diagnostic and prognostic biomarkers. *Cell Death Dis.* **2017**, *8*, e3045. [CrossRef]
90. Zhang, J.H.; Hou, R.; Pan, Y.; Gao, Y.; Yang, Y.; Tian, W.; Zhu, Y.B. A five-microRNA signature for individualized prognosis evaluation and radiotherapy guidance in patients with diffuse lower-grade glioma. *J. Cell Mol. Med.* **2020**, *24*, 7504–7514. [CrossRef]
91. Shen, J.; Hruby, G.W.; McKiernan, J.M.; Gurvich, I.; Lipsky, M.J.; Benson, M.C.; Santella, R.M. Dysregulation of circulating microRNAs and prediction of aggressive prostate cancer. *Prostate* **2012**, *72*, 1469–1477. [CrossRef] [PubMed]
92. Zedan, A.H.; Hansen, T.F.; Assenholt, J.; Madsen, J.S.; Osther, P.J.S. Circulating miRNAs in localized/locally advanced prostate cancer patients after radical prostatectomy and radiotherapy. *Prostate* **2019**, *79*, 425–432. [CrossRef] [PubMed]
93. Cary, K.C.; Cooperberg, M.R. Biomarkers in prostate cancer surveillance and screening: Past, present, and future. *Ther. Adv. Urol.* **2013**, *5*, 318–329. [CrossRef] [PubMed]
94. Chen, D.S.; Mellman, I. Oncology meets immunology: The cancer-immunity cycle. *Immunity* **2013**, *39*, 1–10. [CrossRef]
95. Kirkby, K.J.; Kirkby, N.F.; Burnet, N.G.; Owen, H.; Mackay, R.I.; Crellin, A.; Green, S. Heavy charged particle beam therapy and related new radiotherapy technologies: The clinical potential, physics and technical developments required to deliver benefit for patients with cancer. *Br. J. Radiol.* **2020**, *93*, 20200247. [CrossRef]
96. Lupu-Plesu, M.; Claren, A.; Martial, S.; N'Diaye, P.D.; Lebrigand, K.; Pons, N.; Ambrosetti, D.; Peyrottes, I.; Feuillade, J.; Hérault, J.; et al. Effects of proton versus photon irradiation on (lymph)angiogenic, inflammatory, proliferative and anti-tumor immune responses in head and neck squamous cell carcinoma. *Oncogenesis* **2017**, *6*, e354. [CrossRef]
97. Durante, M.; Formenti, S. Harnessing radiation to improve immunotherapy: Better with particles? *Br. J. Radiol.* **2020**, *93*, 20190224. [CrossRef]

Journal of
Personalized Medicine

Communication

Relative Biological Effectiveness of Carbon Ions for Head-and-Neck Squamous Cell Carcinomas According to Human Papillomavirus Status

Naoto Osu [1,†], Daijiro Kobayashi [2,†], Katsuyuki Shirai [3], Atsushi Musha [4], Hiro Sato [4], Yuka Hirota [1], Atsushi Shibata [5], Takahiro Oike [1,4,*] and Tatsuya Ohno [1,4]

1 Department of Radiation Oncology, Gunma University Graduate School of Medicine, 3-39-22, Showa-machi, Maebashi 371-8511, Japan; m12201018@gunma-u.ac.jp (N.O.); yukahirota@gunma-u.ac.jp (Y.H.); tohno@gunma-u.ac.jp (T.O.)
2 Department of Radiation Oncology, Gunma Prefectural Cancer Center, 617-1, Takahayashi-nishicho, Ota 373-8550, Japan; m07201029@gmail.com
3 Department of Radiology, Jichi Medical University, 3311-1, Yakushiji, Shimotsuke, Tochigi 329-0498, Japan; kshirai@jichi.ac.jp
4 Gunma University Heavy Ion Medical Center, 3-39-22, Showa-machi, Maebashi 371-8511, Japan; musha@gunma-u.ac.jp (A.M.); hiro.sato@gunma-u.ac.jp (H.S.)
5 Signal Transduction Program, Gunma University Initiative for Advanced Research (GIAR), 3-39-22, Showa-machi, Maebashi 371-8511, Japan; shibata.at@gunma-u.ac.jp
* Correspondence: oiketakahiro@gunma-u.ac.jp or oiketakahiro@gmail.com; Tel.: +81-27-220-8383
† These two authors contribute equally to this work.

Received: 29 June 2020; Accepted: 24 July 2020; Published: 25 July 2020

Abstract: Carbon-ion radiotherapy (CIRT) has strong antitumor effects and excellent dose conformity. In head-and-neck squamous cell carcinoma (HNSCC), human papillomavirus (HPV) status is a prognostic factor for photon radiotherapy outcomes. However, the effect of HPV status on the sensitivity of HNSCCs to carbon ions remains unclear. Here, we showed that the relative biological effectiveness (RBE) of carbon ions over X-rays was higher in HPV-negative cells than in HSGc-C5 cells, which are used for CIRT dose establishment, whereas the RBE in HPV-positive cells was modest. These data indicate that CIRT is more advantageous in HPV-negative than in HPV-positive HNSCCs.

Keywords: carbon-ion radiotherapy; head-and-neck tumors; squamous cell carcinoma; radiosensitivity; relative biological effectiveness

1. Introduction

Carbon-ion radiotherapy (CIRT) is a promising modality with a strong antitumor effect even in tumors resistant to conventional photon radiotherapy [1]. CIRT is characterized by a highly conformal dose distribution to targets; this property enables sufficient dose delivery to tumors in the head-and-neck region while sparing the surrounding critical organs at risk (e.g., the salivary glands and the eyes) [2]. In Japan, which has the greatest number of CIRT facilities in the world, non-squamous cell carcinomas have been the major target for CIRT in the head and neck regions. However, radiation oncologists often encounter head-and-neck squamous cell carcinomas (HNSCCs) that show resistance to photon radiotherapy, underscoring the need to establish a strategy for stratifying patients and for switching photon-resistant HNSCC patients to CIRT.

Precision medicine enables the design of personalized treatment strategies according to the biological information about individual tumors [3]. Certain genetic profiles predict radiotherapy outcomes, suggesting that precision medicine can be applied to radiotherapy. For example, we and others showed that the *EGFR* mutational status predicts the sensitivity of non-small cell lung cancers to photon radiotherapy [4,5]. Torres-Roca et al. developed an algorithm based on the mRNA expression levels of ten genes to predict radiotherapy outcomes in various cancers [6]. Human papillomavirus (HPV) infection is a favorable prognostic factor in HNSCC [7], and HPV-negative HNSCCs are more resistant to photon irradiation than HPV-positive HNSCCs [8]. The molecular mechanisms explaining the difference in photon sensitivity between HPV-positive and negative HNSCCs have not been elucidated fully. However, studies suggest p53-associated apoptosis and DNA repair as candidate mechanisms [8]. For the former, it is considered that the function of p53 in inducing apoptosis is retained in HPV-positive head and neck cancer cells, although downregulated by the HPV E6-oncoprotein, whereas HPV-negative head and neck cancer cells harbor genetic alterations in *p53*, contributing to the anti-apoptotic phenotype. For the latter, data suggest that in HPV-positive cancer cells, p16 overexpression impairs the recruitment of RAD51 to DNA damage sites, contributing to decreased homologous recombination activity. HPV negativity thus has potential as a biomarker of photon resistance that can be used to stratify patients with HNSCC and to determine indications for CIRT. However, there is limited information on the sensitivity of HNSCCs to carbon ions. For example, Particle Irradiation Data Ensemble (PIDE, ver. 3.1), a large database of cell lines tested in vitro for sensitivity to particle radiation, contains only three HNSCC cell lines [9]. In addition, the effect of HPV status on the relative biological effectiveness (RBE) of carbon ions remains unclear. To address these issues, we examined the carbon-ion sensitivity of HNSCCs according to HPV status, as well as the RBE of CIRT in this patient population.

2. Materials and Methods

2.1. Cell Line and Cell Culture

Four HPV-positive and six HPV-negative HNSCC cell lines were used in this study (Table 1) [10–14]. UD-SCC-2 was obtained from Dr. Silke Schwarz of Ulm University (Ulm, Germany). UM-SCC-1, UM-SCC-47, and UM-SCC-104 were obtained from Merck (Kenilworth, NJ, USA). UPCI: SCC154 was obtained from Dr. Susanne Gollin of University of Pittsburgh (Pittsburgh, PA, USA). A-253, Detroit 562, Fadu, SCC-9, and SCC-25 were obtained from ATCC (Manassas, VA, USA). Based on the historical context of the development of CIRT, the HSGc-C5 cell line, obtained from JCRB Cell Bank (National Institutes of Biomedical Innovation, Health and Nutrition, Ibaragi, Japan), was used as the reference for the carbon-ion RBE [15]. The cells were cultured in RPMI-1640 (Sigma-Aldrich, St. Louis, MO, USA) supplemented with 10% fetal bovine serum (Life Technologies, Carlsbad, CA, USA).

Table 1. Cell lines used in this study.

Cell Line	HPV Status	Origin	Reference
UD-SCC-2	Positive	Pharynx	[10]
UM-SCC-47	Positive	Tongue	[11]
UM-SCC-104	Positive	Oral cavity	[10]
UPCI:SCC154	Positive	Tongue	[10]
A-253	Negative	Salivary gland	[12]
Detroit 562	Negative	Pharynx	[13]
FaDu	Negative	Pharynx	[13]
SCC-9	Negative	Tongue	[14]
SCC-25	Negative	Tongue	[13]
UM-SCC-1	Negative	Oral cavity	[11]

HPV, human papillomavirus.

2.2. Clonogenic Assays

Clonogenic assays were performed as described previously [16]. Briefly, cells thawed from frozen stocks were cultured over more than two passages and used for experiments after confirming that they were in the logarithmic growth phase. The cells were treated with trypsin (Sigma-Aldrich) for 5 min at 37 °C for detachment, and single-cell suspensions in culture media were prepared in 50 mL conical tubes. The cell numbers were determined using the improved Neubauer hemocytometer with an inverted microscope. Based on the cell count results, the seeding of the cells was performed using final cell suspensions prepared after two one-to-ten serial dilutions (×100 dilution in total). The cells seeded in 6-well plates were incubated for a minimum period to enable cell attachment (6–12 h, according to cell line characteristics) and received X-ray or carbon ion irradiation. After incubation for an additional 10–14 days, the cells were fixed with methanol and then stained with crystal violet. Clumps of equal to or more than 50 cells were recognized as colonies, and the number of colonies per well was determined using an inverted microscope. The surviving fraction for a given dose was calculated by dividing the number of colonies for the dose by the number of seeded cells for the dose, which was further divided by the plating efficiency, calculated based on unirradiated controls. The surviving fractions were fitted to the linear quadratic model [17], and the D_{10} (i.e., the dose that reduces cell survival to 10%) was calculated. The RBE of carbon ions for a given cell line was calculated by dividing the D_{10} value for X-rays by that for carbon ions [2,15]. At least four samples were used for each experiment. The experiments were repeated at least twice.

2.3. Irradiation

X-ray irradiation was performed using a Faxitron RX-650 (100 kVp, 1.14 Gy/min; Faxitron Bioptics, Tucson, AZ, USA) [4]. Carbon-ion irradiation was performed at the Gunma University Heavy Ion Medical Center. The specific parameters were as follows: 290 MeV/nucleon; an average linear energy transfer at the center of a 6 cm spread-out Bragg peak (SOBP) of approximately 50 keV/μm [4].

2.4. Statistics

Differences between two non-paired groups were examined using the non-parametric two-sided Mann–Whitney U-test. Differences between two paired groups were examined using the non-parametric two-sided Wilcoxon paired signed-rank test. The level of significance for the differences was set at p of <0.05. All statistical analyses were done by using Prism8 (GraphPad Software, San Diego, CA, USA).

3. Results

The sensitivity of the four HPV-positive and six HPV-negative HNSCC cell lines to X-rays was tested using clonogenic assays (Table 1). The results showed that resistance to X-rays was higher in HPV-negative than in HPV-positive cell lines (Figure 1a). D_{10} values were significantly higher for HPV-negative cell lines than for HPV-positive cell lines (8.2 ± 2.2 Gy vs. 4.3 ± 1.2 Gy, p = 0.038) (Figure 2a). These data are consistent with the findings of previous studies showing that HPV-negative head-and-neck tumors are resistant to X-rays compared with their HPV-positive counterparts and confirm the robustness of the present experimental system for the assessment of radiosensitivity [8].

Examination of the clonogenic survival of the ten cell lines treated with carbon-ion irradiation showed that carbon ions had a greater cell killing effect than X-rays in all cell lines examined (Figure 1a,b). The D_{10} values were significantly higher for HPV-negative cell lines than for HPV-positive cell lines (3.3 ± 0.7 Gy vs. 2.3 ± 0.3 Gy, p = 0.033) (Figure 2b). However, the D_{10} range was narrower for carbon ions than for X-rays, indicating the high cell killing effect of carbon ions on HNSCC cells regardless of HPV status (Figure 2a,b). The differences in α/β values between X-rays and carbon ions were not statistically significant (p = 0.46) (Table S1).

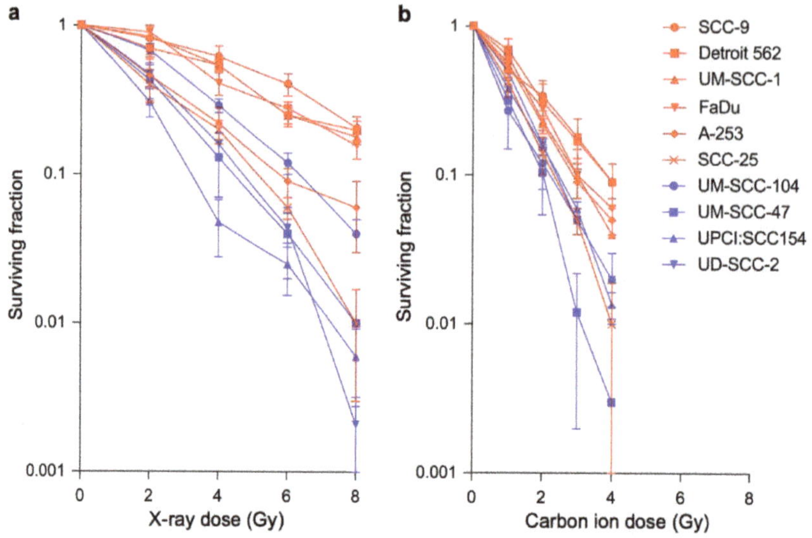

Figure 1. Clonogenic survival of head-and-neck squamous cell carcinoma cell lines treated with X-rays (**a**) or carbon ions (**b**). Human papillomavirus-positive or -negative cell lines are indicated in blue and red, respectively.

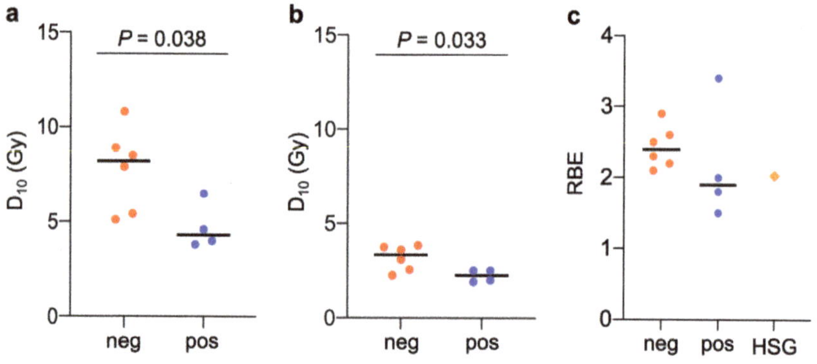

Figure 2. D_{10} for X-rays (**a**), D_{10} for carbon ions (**b**), and relative biological effectiveness (RBE) of carbon ions (**c**) for human papillomavirus-positive (pos) or -negative (neg) head-and-neck squamous cell carcinoma cell lines. RBE data for the HSGc-C5 cell line (HSG) were used as the reference. Black lines show median values. *p*-values as assessed by the Mann–Whitney U-test are shown.

The RBE of carbon ions was calculated in HPV-positive and HPV-negative cell lines (Table 2). The HSGc-C5 cell line was used as the reference for RBE because the clinical dose unit for CIRT, i.e., Gy (RBE), is determined using RBE data obtained with this cell line [15,18]. Under the experimental conditions used, the RBE in HSGc-C5 cells was 2.0 (Figure S1). The RBE was higher in all the six HPV-negative cell lines (i.e., 2.4 ± 0.2) than in the HSGc-C5 cell line (Figure 2c). By contrast, the RBE was lower in three of the four HPV-positive cell lines (i.e., 2.1 ± 0.8) than in HSGc-C5 cells (Figure 2c). These data indicate that CIRT is more effective in HPV-negative HNSCCs than in HPV-positive HNSCCs.

Table 2. D_{10} and RBE in HPV-positive and negative cell lines.

Cell Line	HPV Status	D_{10}-X (Gy)	D_{10}-C (Gy)	RBE
UD-SCC-2	Positive	4.58	2.52	1.81
UM-SCC-47	Positive	3.98	2.01	1.98
UM-SCC-104	Positive	6.52	1.92	3.38
UPCI:SCC154	Positive	3.80	2.52	1.50
A-253	Negative	5.40	2.56	2.10
Detroit 562	Negative	8.48	3.84	2.20
FaDu	Negative	8.85	3.60	2.45
SCC-9	Negative	10.83	3.75	2.88
SCC-25	Negative	5.06	2.25	2.25
UM-SCC-1	Negative	7.90	3.09	2.56

X, X-rays; C, carbon ions.

4. Discussion

We showed that the RBE of carbon ions over X-rays was higher in HPV-negative cells than in the HSGc-C5 cell line, which was used as the reference for CIRT dosing, whereas the RBE of carbon ions was lower in HPV-positive cells. This is the first report analyzing the RBE of carbon ions in relation to HPV status in HNSCC. To the best of our knowledge, this is the largest dataset of cells used for the in vitro testing of the sensitivity of HNSCC to carbon ions.

Full clinical studies for CIRT began in 1994 at the Heavy Ion Medical Accelerator in Chiba (HIMAC) of the National Institute of Radiological Sciences (NIRS) in Japan [1]. The Gesellschaft für Schwerionenforschung (GSI) center in Germany started treating patients with carbon ions in 1997. Two CIRT centers in Japan—i.e., the Hyogo Ion Beam Medical Center (HIBMC) and Gunma University Heavy Ion Medical Center (GHMC)—joined in 2002 and 2010, respectively, and the CIRT facilities are now spreading mainly in Asia and Europe. Nevertheless, compared with proton radiotherapy, another particle therapy modality, it can still be said that CIRT is an extremely limited medical resource because only 13 facilities in the world are in operation as of 2020. Annually, more than 14 million patients are newly diagnosed with cancer worldwide. By contrast, CIRT has the capacity of only a few thousand per year, even if all the facilities in the world were combined. This means that less than one percent of the patients newly diagnosed as having cancer can have the opportunity to be treated with CIRT. The biggest barriers to the development of a new CIRT facility are the high capital costs and the high operational costs: it is estimated that it costs approximately 138.6 million EUR [1]. Without a technological breakthrough to lower the costs' magnitude, the critical shortage of CIRT facilities will remain for the coming decades. From this perspective, the optimization of patient stratification is of high importance to maximize the use efficacy of CIRT. In this context, the tumors located in the head-and-neck regions are ideal targets for CIRT, which possesses high organ-sparing ability, because the head-and-neck regions are one of the anatomical sites where functionally important organs are concentrated, forming a complex structure with each other. In addition to the advantages of carbon ions over photons in terms of dose conformity, high-linear-energy-transfer carbon ions show strong cell-killing effects even for photon-resistant cancer cells. Taking these together, in the present study, we sought to elucidate the RBE of carbon ions for a subset of photon-resistant head-and-neck tumors, to be considered as a candidate for CIRT.

When CIRT was launched at NIRS, the clinical SOBP of HIMAC beams was designed to achieve uniform cell killing across the SOBP width [15]. For this purpose, the a and b parameters in the linear quadratic survival curves corresponding to varying linear energy transfer were obtained by clonogenic assays. The cell line used as the reference in the series of clonogenic assay experiments should represent the responses of tumors to carbon ions. Therefore, HSG cells, which show intermediate radiosensitivity among various cell lines, were chosen. From this standpoint, although the current CIRT employs the dose unit of Gy(RBE), the antitumor effect of the CIRT compared with photon radiotherapy should be different according to the actual RBEs that the individual tumors show. Thus, it is critically important to elucidate the RBE of a subset of tumors that share specific biological features in order to achieve the above-mentioned optimization of patient stratification in CIRT. To this end, in the present study, we sought to elucidate the RBE of HNSCCs according to HPV status by using HSG cells as the reference.

Kagawa et al. reported that the RBE for carbon ions for HSGc-C5 cells was 1.8 at the center of a 6 cm SOBP of 320 MeV/n beams using 4 MV X-rays as the control [18]. Yoshida et al. reported that the RBE for HSGc-C5 cells was 2.0 at the center of an 8 cm SOBP of 350 MeV/n beams using 200 kVp X-rays as the control [19]. The RBE values reported in these studies are broadly consistent with that obtained in the present study (i.e., 2.0 at the center of a 6 cm SOBP of 290 MeV/n beams using 100 kVp as the control), supporting the robustness of our experimental systems for RBE measurements.

Mizoe et al. reported the outcomes of a phase II clinical trial of CIRT in 236 head-and-neck tumors [20]. In that study, 64.0 Gy(RBE) given in 16 fractions over 4 weeks caused modest normal tissue toxicities; i.e., grade 3 skin reactions in 6% and grade 3 mucosal reactions in 10% of the patients in the acute phase, and grade 2 skin reactions in 3% and grade 2 mucosal reactions in 2% of the patients in the late phase. In this study, the RBE values in HPV-negative cells were approximately 10–30% higher than those in HSGc-C5 cells. The clinical Gy(RBE) dose unit is calculated according to the clonogenic survival of HSGc-C5 cells. Therefore, theoretically, it is estimated that CIRT at 64.0 Gy(RBE) exerts antitumor effects equivalent to approximately 70.4–83.2 Gy(RBE) in HPV-negative HNSCCs with moderate tissue toxicities. These data indicate that CIRT may be beneficial in this type of tumor. Clinical trials of CIRT for the treatment of HPV-negative HNSCCs are necessary to validate the results of the present study.

UM-SCC-104 showed an RBE greater than 3, which was exceptionally high for an HPV-positive cell line. In fact, the D_{10} for X-rays for this cell line was intermediate (i.e., 6.5 Gy), ranking it fifth among the ten cell lines examined in this study. By contrast, the D_{10} for carbon ions for this cell line was the lowest among the ten cell lines (i.e., 1.9 Gy). This indicates a specific sensitivity of UM-SCC-104 to carbon ions. Wang et al. reported that in the repair of DNA double-strand breaks (DSBs) induced by heavy ions, only Ku-dependent non-homologous end joining (NHEJ), but not other DSB repair pathways, is impaired [21]. Tang et al. reported that upon the establishment of the UM-SCC-104, this cell line shows strong and diffuse expression of EGFR [22], a protein known to be involved in NHEJ by interacting with the catalytic subunit of DNA-dependent protein kinase [23]. These data together may suggest that UM-SCC-104 relies heavily on NHEJ in the repair of DSBs.

There was obvious difference in photon sensitivity between the HPV-positive and HPV-negative HNSCC lines examined in this study, whereas the difference in carbon ion sensitivity between the two groups was mediocre. It is worth noting that the HPV-positive lines harbored wild-type *p53*, whereas the HPV-negative lines were *p53*-mutant (Table 3) [24–26]. We have previously shown that photon sensitivity is affected by *p53* status; functional deficiency in p53 contributes to photon resistance through the abrogation of radiation-induced apoptosis. By contrast, carbon ions exert cell killing regardless of *p53* status through the efficient induction of mitotic catastrophe [27]. Thus, it can be hypothesized that CIRT shows promising anti-tumor effects for anti-apoptotic p53-mutated HPV-negative HNSCCs, which should be tested in future research.

Table 3. *TP53* mutation status for the cell lines used in this study.

Cell Line	*TP53*	Reference
UD-SCC-2	wild-type	[24]
UM-SCC-47	wild-type	[24]
UM-SCC-104	wild-type	[22]
UPCI:SCC154	wild-type	[25]
A-253	mutant (deletion)	[12]
Detroit 562	mutant (codon 248)	[12]
FaDu	mutant (codon 258)	[12]
SCC-9	mutant (deletion)	[12]
SCC-25	mutant (deletion)	[24]
UM-SCC-1	mutant (splice site)	[26]

One limitation of this study is that we did not analyze the molecular mechanisms underlying the higher RBE for HPV-negative HNSCCs, and this issue warrants future research.

5. Conclusions

We determined the RBE of carbon ions in HPV-positive and HPV-negative HNSCCs. The RBE values were higher in HPV-negative cells than in the reference HSGc-C5 cells, suggesting that CIRT is beneficial for the treatment of HPV-negative HNSCC and that clinical validation is warranted.

Supplementary Materials: The following are available online at http://www.mdpi.com/2075-4426/10/3/71/s1. Table S1: α and β parameters for X-rays or carbon ions for HPV-positive and -negative cell lines. Figure S1: Clonogenic survival of HSGc-C5 cells treated with X-rays or carbon ions.

Author Contributions: Conceptualization, T.O. (Takahiro Oike); formal analysis, N.O., D.K., K.S., A.M., H.S., and Y.H.; writing—original draft preparation, N.O.; writing—review and editing, T.O. (Takahiro Oike); supervision, A.S. and T.O. (Tatsuya Ohno); funding acquisition, N.O. and T.O. (Tatsuya Ohno). All authors have read and agreed to the published version of the manuscript.

Funding: This work was supported by Grants-in-Aid from the Ministry of Education, Culture, Sports, Science, and Technology of Japan for programs for Leading Graduate Schools, Cultivating Global Leaders in Heavy Ion Therapeutics and Engineering. This work was also supported by the Gunma University Heavy Ion Medical Center.

Acknowledgments: We thank Yukari Yoshida of Gunma University for technical assistance.

Conflicts of Interest: The authors declare no conflict of interest.

References

1. Schlaff, C.D.; Krauze, A.; Belard, A.; O'Connell, J.J.; Camphausen, K.A. Bringing the heavy: Carbon ion therapy in the radiobiological and clinical context. *Radiat. Oncol.* **2014**, *9*, 88. [CrossRef] [PubMed]
2. Loeffler, J.S.; Durante, M. Charged particle therapy-optimization, challenges and future directions. *Nat. Rev. Clin. Oncol.* **2013**, *10*, 411–424. [CrossRef] [PubMed]
3. Pauli, C.; Hopkins, B.D.; Prandi, D.; Shaw, R.; Fedrizzi, T.; Sboner, A.; Sailer, V.; Augello, M.; Puca, L.; Rosati, R.; et al. Personalized In Vitro and In Vivo Cancer Models to Guide Precision Medicine. *Cancer Discov.* **2017**, *7*, 462–477. [CrossRef] [PubMed]
4. Amornwichet, N.; Oike, T.; Shibata, A.; Nirodi, C.S.; Ogiwara, H.; Makino, H.; Kimura, Y.; Hirota, Y.; Isono, M.; Yoshida, Y.; et al. The EGFR mutation status affects the relative biological effectiveness of carbon-ion beams in non-small cell lung carcinoma cells. *Sci. Rep.* **2015**, *5*, 11305. [CrossRef]
5. Yagishita, S.; Horinouchi, H.; Katsui Taniyama, T.; Nakamichi, S.; Kitazono, S.; Mizugaki, H.; Kanda, S.; Fujiwara, Y.; Nokihara, H.; Yamamoto, N.; et al. Epidermal growth factor receptor mutation is associated with longer local control after definitive chemoradiotherapy in patients with stage III nonsquamous non-small-cell lung cancer. *Int. J. Radiat. Oncol. Biol. Phys.* **2015**, *91*, 140–148. [CrossRef]
6. Torres-Roca, J.F. A molecular assay of tumor radiosensitivity: A roadmap towards biology-based personalized radiation therapy. *Pers. Med.* **2012**, *9*, 547–557. [CrossRef]
7. Ang, K.K.; Harris, J.; Wheeler, R.; Weber, R.; Rosenthal, D.I.; Nguyen-Tân, P.F.; Westra, W.H.; Chung, C.H.; Jordan, R.C.; Lu, C.; et al. Human papillomavirus and survival of patients with oropharyngeal cancer. *N. Engl. J. Med.* **2010**, *363*, 24–35. [CrossRef]
8. Mirghani, H.; Amen, F.; Tao, Y.; Deutsch, E.; Levy, A. Increased radiosensitivity of HPV-positive head and neck cancers: Molecular basis and therapeutic perspectives. *Cancer Treat. Rev.* **2015**, *41*, 844–852. [CrossRef]
9. Friedrich, T.; Scholz, U.; Elsässer, T.; Durante, M.; Scholz, M. Systematic analysis of RBE and related quantities using a database of cell survival experiments with ion beam irradiation. *J. Radiat. Res.* **2013**, *54*, 494–514. [CrossRef]
10. Olthof, N.C.; Huebbers, C.U.; Kolligs, J.; Henfling, M.; Ramaekers, F.C.; Cornet, I.; van Lent-Albrechts, J.A.; Stegmann, A.P.; Silling, S.; Wieland, U.; et al. Viral load, gene expression and mapping of viral integration sites in HPV16-associated HNSCC cell lines. *Int. J. Cancer* **2015**, *136*, E207–E218. [CrossRef]
11. Brenner, J.C.; Graham, M.P.; Kumar, B.; Saunders, L.M.; Kupfer, R.; Lyons, R.H.; Bradford, C.R.; Carey, T.E. Genotyping of 73 UM-SCC head and neck squamous cell carcinoma cell lines. *Head Neck* **2010**, *32*, 417–426. [CrossRef] [PubMed]

12. St. John, L.S.; Sauter, E.R.; Herlyn, M.; Litwin, S.; Adler-Storthz, K. Endogenous p53 gene status predicts the response of human squamous cell carcinomas to wild-type p53. *Cancer Gene Ther.* **2000**, *7*, 749–756. [CrossRef] [PubMed]
13. Nichols, A.C.; Yoo, J.; Palma, D.A.; Fung, K.; Franklin, J.H.; Koropatnick, J.; Mymryk, J.S.; Batada, N.N.; Barrett, J.W. Frequent mutations in TP53 and CDKN2A found by next-generation sequencing of head and neck cancer cell lines. *Arch. Otolaryngol. Head Neck Surg.* **2012**, *138*, 732–739. [CrossRef] [PubMed]
14. Cooper, T.; Biron, V.L.; Fast, D.; Tam, R.; Carey, T.; Shmulevitz, M.; Seikaly, H. Oncolytic activity of reovirus in HPV positive and negative head and neck squamous cell carcinoma. *J. Otolaryngol. Head Neck Surg.* **2015**, *44*, 8. [CrossRef]
15. Kanai, T.; Endo, M.; Minohara, S.; Miyahara, N.; Koyama-ito, H.; Tomura, H.; Matsufuji, N.; Futami, Y.; Fukumura, A.; Hiraoka, T.; et al. Biophysical characteristics of HIMAC clinical irradiation system for heavy-ion radiation therapy. *Int. J. Radiat. Oncol. Biol. Phys.* **1999**, *44*, 201–210. [CrossRef]
16. Anakura, M.; Nachankar, A.; Kobayashi, D.; Amornwichet, N.; Hirota, Y.; Shibata, A.; Oike, T.; Nakano, T. Radiosensitivity Differences between EGFR Mutant and Wild-Type Lung Cancer Cells are Larger at Lower Doses. *Int. J. Mol. Sci.* **2019**, *20*, 3635. [CrossRef]
17. Oike, T.; Ogiwara, H.; Torikai, K.; Nakano, T.; Yokota, J.; Kohno, T. Garcinol, a histone acetyltransferase inhibitor, radiosensitizes cancer cells by inhibiting non-homologous end joining. *Int. J. Radiat. Oncol. Biol. Phys.* **2012**, *84*, 815–821. [CrossRef]
18. Kagawa, K.; Murakami, M.; Hishikawa, Y.; Abe, M.; Akagi, T.; Yanou, T.; Kagiya, G.; Furusawa, Y.; Ando, K.; Nojima, K.; et al. Preclinical biological assessment of proton and carbon ion beams at Hyogo Ion Beam Medical Center. *Int. J. Radiat. Oncol. Biol. Phys.* **2002**, *54*, 928–938. [CrossRef]
19. Yoshida, Y.; Musha, A.; Kawamura, H.; Kanai, T.; Takahashi, T. Biology research. In *Annual Report for Fiscal Year 2009–2011*; Gunma University Heavy Ion Medical Center, Ed.; Gunma University Heavy Ion Medical Center: Maebashi, Japan, 2013; pp. 83–84.
20. Mizoe, J.E.; Hasegawa, A.; Jingu, K.; Takagi, R.; Bessyo, H.; Morikawa, T.; Tonoki, M.; Tsuji, H.; Kamada, T.; Tsujii, H.; et al. Results of carbon ion radiotherapy for head and neck cancer. *Radiother. Oncol.* **2012**, *103*, 32–37. [CrossRef]
21. Wang, H.; Wang, X.; Zhang, P.; Wang, Y. The Ku-dependent non-homologous end-joining but not other repair pathway is inhibited by high linear energy transfer ionizing radiation. *DNA Repair (Amst)* **2008**, *7*, 725–733. [CrossRef]
22. Tang, A.L.; Hauff, S.J.; Owen, J.H.; Graham, M.P.; Czerwinski, M.J.; Park, J.J.; Walline, H.; Papagerakis, S.; Stoerker, J.; McHugh, J.B.; et al. UM-SCC-104: A new human papillomavirus-16-positive cancer stem cell-containing head and neck squamous cell carcinoma cell line. *Head Neck* **2012**, *34*, 1480–1491. [CrossRef]
23. Das, A.K.; Chen, B.P.; Story, M.D.; Sato, M.; Minna, J.D.; Chen, D.J.; Nirodi, C.S. Somatic mutations in the tyrosine kinase domain of epidermal growth factor receptor (EGFR) abrogate EGFR-mediated radioprotection in non-small cell lung carcinoma. *Cancer Res.* **2007**, *67*, 5267–5274. [CrossRef]
24. Martin, D.; Abba, M.C.; Molinolo, A.A.; Vitale-Cross, L.; Wang, Z.; Zaida, M.; Delic, N.C.; Samuels, Y.; Lyons, J.G.; Gutkind, J.S. The head and neck cancer cell oncogenome: A platform for the development of precision molecular therapies. *Oncotarget* **2014**, *5*, 8906–8923. [CrossRef]
25. Telmer, C.A.; An, J.; Malehorn, D.E.; Zeng, X.; Gollin, S.M.; Ishwad, C.S.; Jarvik, J.W. Detection and assignment of TP53 mutations in tumor DNA using peptide mass signature genotyping. *Hum. Mutat.* **2003**, *22*, 158–165. [CrossRef]
26. Tanaka, N.; Zhao, M.; Tang, L.; Patel, A.A.; Xi, Q.; Van, H.T.; Takahashi, H.; Osman, A.A.; Zhang, J.; Wang, J.; et al. Gain-of-function mutant p53 promotes the oncogenic potential of head and neck squamous cell carcinoma cells by targeting the transcription factors FOXO3a and FOXM1. *Oncogene* **2018**, *37*, 1279–1292. [CrossRef]
27. Amornwichet, N.; Oike, T.; Shibata, A.; Ogiwara, H.; Tsuchiya, N.; Yamauchi, M.; Saitoh, Y.; Sekine, R.; Isono, M.; Yoshida, Y.; et al. Carbon-ion beam irradiation kills X-ray-resistant p53-null cancer cells by inducing mitotic catastrophe. *PLoS ONE* **2014**, *9*, e115121. [CrossRef]

Journal of
Personalized
Medicine

MDPI

Article

Metabolic Profiles of Whole Serum and Serum-Derived Exosomes Are Different in Head and Neck Cancer Patients Treated by Radiotherapy

Anna Wojakowska [1,†], Aneta Zebrowska [2,†], Agata Skowronek [2], Tomasz Rutkowski [2], Krzysztof Polanski [3], Piotr Widlak [2], Lukasz Marczak [1,*] and Monika Pietrowska [2,*]

1 Institute of Bioorganic Chemistry Polish Academy of Sciences, 61-704 Poznan, Poland; astasz@ibch.poznan.pl
2 Maria Sklodowska-Curie National Research Institute of Oncology, Gliwice Branch, 44-101 Gliwice, Poland; aneta7zebrowska@gmail.com (A.Z.); agata.w2012@gmail.com (A.S.); Tomasz.Rutkowski@io.gliwice.pl (T.R.); Piotr.Widlak@io.gliwice.pl (P.W.)
3 Wellcome Sanger Institute, Wellcome Genome Campus, Hinxton, Cambridgeshire CB10 1SA, UK; kp9@sanger.ac.uk
* Correspondence: lukasmar@ibch.poznan.pl (L.M.); Monika.Pietrowska@io.gliwice.pl (M.P.)
† These authors contributed equally.

Received: 15 October 2020; Accepted: 13 November 2020; Published: 13 November 2020

Abstract: Background: In general, the serum metabolome reflects the patient's body response to both disease state and implemented treatment. Though serum-derived exosomes are an emerging type of liquid biopsy, the metabolite content of these vesicles remains under researched. The aim of this pilot study was to compare the metabolite profiles of the whole serum and serum-derived exosomes in the context of differences between cancer patients and healthy controls as well as patients' response to radiotherapy (RT). Methods: Serum samples were collected from 10 healthy volunteers and 10 patients with head and neck cancer before and after RT. Metabolites extracted from serum and exosomes were analyzed by the gas chromatography–mass spectrometry (GC–MS). Results: An untargeted GC–MS-based approach identified 182 and 46 metabolites in serum and exosomes, respectively. Metabolites that differentiated cancer and control samples, either serum or exosomes, were associated with energy metabolism. Serum metabolites affected by RT were associated with the metabolism of amino acids, sugars, lipids, and nucleotides. Conclusions: cancer-related features of energy metabolism could be detected in both types of specimens. On the other hand, in contrast to RT-induced changes observed in serum metabolome, this pilot study did not reveal a specific radiation-related pattern of exosome metabolites.

Keywords: head and neck cancer; exosomes; serum; radiotherapy; metabolomics; GC/MS

1. Introduction

Head and neck cancer (HNC) is the sixth most common malignancy worldwide. The incidence of HNC exceeds half a million annually and accounts for approximately 6% of all cancer cases worldwide [1,2]. Although over the last decade we have observed an improvement in the treatment of HNC, there is still a need for new biomarkers of this type of cancer because, since the tumor location and classical staging remain the major criteria of the treatment selection, and molecular heterogeneity of HNC [3]. Radiotherapy (RT), used either alone or in combination with other treatment modalities (surgery, chemotherapy, or immunotherapy) is the major modality in the HNC treatment. The major benefit of RT is a well established local control of the tumor. However, ionizing radiation induces damage to the adjacent healthy tissues, which is reflected at the systemic level in body fluids [4–7]. Hence, detection in the patient's blood of a molecular fingerprint of the body's response to the treatment is another important aspect of HNC diagnostics, which could potentially enable the monitoring and prediction of radiation toxicity.

Various types of "omics" studies (genomics, transcriptomics, proteomics, metabolomics) using different sources of samples (blood, urine, saliva, tissues) uncovered molecules and genes of potential use as clinical biomarkers [8,9]. Cancer cells' metabolism differs from one of the healthy cells and it is considered as the closest footprint of a cancer phenotype. This is why metabolomics studies are among the fastest-growing areas of cancer research in recent decades. Recent studies revealed disparities in the metabolite profile between diseased and normal states as well as between miscellaneous types of cancer or various stages of the disease. Therefore, altered metabolic pathways in various cancer systems might be used to identify biomarkers in terms of diagnosis, prognosis, or treatment schedule choice [10,11]. The NMR-based metabolomics study revealed an increased level of glucose, ketone bodies, ornithine, asparagine, and 2-hydroxybutyrate while decreased levels of citric acid cycle (TCA cycle) intermediates (citrate, succinate, and formate), lactate, alanine, and other gluconeogenic amino acids in the sera of patients with HNC [12]. Another GC/MS-based metabolomic analysis of serum and tissues of HNC patients revealed different metabolite profiles in patients with different treatment outcomes. In patients with disease relapse, the serum levels of metabolites related to the glycolytic pathway (especially glucose, ribose, fructose) were higher while serum levels of amino acids (lysine and trans-4-hydroxy-L-proline) were lower than in samples of patients without disease relapse [13]. Hence, one could conclude that the altered energy metabolism, mostly the switch from the TCA cycle to aerobic glycolysis known as the Warburg effect, is characteristic for patients with HNC [12–15]. Moreover, a few studies addressed therapy-induced changes in metabolic profiles of HNC, revealing compounds whose levels were associated with the treatment escalation (e.g., of the radiation dose during radiotherapy) or the intensity of treatment toxicity [16–18]. However, the knowledge about molecular mechanisms involved in radiation-induced changes of the patient's metabolome remains limited.

In the present study, the GC/MS approach was applied to profile the serum metabolites of HNC patients who underwent RT to uncover the metabolome changes induced by radiation. Furthermore, we included in the study another emerging biospecimen—exosomes circulating in patients' blood. Exosomes are virus-sized (50–150 nm) vesicles of endosomal origin released by the majority of cell types, either normal and cancerous [19]. Exosomes and other classes of extracellular vesicles (EVs) play an essential role in cancer biology, being the key mediators of communication between cells [20,21]. EVs present in the blood and other biofluids represent an interesting type of so-called liquid biopsy, which is an emerging source of potential biomarkers with applicability in treatment personalization [22,23]. There is a growing evidence for the increased level of EVs in the biofluids of cancer patients as well as the radiation-induced enhancement of exosome secretion [24,25]. Even though literature data support the important role of transcriptome and proteome content of cancer-related EVs, much less is known about their metabolome component [20]. Similarly, the data regarding radiation-induced changes in the EVs' cargo refer mainly to its transcriptome and proteome [26,27]. Hence, through searching for cancer-related and RT-induced changes in the serum metabolome of HNC patients, we aimed to address the metabolite profiles of serum-derived EVs.

2. Materials and Methods

2.1. Samples Collection

Ten patients with squamous cell carcinoma located in pharynx regions (6 males and 4 females, aged between 49 and 71 years) treated by the continuous accelerated irradiation (CAIR) scheme with a daily fraction dose of 1.8 Gy to the total dose of 64–72 Gy were included in the study. Blood samples were collected before RT (cancer pre-treatment sample A) and one month after the end of RT (cancer post-treatment sample B). The control group constituted of ten age- and sex-matched healthy volunteers (control sample C). This study was approved by the appropriate local Ethics Committee (NRIO; approval no. 1/2016) and all participants provided informed consent indicating their conscious and voluntary participation. 5 milliliters of blood was collected into an anticoagulant-free tube (Becton Dickinson, Franklin Lakes, NJ, USA; 367955), incubated for 30 min at 20 °C then centrifuged at 1000× *g* for 10 min at 4 °C. The serum (supernatant) was transferred to clean tubes stored at −80 °C until analysis.

2.2. Exosomes Isolation and Characterization

The method for the isolation of exosomes from small amounts of serum was established and optimized in our laboratory as described previously [28]. Briefly, exosomes were isolated from serum (500 μL) by differential centrifugation (1000× *g* and 10,000× *g* for 10 and 30 min, respectively, at 4 °C) and filtration through a 0.22 μm filter followed by the size exclusion chromatography (SEC). SEC was performed using hand-packed columns (BioRad) filled with 10 mL of Sepharose CL-2B (GE Healthcare), conditioned previously with phosphate buffer saline (PBS). Consecutive fractions (500 μL each) were collected and characterized for EV enrichment (fraction #8 was used for further analyses). The size of vesicles in the SEC fractions was evaluated by the dynamic light scattering (DLS) using Zetasizer Nano-ZS90 instrument (Malvern Instruments, Malvern, UK) and by transmission electron microscopy. Exosome markers CD63 and CD81 were analyzed by Western blots as reported in detail elsewhere [28]. The concentration of proteins in the analyzed samples was assessed using the PierceTM BCA Protein Assay kit (Thermo Fisher Scientific, Waltham, MA, USA; 23225) according to the manufacturer's instructions.

2.3. Metabolite Extraction

Two-hundred microliters of 80% MeOH was added to 25 μL of serum sample. In the case of exosomes, 2 mL of 100% MeOH was added to 500 μL of the selected SEC fraction. The mixture was vortexed and centrifuged for 5 min followed by sonication for 10 min. The mixture was placed at −20 °C for 20 min and after that centrifuged for 10 min at 23,000× *g* at 4 °C. The supernatant was transferred to a new tube and evaporated in a SpeedVac concentrator (CentriVap Concentrator, Labconco, USA). The dried extract was then derivatized with 25 μL of methoxyamine hydrochloride in pyridine (20 mg/mL) at 37 °C for 90 min with agitation. The second step of derivatization was performed by adding 40 μL of MSTFA (*N*-Trimethylsilyl-*N*-methyl trifluoroacetamide) and incubation at 37 °C for 30 min with agitation. Samples were subjected to GC/MS analysis directly after derivatization.

2.4. GC–MS Analysis

The GS/MS analysis was performed using TRACE 1310 gas chromatograph connected with TSQ8000 triple-quad mass spectrometer (Thermo Scientific, Waltham, Massachusetts, USA). A DB-5MS bonded-phase fused-silica capillary column (30 m length, 0.25 mm inner diameter, 0.25 μm film thickness) (J&W Scientific Co., Folsom, California, USA) was used for separation. The GC oven temperature gradient was as follows: 70 °C for 2 min, followed by 10 °C/min up to 300 °C (10 min), 2 min at 70 °C, raised by 8 °C/min to 300 °C and held for 16 min at 300 °C. For sample injection, a PTV (Programmable Temperature Vaporization) injector was used in a range of 60–250 °C, transfer line temperature was set to 250 °C, and source to 250 °C. Spectra were recorded in m/z range of 50–850 in EI+ mode with an electron energy of 70 eV. Raw MS-data were converted to abf format and analyzed using MSDial software package v. 3.96. To eliminate the retention time (Rt) shift and to determine the retention indexes (RI) for each compound, the alkane series mixture (C-10 to C-36) was injected into the GC/MS system. Identified artifacts (alkanes, column bleed, plasticizers, MSTFA, and reagents) were excluded from further analyses. Obtained normalized (using total ion current (TIC) approach) results were then exported to Excel for pre-formatting and then used for statistical analyses.

2.5. Statistical and Chemometric Analyses

Differences between independent samples were assessed using the T-test, Welch test, or U-Mann–Whitney test, dependent on the normality and homoscedasticity of data (assessed via the

Shapiro–Wilk test and Levene test, respectively). For paired samples, the paired *t*-test or Wilcoxon test were used based on the normality of the difference distribution. In each case, the Benjamini–Hochberg protocol was used for the false discovery rate (FDR) correction. However, due to the small sample size, none of the differences remained significant after the FDR correction. Hence, the effect size analysis was employed to overcome this problem [29]. For independent samples, the rank-biserial coefficient of correlation (RBCC; an effect size equivalent of the U-Mann–Whitney test) was applied; the effect sizes ≥ 0.3 and ≥ 0.5 were considered medium and high, respectively [30]. For paired samples, the paired *t*-test derived Cohen's d effect size was applied; the effect sizes ≥ 0.5 and ≥ 0.8 were considered medium and high, respectively [31]. Principal component analysis (PCA) and hierarchical cluster analysis (HCA) based on the Euclidean distance method were performed to illustrate general similarities between samples. Metabolic pathways were associated with differentiating compounds that showed high and medium effect sizes using the quantitative enrichment analysis on the MetaboAnalyst platform (https://www.metaboanalyst.ca/MetaboAnalyst/ModuleView.xhtml). Obtained enriched pathways and their connections together with statistical information were further analyzed in Cytoscape. The DyNet addon was used to compare two networks and find interacting nodes [32]; the fold enrichment and significance of enrichment (FDR) were coded by the size and color of nodes, respectively.

3. Results

Extracellular vesicles (EVs) isolated from serum by size exclusion chromatography were characterized by their size and the presence of specific biomarkers. The SEC fraction #8 was enriched in vesicles, in which size was estimated in a range between 50 and 150 nm by the DLS measurement (with the maximum at 100–120 nm) (Figure 1A). The size of the isolated vesicles was confirmed by transmission electron microscopy (TEM) (Figure 1B). Furthermore, the presence of exosome biomarkers, tetraspanins CD63, and CD81, was confirmed in the same fraction by Western blot analysis (the same proteins remained undetected in the whole serum) (Figure 1C). Considering their specific size and the presence of exosome-specific biomarkers, vesicles present in the analyzed fraction were called exosomes for simplicity, yet other subpopulations of the small EVs could be present in this fraction.

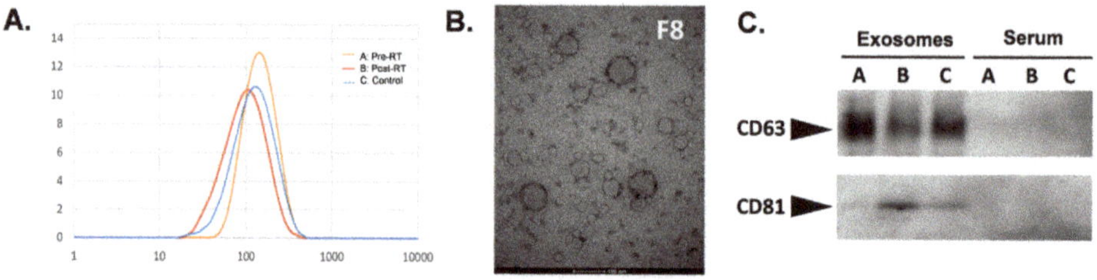

Figure 1. Characterization of serum-derived exosomes. Analysis of the size of vesicles in the size exclusion chromatography (SEC) fraction #8 by the dynamic light scattering (**A**) and transmission electron microscopy (**B**). (**C**) Western blot analysis of CD63 and CD81 in whole serum and serum-derived exosomes (fraction #8) for the three groups of samples (**A**: pre-radiotherapy (RT), **B**: post-RT, **C**: control).

The GC–MS-based approach was used to profile the metabolites in the whole serum and the corresponding serum-derived exosomes of HNC patients, in either pre-treatment (A) and post-treatment (B) samples, or samples of matched healthy controls (C). In general, the untargeted approach allowed to identify 182 metabolites in serum samples and 46 metabolites in exosome samples, of which 33 metabolites overlapped; the complete list of 195 identified compounds is presented in Supplementary Table S1. Figure 2 illustrates the distribution of different classes of small metabolites identified by GC–MS in serum and serum-derived exosome samples. Among the most abundant classes of metabolites common for serum and exosomes were fatty acids, sugar alcohols, and carboxylic acids (22%, 15%, and 12% of all identified compounds, respectively). It is noteworthy that amino acids that were the largest group of metabolites in serum samples that were markedly less frequent in exosome samples (21% vs. 7% of all identified compounds, respectively, which corresponded to 40 and 3 compounds). All identified metabolites were used to perform the unsupervised clustering of samples. The metabolite composition of the whole serum enabled the relatively good separation of all three groups of samples using either the principal component analysis (Figure 3A) or the hierarchical cluster analysis (Figure 4A). Interestingly, control samples C were more similar to cancer pre-treatment samples A than to cancer post-treatment samples B, which indicated the additional putative treatment-related differential component. In contrast, neither the PCA or the HCA type of analysis allowed the separation of corresponding groups when samples of serum-derived exosomes were analyzed (Figures 3B and 4B).

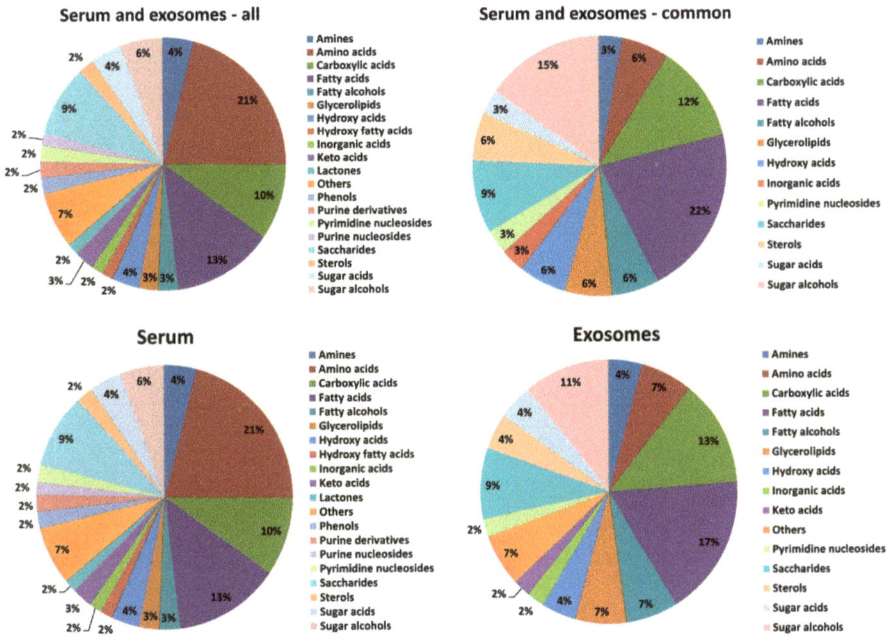

Figure 2. The relative contribution of different classes of metabolites present in serum and serum-derived exosomes (metabolites detected in all types of analyzed samples were considered).

In the next step, we detected specific metabolites for which abundances were significantly different between groups. First, we looked for compounds that differentiated cancer patients (pre-treatment samples A) from healthy individuals (control samples C). There were 27 compounds for which serum levels were markedly different (large effect size; RBCC effect size ≥ 0.5) between control and cancer samples. These included 12 upregulated metabolites (four amino acids, four fatty acids, two purines, one glycerolipid, and lactose) and 15 downregulated metabolites (three carboxylic acids, three purines, three sugars, two fatty acids, serotonin, acetyl-hexosamine, isoleucine, and phosphate) in cancer samples, listed in Table 1. Furthermore, there were 18 cancer-upregulated and 38 cancer-downregulated compounds where differences showed a medium effect size (RBCC effect size ≥ 0.3) (Supplementary Table S1). On the other hand, there were only a few compounds whose abundance was significantly different in serum-derived exosomes from healthy controls and cancer patients. 1-Hexadecanol was markedly upregulated while citric acid, 4-hydroxybenzoic acid, and propylene glycol were markedly downregulated (large effect size) in exosomes from cancer patients (Table 1). Moreover, there were seven metabolites where differences showed no medium effect size, including myo-inositol, linoleic acid, succinic acid, and glyceric acid downregulated in cancer samples (Supplementary Table S1). Metabolites for which levels were different between control and cancer samples (either a large effect size or medium effect size) were annotated with their corresponding metabolic pathways. Interestingly, the overrepresented pathways associated with metabolites discriminating cancer patients and healthy controls (i.e., cancer-specific pattern) in both whole serum and serum-derived exosome samples included ones involved in energy production (citric acid cycle, Warburg effect, pyruvate metabolism, mitochondrial electron transport chain) and inositol metabolism. Pathways associated specifically with serum metabolites included the metabolism of amino acids, sugars, and lipids. On the other hand, pathways associated with metabolites specific for serum-derived exosomes included the oxidation of fatty acids and ketone body metabolism (Figure 5A).

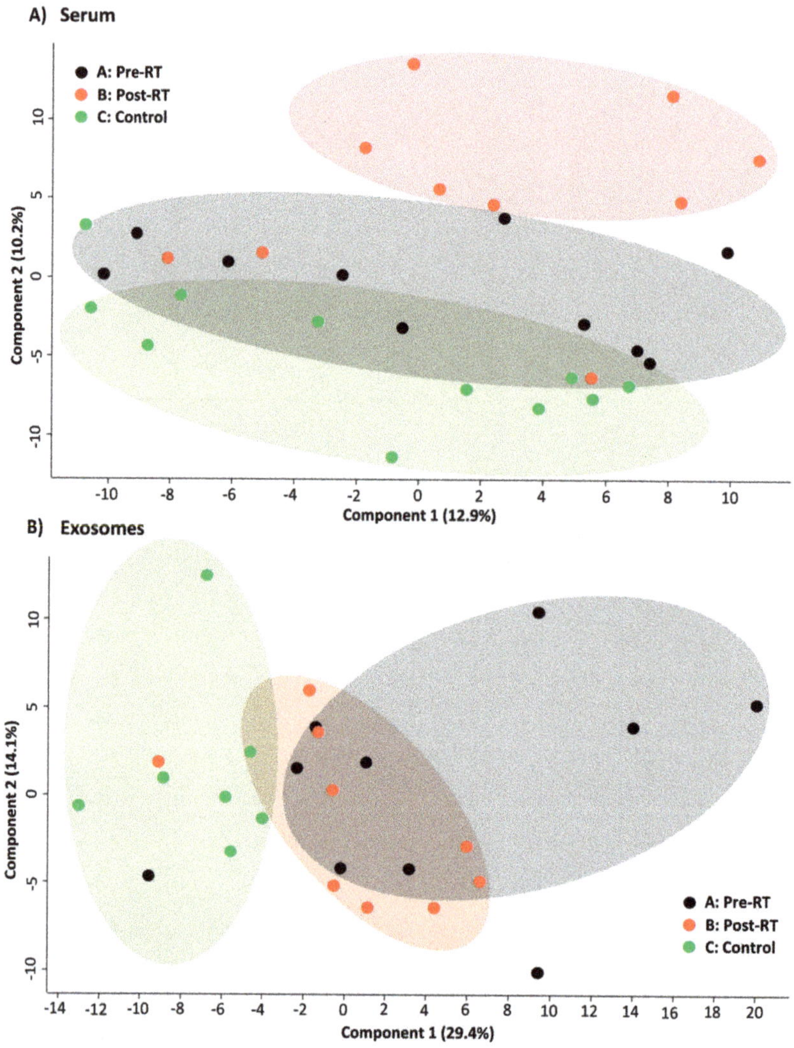

Figure 3. PCA score plots showing the clustering of cancer pre-RT samples A, cancer post-RT samples B, and control samples C. Shown are two the first components responsible for 23.1% of the variability of the serum samples (panel **A**) and 43.5% of the variability for the exosome samples (panel **B**).

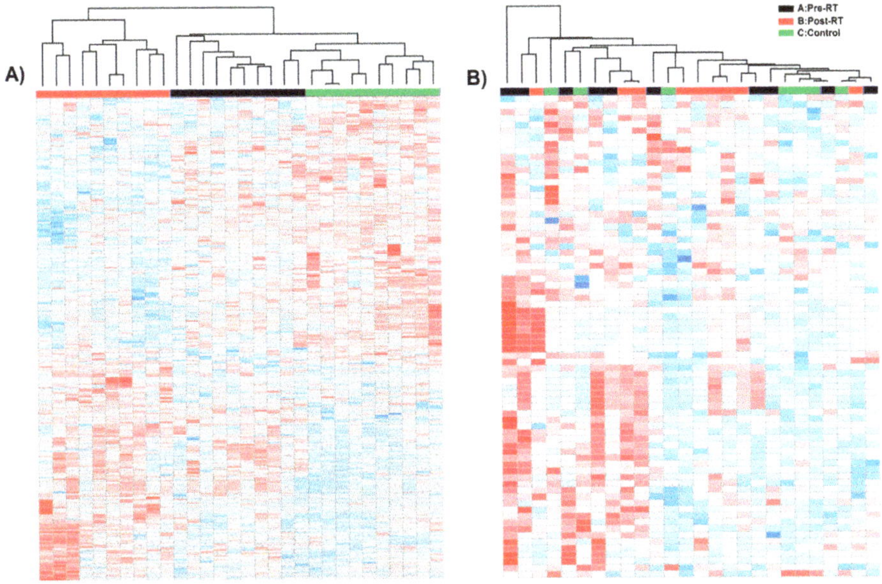

Figure 4. Hierarchical cluster analysis of cancer pre-RT samples A, cancer post-RT samples B, and control samples C. Shown are separate dendrograms for serum samples (panel **A**) and exosome samples (panel **B**).

Then, we looked for metabolites with an abundance that was different in serum and serum-derived exosomes of cancer patients between pre-RT samples A and post-RT samples B, to allow the detection of changes related to radiotherapy. There were 12 compounds with serum levels that were markedly different (large effect size; Cohen's d effect size ≥ 0.8) between pre-RT and post-RT cancer samples. These included four metabolites that were upregulated (including hypotaurine and serotonin) and eight metabolites that were downregulated in post-RT serum samples, listed in Table 2. Furthermore, there were 29 RT-upregulated and 12 RT-downregulated compounds where differences showed a medium effect size (Cohen's d effect size ≥ 0.5) (Supplementary Table S1). In marked contrast, only two metabolites detected in serum-derived exosomes (glycerol and cholesterol) showed reduced levels (medium effect size) in post-RT samples. Finally, metabolites with an abundance different in the pre-RT and post-RT samples (either large effect size or medium effect size) were annotated with their corresponding metabolic pathways. Over represented pathways associated with metabolites with serum level affected by RT included those involved in the metabolism of different classes of compounds (amino acids, sugars, nucleotides, lipids, and biogenic amines), which indicated multifaceted effects of radiation on the serum metabolome profile (Figure 5B).

Table 1. Metabolites that differentiated cancer patients and healthy individuals. Listed are compounds where differences between head and neck cancer (HNC) patients (samples A) and healthy controls (samples C) showed a large effect size (RBCC effect size ≥ 0.5).

Metabolite Name	Class	Mean Abundance in Cancer (Samples A)	Mean Abundance in Control (Samples C)	Significance of Differences between Control and Cancer (RBCC Effect Size)
		Serum Metabolites		
		Upregulated in Cancer		
Myristic acid	Fatty acids	3.90×10^{-3}	3.18×10^{-3}	0.82
Hypoxanthine	Purines	3.48×10^{-4}	1.46×10^{-4}	0.76
L-Glutamic acid	Amino acids	4.97×10^{-3}	2.34×10^{-3}	0.70
Xanthine	Purines	2.96×10^{-5}	2.01×10^{-5}	0.66
beta-Lactose	Saccharides	2.41×10^{-5}	9.82×10^{-6}	0.64
L-Serine	Amino acids	8.19×10^{-3}	6.07×10^{-3}	0.60
Oleic acid monoglyceride	Glycerolipids	2.41×10^{-5}	3.14×10^{-5}	0.60
O-Acetylserine	Amino acids	4.37×10^{-3}	3.60×10^{-3}	0.58
Eicosenoic acid	Fatty acids	3.61×10^{-5}	2.18×10^{-5}	0.58
Palmitoleic acid	Fatty acids	1.02×10^{-3}	3.12×10^{-4}	0.56
Oleamide	Fatty acids	6.71×10^{-5}	1.72×10^{-5}	0.54
L-Aspartic acid	Amino acids	2.02×10^{-3}	1.32×10^{-3}	0.52
		Downregulated in Cancer		
Inosine	Purines	4.55×10^{-5}	4.28×10^{-4}	−1.00
Salicylic acid	Carboxylic acids	6.74×10^{-6}	8.44×10^{-4}	−0.92
Adenosine	Purines	1.27×10^{-5}	5.74×10^{-5}	−0.89
2-Ethylhexanoic acid	Fatty acids	1.14×10^{-4}	2.51×10^{-4}	−0.74
Gentisic acid	Carboxylic acids	6.36×10^{-6}	1.56×10^{-5}	−0.64
D-Threitol	Sugar alcohols	2.01×10^{-4}	2.88×10^{-4}	−0.64
Oxalic acid	Carboxylic acids	2.08×10^{-2}	2.47×10^{-2}	−0.62
Paraxanthine	Purines	1.94×10^{-4}	4.26×10^{-4}	−0.62
Serotonin	Amines	5.43×10^{-5}	1.06×10^{-4}	−0.60
D-Ribose	Saccharides	1.50×10^{-4}	1.51×10^{-4}	−0.60
N-acetyl-d-hexosamine	Amines	6.21×10^{-5}	1.69×10^{-5}	−0.57
Nonanoic acid	Fatty acids	2.23×10^{-4}	2.67×10^{-4}	−0.56
D-Xylonic acid	Sugar acids	3.07×10^{-5}	4.48×10^{-5}	−0.56
Phosphate	Inorganic acids	1.40×10^{-2}	1.64×10^{-2}	−0.54
L-Isoleucine	Amino acids	2.69×10^{-3}	3.30×10^{-3}	−0.52
		Exosome Metabolites		
		Upregulated in Cancer		
1-Hexadecanol	Fatty alcohols	5.81×10^{-5}	3.12×10^{-5}	0.52
		Downregulated in Cancer		
4-Hydroxybenzoic acid	Carboxylic acids	8.05×10^{-7}	2.61×10^{-5}	−0.66
Citric acid	Carboxylic acids	8.58×10^{-6}	3.22×10^{-4}	−0.54
Propylene glycol	Others	2.89×10^{-5}	1.96×10^{-4}	−0.52

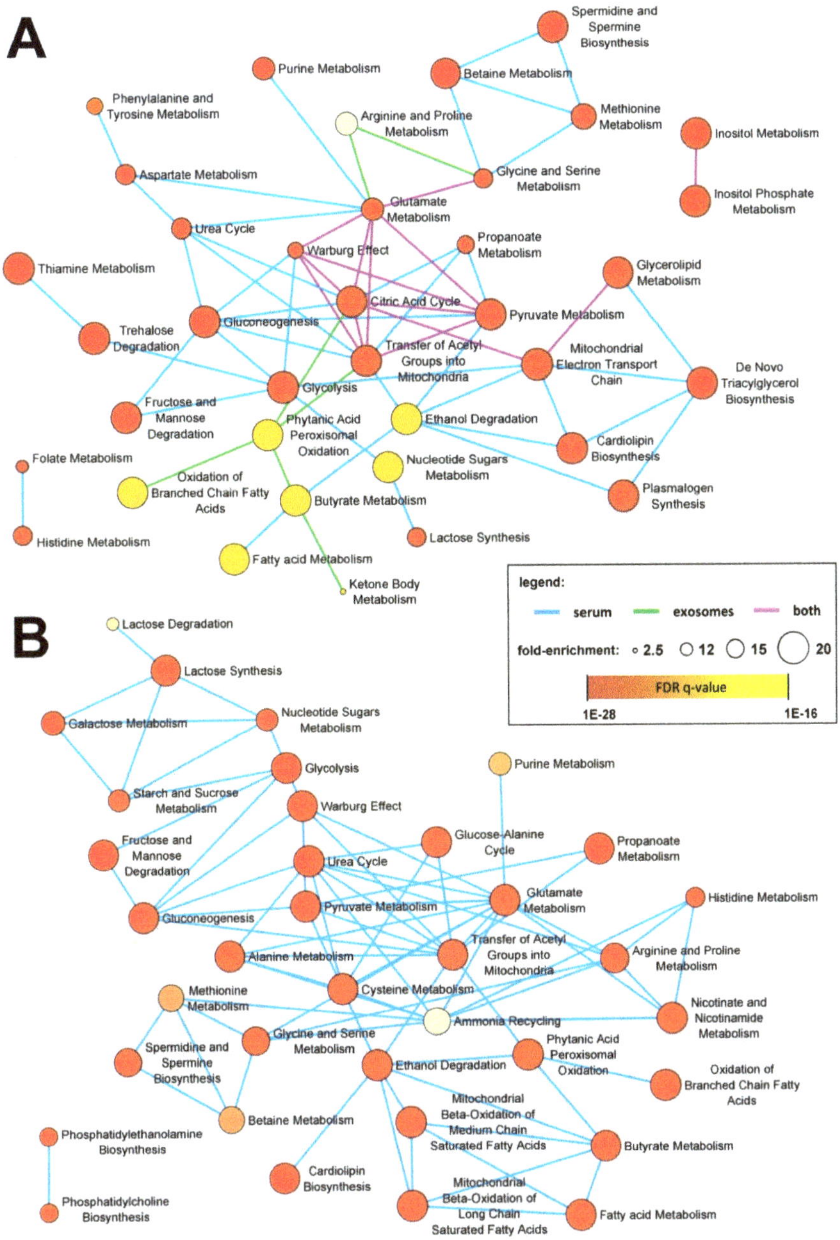

Figure 5. Metabolic pathways associated with specific subsets of compounds detected in the whole serum and serum-derived exosomes. Illustrated are over represented pathways associated with metabolites differentiating between cancer and control samples (panel **A**) and between pre-RT and post-RT samples (panel **B**); metabolites that showed large and medium effect size were included. The size of the network nodes corresponds to the pathway's fold-enrichment while the statistical significance of the over-representation is color coded.

Table 2. Metabolites that were affected by radiotherapy. Listed are compounds where differences between paired pre-RT (samples A) and post-RT (samples C) specimens showed a large effect size (Cohen's d effect size ≥ 0.8).

Metabolite Name	Class	Mean Abundance Pre-RT (Samples A)	Mean Abundance Post-RT (Samples B)	Significance of Differences between Pre-RT and Post-RT (Cohen's D Effect Size)
		Serum Metabolites		
		Upregulated by RT		
Hypotaurine	Others	6.48×10^{-5}	1.09×10^{-4}	−1.16
Glycerol-1-phosphate	Glycerolipids	1.03×10^{-4}	1.46×10^{-4}	−1.06
Oleamide	Fatty acids	6.71×10^{-5}	1.77×10^{-4}	−0.81
Serotonin	Amines	5.43×10^{-5}	6.71×10^{-5}	−0.81
		Downregulated by RT		
1-Methylhistidine	Amino acids	1.13×10^{-4}	7.84×10^{-5}	0.96
Urea	Others	1.81×10^{-4}	4.76×10^{-2}	0.96
Quinic acid	Others	7.48×10^{-5}	5.60×10^{-5}	0.87
2-ketoglucose dimethylacetal	Hydroxy acids	1.68×10^{-4}	7.86×10^{-5}	0.85
4-Deoxyerythronic acid	Sugar acids	4.44×10^{-5}	2.77×10^{-5}	0.85
Galactosylglycerol	Glycerolipids	4.55×10^{-5}	1.69×10^{-5}	0.85
Gentisic acid	Carboxylic acids	6.36×10^{-6}	3.78×10^{-6}	0.85
D-Xylitol	Sugar alcohols	2.29×10^{-4}	1.49×10^{-4}	0.82

4. Discussion

Serum-derived exosomes, an emerging type of liquid biopsy, are a potential source of biomarkers. However, their metabolite compartment is less characterized compared to proteome or miRNome [20]. Here, we compared the metabolite profiles of whole human serum and serum-derived exosomes, and found significantly fewer compounds in the latter specimen. This difference could be caused by both a lower number of compounds present in vesicles per se (i.e., putatively lower molecular complexity) or their lower concentration, which hindered their detection by the method used in our approach. Hence, a direct comparison of metabolic pathways associated with compounds present in the whole serum and serum-derived vesicles could be compromised by this discrepancy. However, it has to be emphasized that the major metabolic hallmark of cancer—the modified energy metabolism could be detected in both specimens. In head and neck cancer, as in many other types of cancers, tumor cells can alter their energy metabolism by switching from the citric acid cycle (TCA cycle) to the aerobic glycolysis and oxidation of fatty acids as a backup mechanism for energy production [16], a phenomenon which is known as the Warburg effect [33]. Our study confirmed that metabolites associated with processes involved in energy metabolism, including glycolysis, gluconeogenesis, Warburg effect, TCA cycle, pyruvate metabolism, and mitochondrial electron transport chain showed different levels in samples of HNC patients and healthy controls. Importantly, features associated with this characteristic cancer phenotype were observed in both whole serum and serum-derived exosomes. Noteworthy, however, different types of cells and tissues, both cancerous and normal, release exosomes circulating in the blood and regulate the metabolome of the whole serum. Nevertheless, pathways associated with metabolites specific for serum-derived exosomes of cancer patients included oxidation of fatty acids and ketone body metabolism. The beta-oxidation of fatty acids and increased lipolysis, which is reflected as the accumulation of ketone bodies, was reported in HNC patients as a potential backup mechanism for energy production [12]. Previous studies reported that molecules involved in fatty acids transport and storage as well as lipolysis and fatty acids oxidation are enriched in EVs and suggested that fatty acid transport from cell to cell and across cell membranes could be mediated by EVs [34,35]. Hence, a specific role of serum EVs in the transmission of mediators associated with cancer-related lipid metabolism deserves further attention.

Our study revealed that RT affected the serum levels of several amino acids, biogenic amines, sugars, nucleotides, lipids, and fatty acids, which mirrored potential RT-induced changes in a plethora of metabolic pathways ongoing in a patients' body. It is noteworthy that different radiation-related mechanisms might contribute to metabolic changes observed in samples collected one month after the end of RT, including toxicity induced by radiation in normal tissues and a reduced number of cancer cells. It was previously reported that the altered metabolism of amino acid plays an important role in the response of HNC patients to RT [36]. For example, Boguszewicz and co-workers [4] demonstrated that a decreased serum level of alanine, the main substrate for gluconeogenesis during fasting and cachexia, correlated with the acute radiation toxicity-associated weight loss in HNC patients undergoing RT. The whole-body response to irradiation frequently involves molecules associated with oxidative stress and inflammation [18]. Hence, it is noteworthy that hypotaurine, which is involved in protection against oxidative stress as an effect of RT [37], was significantly elevated in post-RT serum samples. Moreover, RT-induced changes in the serum level of phospholipids potentially associated with the inflammatory response and disruption of plasma membranes were previously reported in samples of HNC patients [38,39]. Here, we found that compounds associated with lipid metabolism (e.g., phosphatidylethanolamine and phosphatidylcholine biosynthesis) were affected in post-RT serum samples, which confirmed the general RT-related metabolic phenotype. Interestingly, very few RT-related changes were detected in the metabolic profile of serum-derived exosomes. This was in contrast to the significant radiation-induced changes observed at the level of the proteome [40] and miRNome [41] of exosomes released by HNC cells. Exosomes released by irradiated cells are known mediators of radiation bystander effect and other aspects of radiation-related cell-to-cell signaling [42]. Hence, the potential role of metabolites in exosomes-mediated radiation-related signaling should be addressed in further studies.

5. Conclusions

In this pilot study, we compared the metabolite profiles of the whole serum and serum-derived exosomes in healthy controls and patients treated with RT due to a head and neck cancer aiming to reveal cancer-related features (by the comparison of cancer and control samples) and RT-related features (by the comparison of cancer pre-RT and post-RT samples). We found that the metabolite profile of serum-derived exosomes is putatively less complex and consists of fewer components than that of the complete serum. However, cancer-related features of energy metabolism were detected in both types of specimens, which confirmed the feasibility of cancer biomarkers based on exosome metabolites. On the other hand, in contrast to RT-induced changes observed in serum metabolome, this pilot study did not reveal a specific pattern of radiotherapy-related changes in exosome metabolites. Hence, further metabolomics study with a larger cohort of individuals treated with RT is necessary to validate a hypothetical radiation signature of serum exosomes.

Supplementary Materials: The following are available online at http://www.mdpi.com/2075-4426/10/4/229/s1, Table S1: Metabolites identified in human serum and serum-derived exosomes.

Author Contributions: Conceptualization, M.P.; methodology, L.M.; formal analysis, L.M.; investigation, A.Z. and A.S.; resources, T.R.; data curation, A.W., L.M. and K.P.; writing—original draft preparation, A.W., A.Z.; writing—review and editing, P.W.; visualization, A.W. and L.M.; supervision, M.P. All authors have read and agreed to the published version of the manuscript.

Funding: This research was funded by the National Science Centre, Poland, grant no. 2015/17/B/NZ5/01387 (M.P., T.R., P.W.), 2016/22/M/NZ5/00667 (A.Z., A.S., M.P.), and 2017/26/D/NZ2/00964 (A.W., L.M.).

Conflicts of Interest: The authors declare no conflict of interest.

References

1. Gupta, B.; Johnson, N.W.; Kumar, N. Global epidemiology of head and neck cancers: A Continuing Challenge. *Oncology* **2016**, *91*, 13–23. [CrossRef]
2. Budach, V.; Tinhofer, I. Novel prognostic clinical factors and biomarkers for outcome prediction in head and neck cancer: A systematic review. *Lancet Oncol.* **2019**, *20*, e313–e326. [CrossRef]
3. Economopoulou, P.; de Bree, R.; Kotsantis, I.; Psyrri, A. Diagnostic tumor markers in head and neck squamous cell carcinoma (HNSCC) in the clinical setting. *Front. Oncol.* **2019**, *9*, 827. [CrossRef]
4. Boguszewicz, Ł.; Bieleń, A.; Mrochem-Kwarciak, J.; Skorupa, A.; Ciszek, M.; Heyda, A.; Wygoda, A.; Kotylak, A.; Składowski, K.; Sokół, M. NMR-based metabolomics in real-time monitoring of treatment induced toxicity and cachexia in head and neck cancer: A method for early detection of high risk patients. *Metabolomics* **2019**, *15*, 110. [CrossRef]
5. Baskar, R.; Lee, K.A.; Yeo, R.; Yeoh, K.W. Cancer and radiation therapy: Current advances and future directions. *Int. J. Med. Sci.* **2012**, *9*, 193–199. [CrossRef]
6. Darby, S.C.; Cutter, D.J.; Boerma, M.; Constine, L.S.; Fajardo, L.F.; Kodama, K.; Mabuchi, K.; Marks, L.B.; Mettler, F.A.; Pierce, L.J.; et al. Radiation-related heart disease: Current knowledge and future prospects. *Int. J. Radiat. Oncol. Biol. Phys.* **2010**, *76*, 656–665. [CrossRef]
7. Travis, L.B.; Ng, A.K.; Allan, J.M.; Pui, C.H.; Kennedy, A.R.; Xu, X.G.; Purdy, J.A.; Applegate, K.; Yahalom, J.; Constine, L.S.; et al. Second malignant neoplasms and cardiovascular disease following radiotherapy. *Health Phys.* **2014**, *106*, 229–246. [CrossRef]
8. Pinu, F.R.; Beale, D.J.; Paten, A.M.; Kouremenos, K.; Swarup, S.; Schirra, H.J.; Wishart, D. Systems biology and multi-omics integration: Viewpoints from the Metabolomics Research Community. *Metabolites* **2019**, *9*, 76. [CrossRef]
9. Wheelock, C.E.; Goss, V.M.; Balgoma, D.; Nicholas, B.; Brandsma, J.; Skipp, P.J.; Snowden, S.; Burg, D.; D'Amico, A.; Horvath, I.; et al. Application of 'omics technologies to biomarker discovery in inflammatory lung diseases. *Eur. Respir. J.* **2013**, *42*, 802–825. [CrossRef]
10. Patel, S.; Ahmed, S. Emerging field of metabolomics: Big promise for cancer biomarker identification and drug discovery. *J. Pharm. Biomed. Anal.* **2015**, *107*, 63–74. [CrossRef]
11. Armitage, E.G.; Barbas, C. Metabolomics in cancer biomarker discovery: Current trends and future perspectives. *J. Pharm. Biomed. Anal.* **2014**, *87*, 1–11. [CrossRef] [PubMed]
12. Tiziani, S.; Lopes, V.; Günther, U.L. Early stage diagnosis of oral cancer using 1H NMR-Based metabolomics1,2. *Neoplasia* **2009**, *11*, 269–276. [CrossRef] [PubMed]
13. Yonezawa, K.; Nishiumii, S.; Kitamoto-Matsuda, J.; Fujita, T.; Morimoto, K.; Yamashita, D.; Saito, M.; Otsuki, N.; Irino, Y.; Shinohara, M.; et al. Serum and tissue metabolomics of head and neck cancer. *Cancer Genom. Proteom.* **2013**, *10*, 233–238.
14. Hsieh, Y.T.; Chen, Y.F.; Lin, S.C.; Chang, K.W.; Li, W.C. Targeting cellular metabolism modulates head and neck oncogenesis. *Int. J. Mol. Sci.* **2019**, *20*, 3960. [CrossRef]
15. Kasiappan, R.; Kamarajan, P.; Kapila, Y.L. Metabolomics in head and neck cancer: A summary of findings. *Transl. Syst. Med. Oral. Dis.* **2019**, 119–135.
16. Shin, J.M.; Kamarajan, P.; Christopher Fenno, J.; Rickard, A.H.; Kapila, Y.L. Metabolomics of head and neck cancer: A mini-review. *Front. Physiol.* **2016**, *7*, 526. [CrossRef]
17. Rai, V.; Mukherjee, R.; Ghosh, A.K.; Routray, A.; Chakraborty, C. "Omics" in oral cancer: New approaches for biomarker discovery. *Arch. Oral Biol.* **2018**, *87*, 15–34. [CrossRef]
18. Jelonek, K.; Pietrowska, M.; Widlak, P. Systemic effects of ionizing radiation at the proteome and metabolome levels in the blood of cancer patients treated with radiotherapy: The influence of inflammation and radiation toxicity. *Int. J. Radiat. Biol.* **2017**, *93*, 683–696. [CrossRef]
19. Doyle, L.; Wang, M. Overview of extracellular vesicles, their origin, composition, purpose, and methods for exosome isolation and analysis. *Cells* **2019**, *8*, 727. [CrossRef]
20. Zebrowska, A.; Skowronek, A.; Wojakowska, A.; Widlak, P.; Pietrowska, M. Metabolome of exosomes: Focus on vesicles released by cancer cells and present in human body fluids. *Int. J. Mol. Sci.* **2019**, *20*, 3461. [CrossRef]

21. Tian, W.; Liu, S.; Li, B. Potential role of exosomes in cancer metastasis. *Biomed. Res. Int.* **2019**, *2019*, 4649705. [CrossRef] [PubMed]
22. Pang, B.; Zhu, Y.; Ni, J.; Thompson, J.; Malouf, D.; Bucci, J.; Graham, P.; Li, Y. Extracellular vesicles: The next generation of biomarkers for liquid biopsy-based prostate cancer diagnosis. *Theranostics* **2020**, *10*, 2309–2326. [CrossRef] [PubMed]
23. Marrugo-Ramírez, J.; Mir, M.; Samitier, J. Blood-based cancer biomarkers in liquid biopsy: A promising non-invasive alternative to tissue biopsy. *Int. J. Mol. Sci.* **2018**, *19*, 2877. [CrossRef] [PubMed]
24. Jelonek, K.; Widlak, P.; Pietrowska, M. The influence of ionizing radiation on exosome composition, secretion and intercellular communication. *Protein Pept. Lett.* **2016**, *23*, 656–663. [CrossRef]
25. Jabbari, N.; Nawaz, M.; Rezaie, J. Ionizing radiation increases the activity of exosomal secretory pathway in MCF-7 human breast cancer cells: A possible way to communicate resistance against radiotherapy. *Int. J. Mol. Sci.* **2019**, *20*, 3649. [CrossRef]
26. Zorrilla, S.R.; García, A.G.; Carrión, A.B.; Vila, P.G.; Martín, M.S.; Torreira, M.G.; Sayans, M.P. Exosomes in head and neck cancer. Updating and revisiting. *J. Enzyme Inhib. Med. Chem.* **2019**, *34*, 1641–1651. [CrossRef]
27. Xiao, C.; Song, F.; Zheng, Y.L.; Lv, J.; Wang, Q.F.; Xu, N. Exosomes in head and neck squamous cell carcinoma. *Front. Oncol.* **2019**, *9*, 894. [CrossRef]
28. Smolarz, M.; Pietrowska, M.; Matysiak, N.; Mielańczyk, Ł.; Widłak, P. Proteome profiling of exosomes purified from a small amount of human serum: The problem of co-purified serum components. *Proteomes* **2019**, *7*, 18. [CrossRef]
29. Sullivan, G.M.; Feinn, R. Using effect size—Or why the p value is not enough. *J. Grad. Med. Educ.* **2012**, *4*, 279–282. [CrossRef]
30. Cureton, E.E. Rank-biserial correlation. *Psychometrika* **1956**, *21*, 287–290. [CrossRef]
31. Rosenthal, R. Parametric measures of effect size. In *The Handbook of Research Synthesis*; Cooper, H., Hedges, L.V., Valentine, J.C., Eds.; Russell Sage Foundation: New York, NY, USA, 1994; pp. 231–244, References-Scientific Research Publishing; Available online: https://www.scirp.org/(S(351jmbntvnsjt1aadkposzje))/reference/ReferencesPapers.aspx?ReferenceID=1985786 (accessed on 13 July 2020).
32. Goenawan, I.H.; Bryan, K.; Lynn, D.J. DyNet: Visualization and analysis of dynamic molecular interaction networks. *Bioinformatics* **2016**, *32*, 2713–2715. [CrossRef] [PubMed]
33. Warburg, O. On the origin of cancer cells. *Science* **1956**, *123*, 309–314. [CrossRef] [PubMed]
34. Lazar, I.; Clement, E.; Attane, C.; Muller, C.; Nieto, L. Thematic review series: Exosomes and microvesicles: Lipids as key components of their biogenesis and functions: A new role for extracellular vesicles: How small vesicles can feed tumors' big appetite. *J. Lipid Res.* **2018**, *59*, 1793–1804. [CrossRef] [PubMed]
35. Record, M.; Carayon, K.; Poirot, M.; Silvente-Poirot, S. Exosomes as new vesicular lipid transporters involved in cell–cell communication and various pathophysiologies. *Biochim. Biophys. Acta Mol. Cell Biol. Lipids.* **2014**, *1841*, 108–120. [CrossRef]
36. Kim, E.J.; Lee, M.; Kim, D.Y.; Kim, K., II; Yi, J.Y. Mechanisms of energy metabolism in skeletal muscle mitochondria following radiation exposure. *Cells* **2019**, *8*, 950. [CrossRef]
37. Gossai, D.; Lau-Cam, C.A. The effects of taurine, taurine homologs and hypotaurine on cell and membrane antioxidative system alterations caused by type 2 diabetes in rat erythrocytes. *Adv. Exp. Med. Biol.* **2009**, *643*, 359–368.
38. Jelonek, K.; Pietrowska, M.; Ros, M.; Zagdanski, A.; Suchwalko, A.; Polanska, J.; Marczyk, M.; Rutkowski, T.; Skladowski, K.; Clench, M.R.; et al. Radiation-induced changes in serum lipidome of head and neck cancer patients. *Int. J. Mol. Sci.* **2014**, *15*, 6609–6624. [CrossRef]
39. Jelonek, K.; Krzywon, A.; Jablonska, P.; Slominska, E.M.; Smolenski, R.T.; Polanska, J.; Rutkowski, T.; Mrochem-Kwarciak, J.; Skladowski, K.; Widlak, P. Systemic effects of radiotherapy and concurrent chemo-radiotherapy in head and neck cancer patients—Comparison of serum metabolome profiles. *Metabolites* **2020**, *10*, 60. [CrossRef]
40. Abramowicz, A.; Wojakowska, A.; Marczak, L.; Lysek-Gladysinska, M.; Smolarz, M.; Story, M.D.; Polanska, J.; Widlak, P.; Pietrowska, M. Ionizing radiation affects the composition of the proteome of extracellular vesicles released by head-and-neck cancer cells in vitro. *J. Radiat. Res.* **2019**, *60*, 289–297. [CrossRef]

41. Abramowicz, A.; Łabaj, W.; Mika, J.; Szołtysek, K.; Ślęzak-Prochazka, I.; Mielańczyk, Ł.; Story, M.D.; Pietrowska, M.; Polański, A.; Widłak, P. MicroRNA profile of exosomes and parental cells is differently affected by ionizing radiation. *Radiat. Res.* **2020**, *194*, 133–142. [CrossRef]
42. Kumar Jella, K.; Rani, S.; O'Driscoll, L.; McClean, B.; Byrne, H.J.; Lyng, F.M. Exosomes are involved in mediating radiation induced bystander signaling in human keratinocyte cells. *Radiat. Res.* **2014**, *181*, 138–145. [CrossRef] [PubMed]

Journal of
Personalized
Medicine

MDPI

Communication

Induction of Micronuclei in Cervical Cancer Treated with Radiotherapy

Daijiro Kobayashi [1], Takahiro Oike [2,*], Kazutoshi Murata [3], Daisuke Irie [2], Yuka Hirota [2], Hiro Sato [2], Atsushi Shibata [4] and Tatsuya Ohno [2,5]

1 Department of Radiation Oncology, Gunma Prefectural Cancer Center, Gunma 373-8550, Japan; m07201029@gmail.com
2 Department of Radiation Oncology, Gunma University Graduate School of Medicine, Gunma 371-8511, Japan; daisuke_i@gunma-u.ac.jp (D.I.); yukahirota@gunma-u.ac.jp (Y.H.); hiro.sato@gunma-u.ac.jp (H.S.); tohno@gunma-u.ac.jp (T.O.)
3 QST Hospital, National Institute for Quantum and Radiological Science and Technology, Chiba 263-8555, Japan; murata.kazutoshi@qst.go.jp
4 Gunma University Initiative for Advanced Research (GIAR), Gunma University, Gunma 371-8511, Japan; shibata.at@gunma-u.ac.jp
5 Gunma University Heavy Ion Medical Center, Gunma 371-8511, Japan
* Correspondence: oiketakahiro@gunma-u.ac.jp; Tel.: +81-27-220-8383; Fax: +81-27-220-8397

Received: 11 August 2020; Accepted: 1 September 2020; Published: 3 September 2020

check for updates

Abstract: Micronuclei (MN) trigger antitumor immune responses via the cyclic GMP-AMP synthase-signaling effector stimulator of interferon genes (cGAS-STING) pathway. Radiotherapy induces MN in peripheral blood lymphocytes. However, data for solid tumors are lacking. Here, we analyzed MN post-radiotherapy in solid tumor samples. Tumor biopsy specimens were obtained from seven prospectively recruited patients with cervical cancer, before treatment and after receiving radiotherapy at a dose of 10 Gy (in five fractions). The samples were stained with 4′,6-diamidino-2-phenylindole dihydrochloride, and 200 nuclei per sample were randomly identified and assessed for the presence of MN or apoptosis, based on nuclear morphology. The median number of MN-harboring nuclei was significantly greater in samples from patients treated with radiotherapy than in pre-treatment samples (151 (range, 16–327) versus 28 (range, 0–61); $p = 0.015$). No significant differences in the number of apoptotic nuclei were observed between pre-treatment and 10 Gy samples (5 (range, 0–30) versus 12 (range, 2–30); $p = 0.30$). This is the first report to demonstrate MN induction by radiotherapy in solid tumors. The results provide clinical evidence of the activation of antitumor immune responses by radiotherapy.

Keywords: micronuclei; uterine cervical cancer; radiotherapy; cGAS; STING; abscopal effect; immunotherapy

---

1. Introduction

Immunotherapy is rapidly becoming a promising strategy for cancer treatment. Recent reports on the combination use of immunotherapy with radiotherapy (RT) are overwhelming [1,2]. However, this kind of treatment strategy is hampered by the fact that its efficacy is unpredictable [1]. The cost for cancer immunotherapy is unsustainably high [1], therefore, a stratification of the patients who benefit from the combination treatment is needed. To this end, at the present, identification of reliable biomarkers of response to cancer immunotherapy combined with radiotherapy represents one of the mainstream immune-oncology research lines [1].

Micronuclei (MN) are induced following aberrant mitotic events in response to ionizing radiation, and are identified as one or a few smaller nuclei independent from the main nucleus [3,4].

After irradiation, cyclic GMP-AMP (cGAMP) synthase (cGAS) localizes to MN and binds to double-stranded DNAs (dsDNAs) that activate the stimulator of interferon genes (STING), an endoplasmic reticulum adaptor protein [5,6]. This induces GAMP-driven proinflammatory response [7,8], leading to type-1 interferon secretion [9]. As such, MN formation is directly related to the activation of cGAS-STING pathway that is the key axis of antitumor immune responses following radiation [7,8,10,11].

Taken together, RT-induced intratumoral MN may be used as a biomarker of the response to cancer immunotherapy combined with radiotherapy. Induction of MN by RT has been demonstrated in peripheral blood lymphocytes obtained from individuals treated with RT [12–15]. However, the induction of MN by RT in solid tumors has not been reported. This study aimed to obtain proof of principle for the induction of MN by RT in solid tumors. To this end, we evaluated tumor specimens obtained at pre-treatment and intra-RT time points from the same patients with cervical cancer.

2. Materials and Methods

2.1. Patients

Patients with cervical cancer were prospectively enrolled in the study if they met the following criteria: (a) pathologically-confirmed newly diagnosed cervical cancer; (b) treated with definitive RT at Gunma University Hospital between November 2017 and November 2018; (c) staged as IB1–IVA according to the 2009 International Federation of Gynecology and Obstetrics staging system; and (d) no previous exposure to radiotherapy or cytotoxic agents.

This study was approved by the Ethical Review Board Committee of Gunma University Hospital (approval number, 1109). Written consent was obtained from all participants.

2.2. Treatment

Patients were treated with concurrent chemoradiotherapy using standardized protocols [16]. Briefly, RT consisted of EBRT using 10 MV X-rays and computed tomography-based high dose-rate image-guided brachytherapy (IGBT). For EBRT, whole pelvic irradiation was delivered at a dose of 50 Gy in 25 fractions, and a central shielding technique was used for the latter 10–30 Gy. IGBT was performed with a ^{192}Ir Remote-After-Loading System (microSelectron, Elekta, Stockholm, Sweden), using tandem and ovoid applicators. A total of 24 Gy was delivered in four fractions, one fraction per week. Cisplatin (40 mg/m^2) was administered weekly during the RT treatment period, with the first course administered on day 1. Patients $\geq$ 75 years old did not receive chemotherapy.

2.3. Sample Collection and Nuclear Morphology Assessment

Specimens were obtained by punch biopsy from the center of tumors of the uterine cervix before the initiation of RT and after RT at 10 Gy. The nuclei contained in the tumor specimens were stained with DAPI (Sigma-Aldrich, St. Louis, MO, USA), as described previously [17]. Briefly, the biopsy specimens were kept in ice-cold phosphate buffered saline (PBS) and transported immediately from the hospital to the laboratory. Within 10 min from the biopsy, the tumor was minced using a surgical knife and incubated in a solution containing 0.25% trypsin (Thermo Scientific, Waltham, MA, USA) and 1 mM ethylenediaminetetraacetic acid (Sigma-Aldrich) at 37 °C for 5 min. The samples were then passed through a 70-micron nylon mesh cell strainer (Falcon, New York, NY, USA) in 5 mL PBS. Strained cells were collected by centrifugation at 1500× *g* rpm for 5 min and suspended in 0.4 mL PBS. A Cytospin™ 4 Cytocentrifuge (Thermo Scientific) was used to spread 0.1 mL of the cell suspension in a monolayer on slide glasses. The cells were then fixed with 3% paraformaldehyde-2% sucrose solution for 10 min. Fixed cells were incubated with 0.7% Triton X-100 (Sigma-Aldrich) and stained with DAPI. Coverslips were mounted in Vectashield (Vector Laboratories, Burlingame, CA, USA).

Microscopic images were obtained under a fluorescence microscope (Eclipse Ni, Nikon, Tokyo, Japan), using the settings for conventional image capture with a 40× objective lens. In continuous fields, 200 nuclei were identified and the nuclear events (i.e., MN and apoptosis) for each nucleus were recorded. MN were determined by the presence of small fragments separate from the main nuclei (Figure 1b) [8]. Apoptosis was determined by the presence of apoptotic bodies, nuclear condensation, or nuclear fragmentation (Figure 1c) [18].

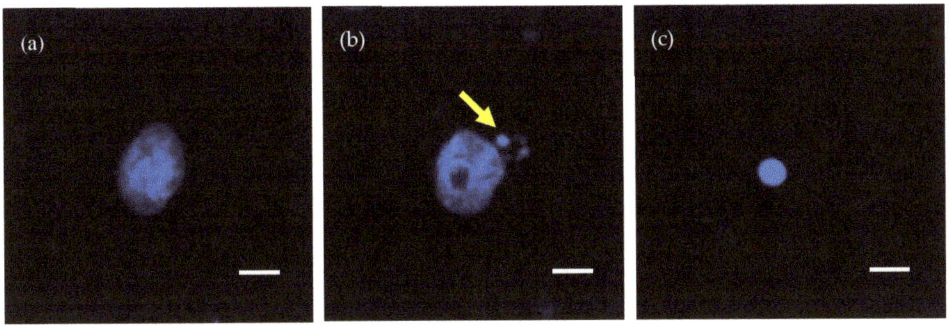

Figure 1. Representative images of nuclei stained with 4′,6-diamidino-2-phenylindole dihydrochloride. (**a**) Normal nucleus. (**b**) Nucleus harboring micronuclei (arrow). (**c**) Apoptosis. Scale bar = 10 µm.

2.4. Statistical Analysis

Differences in the prevalence of nuclear events between pre-RT and post-RT samples in the same patient were examined by paired non-parametric Wilcoxon test. Differences in the induction rate of nuclear events between the CCRT group and the RT group alone were examined by unpaired non-parametric Mann–Whitney test. Correlations of the interval between two biopsies with the induction rate of nuclear events were examined by Spearman's rank order test. Differences were considered statistically significant at $p < 0.05$. Statistical analysis was performed using Prism8 (GraphPad, San Diego, CA, USA).

3. Results

Seven patients were enrolled in this study (Table 1). The median age was 57 (42–82) years. Four patients received concurrent chemoradiotherapy (CCRT) with weekly cisplatin (40 mg/m^2), and the remaining three patients received RT alone because of older age (i.e., ≥ 75 years). The median total dose of external beam radiotherapy (EBRT) was 55.6 (50.0–58.0) Gy. We confirmed that more than 95% of the planned doses were appropriately delivered to tumors (Figure 2).

Tumor biopsy was performed before the initiation of RT and after exposure to 10 Gy in the same patients. The median interval between first biopsy and second biopsy was 7 days (range, 4–10 days). Two patients with a 4-day interval underwent biopsies on Monday and Friday of the same week. The patient with a 10-day interval underwent biopsy before and after the year-end holiday. The other four patients underwent biopsies on Monday of the first week and Monday or Tuesday of the following week (i.e., 7- and 8-day intervals, respectively).

MN and apoptosis in each sample were determined by morphological assessment of nuclei stained with 4′,6-diamidino-2-phenylindole, dihydrochloride (DAPI) (see Section 2.3 for detailed methods). Representative images of MN and apoptosis are shown in Figure 1.

A random 200 nuclei were evaluated for each experimental setting; the median number of nuclei harboring MN was 28 (range, 0–61) pre-RT and 151 (range, 16–327) after RT, at a dose of 10 Gy. The number of MN-harboring nuclei was significantly greater in 10 Gy samples than in pre-RT samples ($p = 0.015$) (Figure 3). In contrast to MN, the number of apoptotic nuclei did not differ significantly between the pre-RT samples and the 10 Gy samples (5 (range, 0–30) versus 12 (range, 2–30); $p = 0.30$).

Table 1. Patient characteristics.

Characteristics	Median (Range)
Age (years)	57 (42–82)
Age ≤ 50 vs. > 50	3 vs. 4
Menstrual status (premenopausal vs. postmenopausal)	2 vs. 5
Follow-up (months)	11 (1–21)
FIGO stage	
IB	0
II	4
III	2
IVA	1
Histology	
Squamous cell carcinoma	7
Tumor diameter (cm)	61.3 (41.1–80.1)
Serum tumor marker	
CEA (ng/mL)	4.4 (0.9–7.4)
SCC (ng/mL)	8.9 (0.9–28.3)
Treatment method	
Chemoradiotherapy	4
Radiotherapy alone	3
EBRT dose	55.6 Gy/29 fr.
IGBT dose	24 Gy/4 fr.
Interval between first and second biopsy (days)	7 (4–10)
Response at the end of EBRT (absence of gross residual tumor vs. presence of gross residual tumor)	1 vs. 6

FIGO, International Federation of Gynecology and Obstetrics; CEA, carcinoembryonic antigen; SCC, squamous cell carcinoma antigen; EBRT, external beam radiotherapy; IGBT, image-guided brachytherapy; fr., fraction.

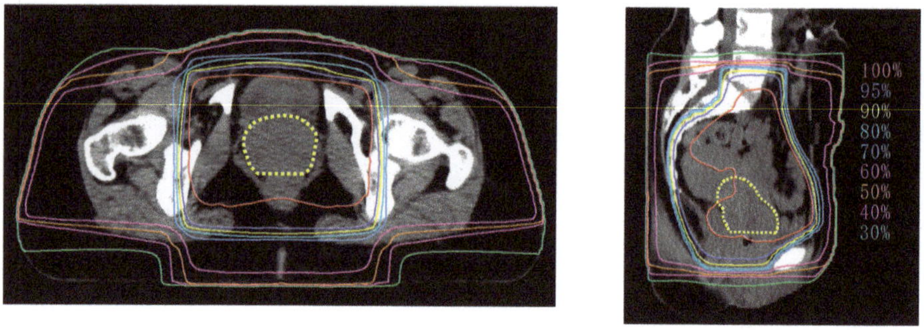

(**a**) (**b**)

Figure 2. Representative images of dose distribution of external beam radiotherapy. Dashed line indicates tumor (yellow). (**a**) Axial plane; (**b**) sagittal plane.

To analyze the influence of chemotherapy administered concurrently with RT on MN induction, we compared the rate of MN-harboring nuclei at 10 Gy relative to that for pre-RT settings (i.e., MN induction rate) between the CCRT group (n = 4) and the RT alone group (n = 3) (Figure 4a). The median MN induction rate was 21.5% (4.0–46.5%) in patients treated with RT alone and 58.5% (11.5–163.5%) in those treated with CCRT; there was no significant difference in MN induction rate between the two groups (p = 0.22). The interval between the first and second biopsies was not significantly correlated with the MN induction rate (p = 0.29, R^2 = 0.22) (Figure 4b).

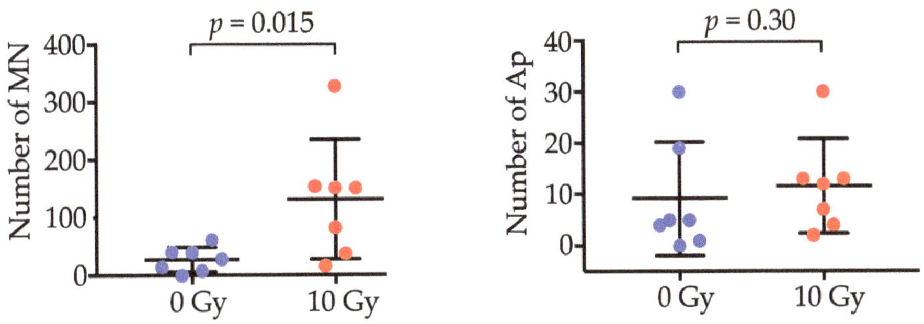

(**a**) micronuclei (**b**) apoptosis

Figure 3. The number of nuclei harboring micronuclei (MN) (**a**) and those undergoing apoptosis (Ap) (**b**) pre-radiotherapy or after 10 Gy RT. *p* values were assessed by the paired non-parametric Wilcoxon test.

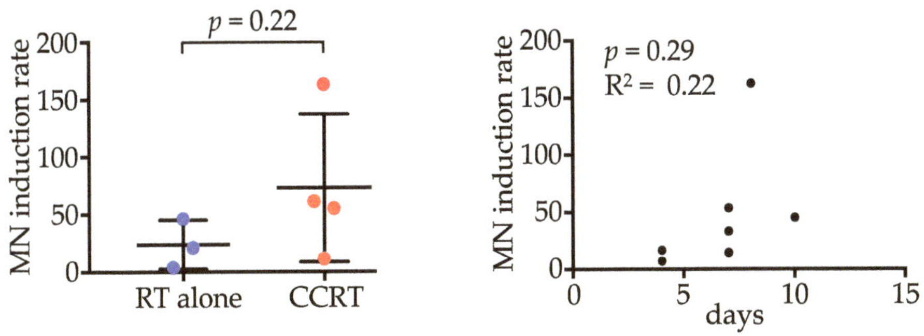

(**a**) (**b**)

Figure 4. Induction rate of micronuclei (MN) at 10 Gy, relative to pre-RT settings. (**a**) Comparison between patients treated with radiotherapy (RT) alone and those receiving concurrent chemoradiotherapy (CCRT). *p* value was assessed by the Mann–Whitney test. (**b**) Correlation between the interval between two biopsies and the induction rate of MN. *p* value and R square value were assessed by Spearman's Rank Order test.

4. Discussion

This study examined the induction of MN by radiotherapy, using cervical biopsy samples obtained before and after radiotherapy. Intratumoral MN showed a 5.4-fold increase after RT for 10 Gy in 5 fractions compared with pre-treatment setting. The increase in MN after irradiation was comparable with that reported previously in peripheral blood lymphocytes [12–15]. The novelty of this study is that, for the first time, we demonstrated the induction of MN in primary tumors treated with clinical radiation beams. In contrast to MN, there was no significant difference in the rate of apoptosis before and after irradiation. In a previous in vitro study, we investigated the nuclear morphology of cell death after X-ray irradiation at 4 Gy [19]. In that study, the most common mode of clonogenic cell death induced by X-rays was mitotic catastrophe, and the median rate of apoptosis was approximately 1%. MN represent an increase in genetic instability, and they are a hallmark of mitotic catastrophe [20–22], which is consistent with the results of this study. In addition, it is worth noting that a previous study showed that excessive expression of Trex1 by high dose irradiation in a single fraction decreases cytosolic dsDNA [11]. These data indicate that the fractionated RT schedule employed in the present study (i.e., 2 Gy per fraction and five fractions per week) might be effective in inducing MN.

Advances in radiotherapy techniques have improved the outcomes of patients with newly diagnosed uterine cervical cancer [16]. However, the platinum-based combinations used in first-line chemotherapy for metastatic or recurrent tumors rarely provide durable disease control [23]. McLachlan et al. reported the outcome of second-line chemotherapy in the patients with recurrent or metastatic cervical cancer [24]. In that report, they showed the response rate was insufficient as the median overall survival was 9.3 months. As such, better treatments are still needed for patients with recurrent or metastatic cervical cancer, and patients should be considered for clinical trials whenever feasible, including novel targeted agents and immunotherapy.

Almost all cases of uterine cervical cancer are caused by high-risk human papillomavirus (HPV) infection [25] and HPV expresses foreign antigens within host cells. Although immunotherapy has the potential to improve the survival of uterine cervical cancer patients, the response rate of uterine cervical cancer to checkpoint immunotherapy is 10–25% [26]. Previous studies suggest the differences in the immunological microenvironments and escape mechanisms by histological subtypes. Reddy et al. showed that the expression of programmed cell death-ligand 1 (PD-L1) was higher in squamous cell carcinoma than in adenocarcinoma [27]. Boussios et al. showed that diffuse PD-L1 expression in squamous cell carcinoma is correlated with poor disease-free survival and disease-specific survival compared to the cases with marginal PD-L1 expression; in adenocarcinoma, survival benefit was observed for the patients with tumors lacking PD-L1-positive tumor-associated macrophages [28,29]. The cohort of the present study solely consisted of squamous cell carcinoma. From these perspectives, future studies should compare post-RT MN induction between squamous cell carcinoma and adenocarcinoma.

The abscopal effect is an anti-tumor effect observed in the unirradiated sites of RT-treated patients. Abscopal effect "comes by chance, not through seeking", i.e., not observed in all RT-treated cases and the methods for its prediction has not been established, despite a number of clinical trials as summarized by Wang and colleagues [30]. This heterogeneity in the induction of abscopal effect post-RT can be attributable to the variance in the strength of post-RT antitumor immune responses. cGAS-STING pathway may be the mediator of post-RT abscopal effect, and MN may be the predictive biomarker. This possibility warrants further investigation in future.

In this study, we selected the time point corresponding to a dose of 10 Gy irradiation. Gamulin et al. reported that the number of MN increases gradually during RT, reaching the highest value after the administration of the last RT fraction [31]. Nevertheless, we thought, from clinical experience of rapid shrinkage of uterine cervical tumors during RT course, that sufficient samples of viable cells may not be available at later time points; therefore, we chose 10 Gy for sample collection in this study.

5. Conclusions

MN trigger antitumor immune responses via the cGAS-STING pathway. For the first time, we present clinical evidence of MN induction by RT in solid tumors. The present data provide an important insight into the activation of antitumor immune responses by RT.

Author Contributions: Conceptualization, D.K.; data acquisition, D.K., D.I., K.M., and Y.H.; formal analysis, D.K.; writing—original draft preparation, D.K.; writing—review and editing, H.S.; T.O. (Takahiro Oike); supervision, A.S., T.O. (Takahiro Oike), and T.O. (Tatsuya Ohno); funding acquisition, D.K. All authors have read and agreed to the published version of the manuscript.

Funding: This research was supported by Grants-in-Aid from the Japan Society for the Promotion of Science for Exploratory Research KAKENHI [19K17260]. This work was also supported by Gunma University Heavy Ion Medical Center.

Conflicts of Interest: The authors declare no conflict of interest.

Abbreviations

CCRT	Concurrent chemoradiotherapy
cGAS	Cyclic GMP-AMP synthase
DAPI	4′,6-diamidino-2-phenylindole, dihydrochloride
EBRT	External beam radiotherapy
IGBT	Image-guided brachytherapy
IMRT	Intensity modulated radiotherapy
MN	Micronuclei
PBS	Phosphate buffer saline
PD-L1	Programmed cell death-ligand 1
RT	Radiotherapy
STING	Stimulator of interferon genes

References

1. Nardone, V.; Pastina, P.; Giannicola, R.; Agostino, R.; Croci, S.; Tini, P.; Pirtoli, L.; Giordano, A.; Tagliaferri, P.; Correale, P. How to increase the efficacy of immunotherapy in NSCLC and HNSCC: Role of radiation therapy, chemotherapy, and other strategies. *Front. Immunol.* **2018**, *9*, 2941. [CrossRef]
2. Whiteside, T.L.; Demaria, S.; Rodriguez-Ruiz, M.E.; Zarour, H.M.; Melero, I. emerging opportunities and challenges in cancer immunotherapy. *Clin. Cancer Res.* **2016**, *22*, 1845–1855. [CrossRef]
3. Fenech, M. Cytokinesis-block micronucleus cytome assay. *Nat. Protoc.* **2007**, *2*, 1084–1104. [CrossRef]
4. Utani, K.; Kohno, Y.; Okamoto, A.; Shimizu, N. Emergence of micronuclei and their effects on the fate of cells under replication stress. *PLoS ONE* **2010**, *5*, e10089. [CrossRef]
5. Gao, D.; Li, T.; Li, X.D.; Chen, X.; Li, Q.Z.; Wight-Carter, M.; Chen, Z.J. Activation of cyclic GMP-AMP synthase by self-DNA causes autoimmune diseases. *Proc. Natl. Acad. Sci. USA* **2015**, *112*, E5699–E5705. [CrossRef]
6. Zhang, X.; Shi, H.; Wu, J.; Zhang, X.; Sun, L.; Chen, C.; Chen, Z.J. Cyclic GMP-AMP containing mixed phosphodiester linkages is an endogenous high-affinity ligand for STING. *Mol. Cell.* **2013**, *51*, 226–235. [CrossRef]
7. Harding, S.M.; Benci, J.L.; Irianto, J.; Discher, D.E.; Minn, A.J.; Greenberg, R.A. Mitotic progression following DNA damage enables pattern recognition within micronuclei. *Nature* **2017**, *548*, 466–470. [CrossRef]
8. Mackenzie, K.J.; Carroll, P.; Martin, C.A.; Murina, O.; Fluteau, A.; Simpson, D.J.; Olova, N.; Sutcliffe, H.; Rainger, J.K.; Leitch, A.; et al. cGAS surveillance of micronuclei links genome instability to innate immunity. *Nature* **2017**, *548*, 461–465. [CrossRef]
9. Deng, L.; Liang, H.; Xu, M.; Yang, X.; Burnette, B.; Arina, A.; Li, X.D.; Mauceri, H.; Beckett, M.; Darga, T.; et al. STING-dependent cytosolic DNA sensing promotes radiation-induced type I interferon-dependent antitumor immunity in immunogenic tumors. *Immunity* **2014**, *41*, 843–852. [CrossRef]
10. Gekara, N.O. DNA damage-induced immune response: Micronuclei provide key platform. *J. Cell Biol.* **2017**, *216*, 2999–3001. [CrossRef]
11. Vanpouille-Box, C.; Alard, A.; Aryankalayil, M.J.; Sarfraz, Y.; Diamond, J.M.; Schneider, R.J.; Inghirami, G.; Coleman, C.N.; Formenti, S.C.; Demaria, S. DNA exonuclease Trex1 regulates radiotherapy-induced tumour immunogenicity. *Nat. Commun.* **2017**, *8*, 15618. [CrossRef]
12. Lee, T.K.; O'Brien, K.F.; Naves, J.L.; Christie, K.I.; Arastu, H.H.; Eaves, G.S.; Wiley, A.L., Jr.; Karlsson, U.L.; Salehpour, M.R. Micronuclei in lymphocytes of prostate cancer patients undergoing radiation therapy. *Mutat. Res.* **2000**, *469*, 63–70. [CrossRef]
13. Tichy, A.; Kabacik, S.; O'Brien, G.; Pejchal, J.; Sinkorova, Z.; Kmochova, A.; Sirak, I.; Malkova, A.; Beltran, C.G.; Gonzalez, J.R.; et al. The first in vivo multiparametric comparison of different radiation exposure biomarkers in human blood. *PLoS ONE* **2018**, *13*, e0193412. [CrossRef]
14. Unal, D.; Kiraz, A.; Avci, D.; Tasdemir, A.; Unal, T.D.; Cagli, S.; Eroglu, C.; Yuce, I.; Ozcan, I.; Kaplan, B. Cytogenetic damage of radiotherapy in long-term head and neck cancer survivors. *Int. J. Radiat. Biol.* **2016**, *92*, 364–370. [CrossRef]

15. Werbrouck, J.; Ost, P.; Fonteyne, V.; De Meerleer, G.; De Neve, W.; Bogaert, E.; Beels, L.; Bacher, K.; Vral, A.; Thierens, H. Early biomarkers related to secondary primary cancer risk in radiotherapy treated prostate cancer patients: IMRT versus IMAT. *Radiother. Oncol.* **2013**, *107*, 377–381. [CrossRef]
16. Ohno, T.; Noda, S.E.; Okonogi, N.; Murata, K.; Shibuya, K.; Kiyohara, H.; Tamaki, T.; Ando, K.; Oike, T.; Ohkubo, Y.; et al. In-room computed tomography-based brachytherapy for uterine cervical cancer: Results of a 5-year retrospective study. *J. Radiat. Res.* **2017**, *58*, 543–551. [CrossRef]
17. Kobayashi, D.; Shibata, A.; Oike, T.; Nakano, T. One-step protocol for evaluation of the mode of radiation-induced clonogenic cell death by fluorescence microscopy. *J. Vis. Exp.* **2017**, 56338. [CrossRef]
18. Amornwichet, N.; Oike, T.; Shibata, A.; Ogiwara, H.; Tsuchiya, N.; Yamauchi, M.; Saitoh, Y.; Sekine, R.; Isono, M.; Yoshida, Y.; et al. Carbon-ion beam irradiation kills X-ray-resistant p53-null cancer cells by inducing mitotic catastrophe. *PLoS ONE* **2014**, *9*, e115121. [CrossRef]
19. Kobayashi, D.; Oike, T.; Shibata, A.; Niimi, A.; Kubota, Y.; Sakai, M.; Amornwhichet, N.; Yoshimoto, Y.; Hagiwara, Y.; Kimura, Y.; et al. Mitotic catastrophe is a putative mechanism underlying the weak correlation between sensitivity to carbon ions and cisplatin. *Sci. Rep.* **2017**, *7*, 40588. [CrossRef] [PubMed]
20. Eom, Y.W.; Kim, M.A.; Park, S.S.; Goo, M.J.; Kwon, H.J.; Sohn, S.; Kim, W.H.; Yoon, G.; Choi, K.S. Two distinct modes of cell death induced by doxorubicin: Apoptosis and cell death through mitotic catastrophe accompanied by senescence-like phenotype. *Oncogene* **2005**, *24*, 4765–4777. [CrossRef]
21. Gascoigne, K.E.; Taylor, S.S. How do anti-mitotic drugs kill cancer cells? *J. Cell Sci.* **2009**, *122*, 2579–2585. [CrossRef] [PubMed]
22. Roninson, I.B.; Broude, E.V.; Chang, B.D. If not apoptosis, then what? Treatment-induced senescence and mitotic catastrophe in tumor cells. *Drug Resist. Updat.* **2001**, *4*, 303–313. [CrossRef] [PubMed]
23. Ramondetta, L. What is the appropriate approach to treating women with incurable cervical cancer? *J. Natl. Compr. Cancer Netw.* **2013**, *11*, 348–355. [CrossRef] [PubMed]
24. McLachlan, J.; Boussios, S.; Okines, A.; Glaessgen, D.; Bodlar, S.; Kalaitzaki, R.; Taylor, A.; Lalondrelle, S.; Gore, M.; Kaye, S.; et al. The impact of systemic therapy beyond first-line treatment for advanced cervical cancer. *Clin. Oncol.* **2017**, *29*, 153–160. [CrossRef] [PubMed]
25. Gillison, M.L.; Chaturvedi, A.K.; Lowy, D.R. HPV prophylactic vaccines and the potential prevention of noncervical cancers in both men and women. *Cancer* **2008**, *113*, 3036–3046. [CrossRef]
26. Otter, S.J.; Chatterjee, J.; Stewart, A.J.; Michael, A. The role of biomarkers for the prediction of response to checkpoint immunotherapy and the rationale for the use of checkpoint immunotherapy in cervical cancer. *Clin. Oncol.* **2019**, *31*, 834–843. [CrossRef]
27. Reddy, O.L.; Shintaku, P.I.; Moatamed, N.A. Programmed death-ligand 1 (PD-L1) is expressed in a significant number of the uterine cervical carcinomas. *Diagn. Pathol.* **2017**, *12*, 45. [CrossRef]
28. Boussios, S.; Seraj, E.; Zarkavelis, G.; Petrakis, D.; Kollas, A.; Kafantari, A.; Assi, A.; Tatsi, K.; Pavlidis, N.; Pentheroudakis, G. Management of patients with recurrent/advanced cervical cancer beyond first line platinum regimens: Where do we stand? A literature review. *Crit. Rev. Oncol. Hematol.* **2016**, *108*, 164–174. [CrossRef]
29. Heeren, A.M.; Punt, S.; Bleeker, M.C.; Gaarenstroom, K.N.; van der Velden, J.; Kenter, G.G.; de Gruijl, T.D.; Jordanova, E.S. Prognostic effect of different PD-L1 expression patterns in squamous cell carcinoma and adenocarcinoma of the cervix. *Mod. Pathol.* **2016**, *29*, 753–763. [CrossRef]
30. Wang, D.; Zhang, X.; Gao, Y.; Cui, X.; Yang, Y.; Mao, W.; Li, M.; Zhang, B.; Yu, J. Research progress and existing problems for abscopal effect. *Cancer Manag. Res.* **2020**, *12*, 6695–6706. [CrossRef]
31. Gamulin, M.; Kopjar, N.; Grgic, M.; Ramic, S.; Bisof, V.; Garaj-Vrhovac, V. Genome damage in oropharyngeal cancer patients treated by radiotherapy. *Croat. Med. J.* **2008**, *49*, 515–527. [CrossRef] [PubMed]

Journal of *Personalized Medicine*

Article

The Cytokinesis-Block Micronucleus Assay on Human Isolated Fresh and Cryopreserved Peripheral Blood Mononuclear Cells

Simon Sioen, Karlien Cloet, Anne Vral and Ans Baeyens *

Radiobiology, Department of Human Structure and Repair, Ghent University, Corneel Heymanslaan 10, 9000 Gent, Belgium; Simon.Sioen@ugent.be (S.S.); Karlien.Cloet@gmail.com (K.C.); Anne.Vral@ugent.be (A.V.)

* Correspondence: Ans.Baeyens@ugent.be; Tel.: +32-3324919

Received: 23 July 2020; Accepted: 11 September 2020; Published: 14 September 2020

Abstract: The cytokinesis-block micronucleus (CBMN) assay is a standardized method used for genotoxicity studies. Conventional whole blood cultures (WBC) are often used for this assay, although the assay can also be performed on isolated peripheral blood mononuclear cell (PBMC) cultures. However, the standardization of a protocol for the PBMC CBMN assay has not been investigated extensively. The aim of this study was to optimize a reliable CBMN assay protocol for fresh and cryopreserved peripheral blood mononuclear cells (PBMCS), and to compare micronuclei (MNi) results between WBC and PBMC cultures. The G_0 CBMN assay was performed on whole blood, freshly isolated, and cryopreserved PBMCS from healthy human blood samples and five radiosensitive patient samples. Cells were exposed to 220 kV X-ray in vitro doses ranging from 0.5 to 2 Gy. The optimized PBMC CBMN assay showed adequate repeatability and small inter-individual variability. MNi values were significantly higher for WBC than for fresh PBMCS. Additionally, cryopreservation of PBMCS resulted in a significant increase of MNi values, while different cryopreservation times had no significant impact. In conclusion, our standardized CBMN assay on fresh and cryopreserved PBMCS can be used for genotoxicity studies, biological dosimetry, and radiosensitivity assessment.

Keywords: PBMCS; micronucleus assay; biological dosimetry; human blood; genotoxicity tests; radiosensitivity

1. Introduction

Chromosomal damage can be assessed using various cytogenetic assays. These assays are often used in environmental biomonitoring studies, for example studies evaluating the genotoxic impact of nanoparticles on chromosomal damage, and in occupational genotoxicity studies, such as the influence of anesthetic gases in medical workers or the effect of cadmium exposure on battery manufacture workers [1–4]. Next to this, mutagen sensitivity phenotyping, measured by quantifying genotoxic events induced by chemical or physical agents, has been used as an indirect measure of cancer susceptibility [5,6]. Furthermore, the measurement of chromosomal damage induced by ionizing radiation is frequently used for radiation protection (e.g., biological dosimetry), as well as for radiobiological research (e.g., in vitro chromosomal radiosensitivity studies and prediction, or the follow up of radiation side effects) [3,7,8].

Ionizing radiation affects cells directly and indirectly, and can lead to an increase of the frequency of biological phenomena such as cell death, malignant transformations and chromosomal aberrations [9–11]. Cytogenetic biological dosimetry measures radiation-induced chromosomal aberrations as a proxy to estimate a received dose [12,13]. Over the past few decades, the use of chromosomal damage biomarkers has proven to be of value for dose assessments, especially when physical dosimetry data is insufficiently available [13].

The cytokinesis-block micronucleus (CBMN) assay, developed by Fenech and Moreley, is one of the most important in vivo and in vitro cytogenetic methods, next to the comet assay and the dicentric chromosome assay [3,14,15]. Micronuclei (MNi) are small, extra nuclear bodies, that form as a result of whole chromosomes that lag behind during mitosis or as a result of chromosome fragments that are not incorporated into the main daughter nuclei. During the CBMN assay, cytokinesis is blocked by the addition of cytochalasin B, resulting in the formation of binucleated (BN) cells. In these BN cells, which have gone through a single division, the MNi are counted [7,15,16]. The CBMN assay is faster and requires less specialized skills than most cytogenetic methods. This makes the CBMN assay a highly suitable high-throughput method for the biomonitoring of large populations exposed to genotoxic agents in both occupational and environmental settings [3,15].

The CBMN assay, performed on whole blood, is a well-established technique. Samples can be easily obtained through venipuncture, and whole blood cultures require minimal effort to set up, which leads to a reduction in time and cost [3]. One disadvantage of working with fresh whole blood samples is that in most cases only a small amount of blood can be collected. Therefore, repeating the assay is not easy without further blood sampling [17]. Furthermore, fresh blood samples need to be processed within 48 h after collection [18]. To counter these drawbacks, the CBMN assay is now more commonly performed on peripheral blood mononuclear cells (PBMCS) [19,20]. PBMCS, including monocytes and lymphocytes, can be isolated in bulk (1–2 × 10^6 PBMCS/mL) from anticoagulated blood. One fraction can be used immediately for multiple assays while another fraction can be frozen for future tests [21–24]. While freshly isolated PBMCS samples are optimal for many downstream applications, the cryopreservation of PBMCS allows for batching and analysis within a chosen time frame [24,25]. Moreover, the use of cryopreserved PBMCS allows the analysis of sequential samples from the same patient isochronously [23].

Despite the frequent use of PBMCS, there has not been a thorough comparative analysis of CBMN assay results, between whole blood cultures, cryopreserved PBMCS, and freshly isolated PBMCS. In this study, the CBMN assay methodology for fresh and cryopreserved PBMCS was optimized and results were compared to whole blood CBMN assay results. Furthermore, the peripheral blood mononuclear cell (PBMC) CBMN assay was applied for radiosensitivity assessments and retrospective biological dosimetry.

2. Materials and Methods

2.1. Study Population and Blood Sampling

For the comparison of the whole blood and PBMC CBMN assays, blood samples from ten healthy volunteers (five men and five women; 22–53 years) were collected. To investigate the effect of cryopreservation of PBMCS on MNi counts; blood samples from three extra volunteers (two women and one man; 24–44 years) were collected. To validate the PBMC micronucleus assay for radiosensitivity assessment, blood samples from two patients with a known ataxia telangiectasia mutation (ATM), one patient with a heterozygote ATM mutation, one patient with a BRCA2 mutation and one with an unknown mutation, were collected. Repeatability of the optimized PBMC CBMN assay was verified using blood samples from 6 volunteers (3 men and 3 women; 24–43). To test the minimal blood volume for the PBMC MN assay, blood samples from 3 volunteers were collected (1 man and 2 women; 24–46). Lastly, the suitability of the PBMC CBMN assay for biological dosimetry was examined using blood samples from three extra volunteers (1 man and 2 women; 24–26 years).

All peripheral blood samples were collected by venipuncture in lithium heparinized tubes, without the use of extra stabilizers. Each sample was stored at room temperature (20 °C) and was processed within two hours of collection. Informed consent for inclusion was received from all patients and volunteers before participating in the study. The study was conducted in accordance with the Declaration of Helsinki, and the protocol was approved by the Ethics Committee of Ghent University (code: 2017/1621 and 2019/0461). None of the blood donors in this study had any known prior exposure to chemicals, radiotherapy, medication, or other substances that could affect MNi frequencies.

2.2. Isolation and Cryopreservation of Peripheral Blood Mononuclear Cells

2.2.1. Isolation by Density Gradient Centrifugation

Peripheral blood samples were isolated using density-gradient centrifugation (2300 rpm, 20 min, 20 °C, no brakes, Eppendorf, Hamburg, Germany) of diluted blood (1/2 in phosphate buffered saline (PBS) (20 °C)), gently added on to Lymphoprep^{TM} (density: 1.077 g/mL, 20 °C, Axis-Shield, Dundee, UK). The yield and viability of the isolated PBMCS were verified using trypan blue (Gibco, Thermo Fisher Scientific Ltd., Waltham, MA, USA) and a Bürker cell counting chamber (Superior Marienfield, Lauda-Königshofen, Germany). A viability of 95–100% was attained, prior to culturing or cryopreservation. On average 1 mL blood resulted in 1.15×10^6 isolated PBMCS.

2.2.2. Cryopreservation and Thawing Procedures

PBMCS were cryopreserved in fetal calf serum (FCS) (4°, Gibco, Thermo Fisher Scientific Ltd., Waltham, MA, USA) supplemented with 10% dimethylsulfoxide (DMSO) (4 °C, Sigma-Aldrich, Saint Louis, MO, USA), at a concentration of 1.5×10^6 cells/mL. After 24 h in a Mr. Frosty container (Sigma-Aldrich) at −80 °C, cryovials were transferred to liquid nitrogen (−196 °C).

Cells were cryopreserved for 2; 5; 10; 20 and 25 w. Thawing of cells was performed by submerging the cryovials in sterile H_2O (37 °C) until only little pieces of ice remained. Then, the cell suspension was transferred to complete RPMI (cRPMI) [37 °C, RPMI 1640 (Gibco, Thermo Fisher Scientific Ltd., Waltham, MA, USA) with antibiotics (50 U/mL penicillin and 50 mg/mL streptomycin, Gibco)], supplemented with 10% FCS at 37 °C. This was followed by rinsing the cryovials with 1 mL of pre-warmed FCS (37 °C). Lastly, the cells were washed three times with cRPMI medium (1500 rpm, 10 min, 37 °C).

All pre-analytical factors used for PBMC-based assays are documented according to the recent standards determined by Betsou et al. [23].

2.3. Whole Blood Cytokinesis-Block Micronucleus Assay

The whole blood CBMN assay was performed according to a standardized protocol of our laboratory [7] (Figure 1A,B). For each culture, 0.5 mL of blood was added to 4.5 mL of pre-warmed culture medium [cRPMI + 10% FCS, 37 °C]. Following a 1-h incubation step (37 °C, 5% CO_2), cells were irradiated with 0.5; 1 and 2 Gy X-rays in a T25 culture flask. A sham-irradiated control (0 Gy) was included to measure spontaneously occurring MNi. Duplicate cultures were set up for each dose point.

After irradiation, 20 µL/mL of phytohaemagglutanin-L (PHA-L, stock solution 1 mg/mL, Sigma-Aldrich, Saint Louis, MO, USA) was added to stimulate cell division in lymphocytes. At 23 h post-stimulation, 6 µg/mL cytochalasin B (stock solution 1.5 mg/mL, Sigma-Aldrich) was added to block cytokinesis. 70 h post-stimulation, cells were exposed to a cold hypotonic shock using 7 mL of KCl (4 °C, 0.075M, Sigma-Aldrich) and fixed using a methanol: glacial acetic acid: ringer solution (4 °C, 4:1:5, Chem-lab, Zedelgem, Belgium). After overnight storage at 4 °C, cells were fixed two more times using a methanol: glacial acetic acid solution (4:1, 4 °C). Lastly, the cells were dropped on to isopropanol cleaned slides and stained with acridine orange (10 µg/mL, Sigma-Aldrich).

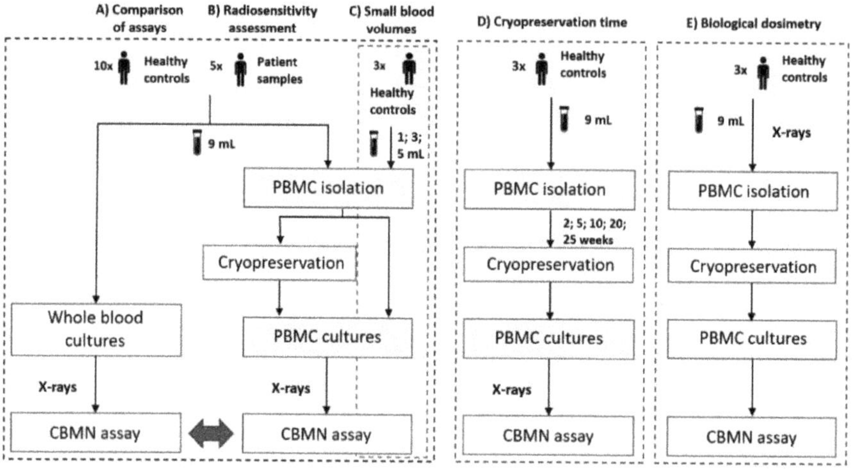

Figure 1. Schematic overview of experiments: comparison between the whole blood and peripheral blood mononuclear cells (PBMC) cytokinesis-block micronucleus (CBMN) assays, performed on (**A**) healthy controls and (**B**) patient samples. (**C**) Effect of different blood volumes on CBMN assay results. (**D**) The effect of different cryopreservation times on CBMN assay results. (**E**) The PBMC CBMN assay performed in a biological dosimetry setting.

2.4. PBMC Cytokinesis-Block Micronucleus Assay

Fresh or thawed PBMCS were resuspended in culture medium [cRPMI, 10% FCS, 1% sodiumpyruvate (100 mM, Gibco, Thermo Fisher Scientific Ltd., Waltham, MA, USA), 0.1% β-mercaptoethanol (50 mM, Gibco), 37 °C] at a concentration of 500 000 cells/mL, and were cultured in 500 μL in a 48-well cell suspension plate (Greiner Cellstar®, Sigma-Aldrich, Saint Louis, MO, USA) (Figure 1A–E). Following a 1-h incubation step (37 °C, 5% CO_2), the cells were exposed to 0.5; 1 and 2 Gy X-rays. A sham-irradiated control (0 Gy) was included. For each dose point, duplicate cultures were set up.

Immediately after irradiation, 5 μL/mL of PHA-L (stock solution 1 mg/mL) was added. At 23 h post-stimulation, 6 μg/mL cytochalasin B (stock solution 1.5 mg/mL) was added. For harvesting and fixing 70 h post-stimulation, the cell suspension was transported to a 1.5 mL Eppendorf tube (Greiner Bio-one, Kremsmünster, Austria) and the well was rinsed with 0.5 mL PBS, to prevent loss of cells.

After centrifugation (8 min, 300 g, Eppendorf, Hamburg, Germany) and supernatant removal, 450 μL KCl (4 °C, 0.075M) was added to induce a cold hypotonic shock. Next, cells were fixed in a methanol: glacial acetic acid: ringer solution (3:1:4, 4 °C). After overnight storage at 4 °C, the cells were fixed two more times using a methanol: glacial acetic acid solution (3:1, 4 °C). Addition of the fixatives was always performed drop by drop while vortexing. The cells were dropped on to isopropanol cleaned slides and stained with acridine orange stain (10 μg/mL, Sigma-Aldrich, Saint Louis, MO, USA). To assure an optimal cell size for scoring MNi, fixating twice with the methanol: glacial acetic acid solution (3:1, 4 °C) is crucial.

To analyze repeatability, the PBMC CBMN assay (freshly and cryopreserved) was performed on 6 parallel cultures from three donors.

2.5. PBMC Cytokinesis-Block Micronucleus Assay in a Biodosimetry Setting

5 mL of whole blood was irradiated in vitro with 0; 0.5; 1 and 2 Gy X-Rays, in a T25 culture flask (Figure 1E). A sham-irradiated control (0 Gy) was included. For each dose point, duplicate cultures were set up. After a 2-h incubation step (37 °C, 5% CO_2), PBMC isolation, cryopreservation,

and thawing procedures were performed as described in Section 2.2. Subsequently, the CBMN assay was performed as described in Section 2.4, excluding the irradiation step.

2.6. In Vitro Irradiation Procedure

In vitro irradiations were performed at the 'Small Animal Radiation Research Platform' (SARRP, XStrahl, Camberley, UK) at Infinity Lab, Ghent University. X-rays (220 kVp, 13 mA), were filtered using 0.15 mm copper and a square field collimator (100 × 100 mm at 35 cm FSD) was used. The applied dose rate was 3.046 Gy/min.

2.7. Scoring Procedure

2.7.1. Micronuclei Scoring

MNi were scored in 500 BN cells by using a fluorescence microscope (200x magnification). A total of 1000 BN cells were scored per sample as duplicated cultures were set up. Each sample was scored by two independent scorers.

2.7.2. Binucleated Yield and Nuclear Division Index

To assure a sufficient proliferative capacity, the nuclear division index (NDI) was calculated. For each culture 500 viable cells (Ntotal) were scored to evaluate the number of mononucleate (N1), binucleate (N2), trinucleate (N3), and polynucleate (N4) cells. The formula used to calculate NDI: NDI= (N1 + 2N2 + 3N3 + 4N4)/Ntotal. All cultures attained NDI's between 1.2 and 2.0.

2.8. Statistical Analysis

Statistical analysis was performed using the Graphpad Prism 6 software (GraphPad Software Inc., San Diego, CA, USA)and MEDCALC® software (MedCalc Software Ltd., Ostend, Belgium). The confidence level of the statistical tests was 95% and statistical significance was set at $p < 0.05$. For the comparison of MNi values between different groups, the paired t test was used. Effects of cryopreservation time on MNi values were analyzed by the Friedman test. Comparison of differences in coefficients of variation (CVs) were analyzed according to Forkman [26].

3. Results

3.1. Comparison of CBMN Assay Results of Whole Blood, Fresh and Cryopreserved PBMCS

The CBMN assay was performed on WBC, fresh PBMC and cryopreserved (2 w and 25 w) PBMC samples (Figure 1A). The results are presented in Table 1 and Figure 2. The mean MNi response of WBC was significantly higher compared to fresh PBMCS (paired *t*-test, $p < 0.0001$). Moreover, the mean MNi response of fresh PBMCS was significantly lower compared to both 2 w and 25 w cryopreserved PBMC samples (paired *t*-test, $p = 0.0111$ and $p = 0.0104$). When comparing both 2 w and 25 w cryopreserved PBMC samples, no significant differences were observed.

To evaluate inter-individual variability, the CV values were analyzed and compared. Although high CV-values were observed in sham-irradiated samples, due to low counted MNi values, low CV values were observed in irradiated samples. No major significant differences in CV values between the different assays were found, for each dose point (Table 1, Forkman test). However, a significant difference in inter-individual variability was noted for the 25 w cryopreserved PBMCS 1 Gy dose, compared to fresh PBMCS. In addition, the repeatability of the newly optimized PBMC CBMN assay was examined by performing the CBMN assay (2Gy) on 6 parallel cultures of three donors. The coefficient of variation for the repeats ranged between 9.8 and 11.8% for the fresh PBMC CBMN assay and between 5.7 and 10.5% for the cryopreserved PBMC CBMN assay. This indicated a good repeatability of both assays.

Table 1. Overview of the micronuclei (MNi) results of the different MN assays. Mean, SD and range values represent number of MNi/1000 binucleated (BN) cells. CVs represent the inter-individual variability.

	WBC (n = 10)				Fresh PBMCS (n = 10)			
Dose (Gy)	0	0.5	1	2	0	0.5	1	2
Mean	25	113	251	650	17	98	199	507
SD	16	18	47	95	10	23	24	55
CV (%)	63	16	19	15	57	24	12	11
Range	13–66	93–155	179–348	506–815	3–33	73–142	166–232	401–594
	Cryopreserved (2 w) PBMCS (n = 10)				**Cryopreserved (25 w) PBMCS (n = 9)**			
Dose (Gy)	0	0.5	1	2	0	0.5	1	2
Mean	9	86	241	630	17	114	232	608
SD	6	17	44	129	6	18	59	123
CV (%)	71	20	18	21	39	16	26 *	20
Range	2–22	67–115	190–338	494–943	11–29	82–135	158–350	424–793

* Significant p value (<0.05, Forkman) for the comparison of WBC to fresh PBMCS or fresh PBMCS compared to cryopreserved PBMCS.

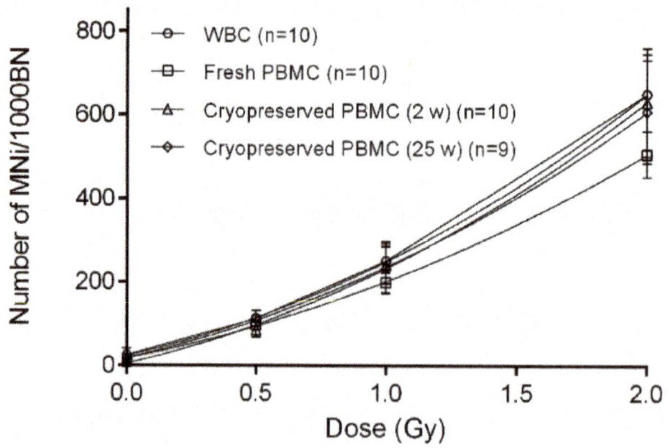

Figure 2. Comparison of the number of micronuclei (MNi) per 1000 binucleated (BN) cells for whole blood cultures (WBC), fresh, 2 weeks, and 25 weeks cryopreserved peripheral blood mononuclear cells (PBMCS) after 0, 0.5, 1 and 2 Gy exposure. The error bars represent SD of the mean.

3.2. Effect of Cryopreservation Time on PBMC CBMN Assay Results

The influence of cryopreservation time on MNi values was investigated as significantly higher MNi values were observed for cryopreserved PBMCS compared to fresh PBMCS. The CBMN assay was performed on cryopreserved PBMCS (2, 5, 10, 20 and 25 weeks) from three healthy donors (Figure 1D). In Figure 3, the numbers of MNi per 1000 BN cells are plotted in function of the cryopreservation time. No significant differences between 2, 5, 10, 20 and 25 w of cryopreservation were found for each dose point.

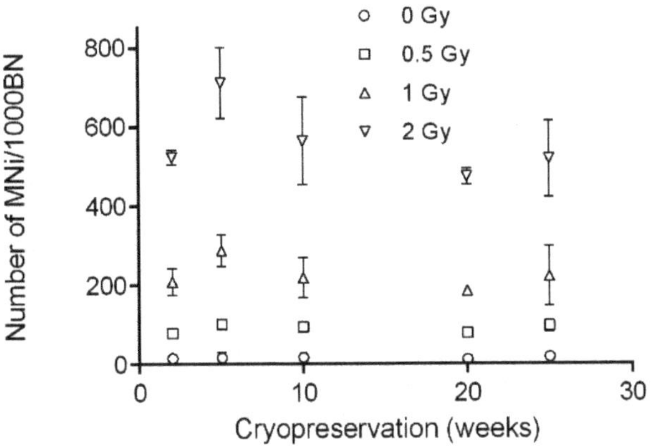

Figure 3. Effect of cryopreservation time (2, 5, 10, 20 and 25 weeks) on the number of micronuclei (MNi) per 1000 binucleated (BN) cells in peripheral blood mononuclear cells (PBMCS). The error bars represent SD of the mean.

3.3. *Radiosensitivity Assessment of Patient Samples Using the PBMC CBMN Assay*

To investigate whether the CBMN assay on freshly isolated and on 25 w cryopreserved PBMCS can be utilized for radiosensitivity assessment, five blood samples of patients were analyzed using the CBMN assay on WBC, freshly isolated (n = 3), and cryopreserved (n = 5; 25 w) PBMCS (Figure 1B). When evaluating WBC in a clinical setting, patients are regarded as being radiosensitive when their MNi values exceed the mean +3SD of a healthy control group, for each dose. The MNi results obtained from the freshly isolated and cryopreserved (25 w) PBMC CBMN assay were plotted against the mean ±3SD linear quadratic fits of their corresponding healthy controls (Figure 4A,B). Based on the clinical data, Patients 1 and 2 were considered radiosensitive while Patients 3, 4 and 5 were not radiosensitive. These diagnoses were confirmed by the results of our optimized PBMC CBMN assay, performed on both freshly isolated and cryopreserved (25 w) PBMCS. These results demonstrate the ability of the PBMC CBMN assay to correctly assess radiosensitivity.

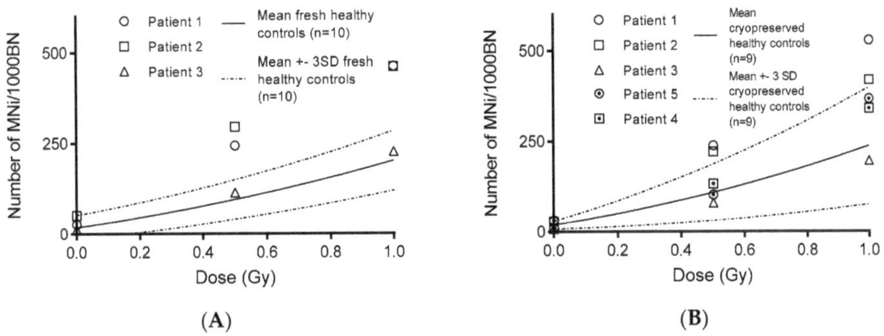

Figure 4. Radiosensitivity assessment of (**A**) fresh and (**B**) 25 weeks cryopreserved peripheral blood mononuclear cells (PBMCS) of 5 patients, exposed to 0, 0.5 and 1 Gy. Patients are regarded as being radiosensitive when their micronuclei (MNi) values exceed the mean +3 SD of a healthy control group, for each dose. According to clinical data, Patients 1 and 2 were considered radiosensitive while Patients 3, 4 and 5 were not radiosensitive.

3.4. The CBMN Assay on PBMCs, Isolated from Small Blood Volumes

The blood volume required for a PBMC CBMN assay was evaluated, as small blood volumes are often preferred in pediatric patients (Figure 5). PBMC isolation was performed on 1 mL, 3 mL and 5 mL of blood and the obtained PBMCS were subsequently used for the CBMN assay (Figure 1C). PBMC isolation on all blood volumes was successful. Moreover, no significant differences in MNi values were observed between the different blood volumes.

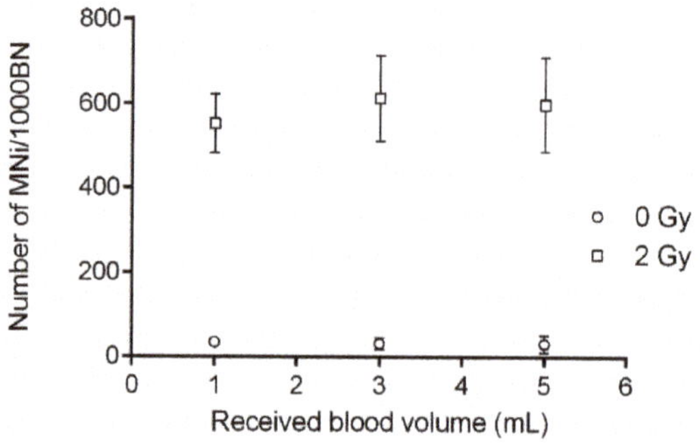

Figure 5. Evaluation of the volume of blood required for a peripheral blood mononuclear cell (PBMC) cytokinesis-block micronucleus (CBMN) assay. PBMC isolation was performed on 1 mL, 3 mL and 5 mL of blood and the obtained PBMCS were subsequently used for the CBMN assay.

3.5. The CBMN Assay on PBMCS in a Biodosimetry Setting

In cytogenetic biological dosimetry, a received dose of ionizing radiation based on the measurement of radiation-induced biological effects, is estimated retrospectively [12,13]. In the given situation, PBMCS are irradiated in whole blood and can only be isolated afterwards. Therefore, a simulation of this scenario was performed to test the PBMC CBMN assay (Figure 1E). Results indicate that, in a biodosimetry setting, the CBMN assay is reliable to estimate the received dose (Figure 6). The MNi response of 2 w cryopreserved PBMCS fit within the mean ± SD of 10 cryopreserved (2 w) controls, for each dose point.

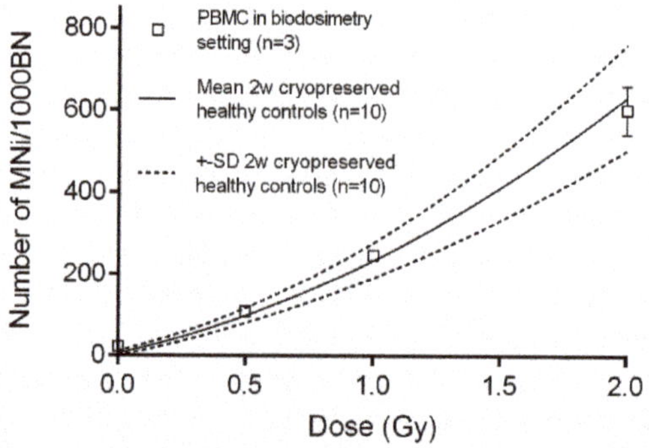

Figure 6. Whole blood was exposed to 0.5, 1 and 2 Gy, before peripheral blood mononuclear cell (PBMC) isolation. The micronuclei (MNi) mean ± SD of three donors is plotted against the linear quadratic fit of the mean ± SD of ten cryopreserved (2 w) PBMC controls.

4. Discussion

While WBC are commonly used for cytogenetic assays, isolated PBMCS are also finding their way in chromosomal damage research [21–23]. The potential for cryopreservation of PBMCS makes this an exceptionally suitable cell type for cytogenetic assays, as it has several major advantages: (1) the ability to obtain a bulk of cells; (2) no need for further blood sampling; (3) the potential for batching and (4) the ability to perform the analysis within a chosen time frame. However, the use of cryopreserved PBMC samples for cytogenetic assays, such as the CBMN assay, has not yet been standardized and extensively studied. In this study, the CBMN assay was optimized for freshly isolated and cryopreserved PBMCS. The repeatability, inter-individual variability and sensitivity of the optimized PBMC CBMN assay was investigated. Furthermore, a thorough comparison was performed between the conventional whole blood CBMN assay and the optimized PBMC CBMN assay, on both freshly isolated and cryopreserved PBMCS.

Our results showed a significantly higher MNi responses in WBC compared to fresh PBMCS. These results may indicate the occurrence of changes in DNA damage response resulting from different culturing methods. Compared to whole blood cultures, PBMC cultures do not contain blood serum (including micronutrients), erythrocytes, platelets, or granulocytes, and they have a different cytokine composition. These differences can contribute to higher MNi values observed in whole blood [27–30]. In addition, the use of 0.1% β-mercaptoethanol in PBMC cultures might lead to a decrease in radiation-induced reactive oxygen species and consequently less DNA damage.

Importantly, as no significant differences were observed in the repeatability and inter-individual variability of both CBMN assays, the difference in MNi response has no direct impact on the reliability of the optimized PBMC CBMN assay. Interestingly, a significant increase in the MNi response of cryopreserved PBMCS was observed when exposed to irradiation. This increase, however, was independent of the cryopreservation time. Moreover, the repeatability and inter-individual variability did not vary significantly after cryopreservation, indicating no significant change in the reliability of the assay. In current literature, several studies have investigated the link between the cryopreservation of human lymphocytes and DNA damage induction and repair. Both Ho et al. and Koppen et al. reported no significant differences in DNA damage induction between fresh and cryopreserved PBMCS or whole blood samples, which is in line with our results [31,32]. Duthie et al. demonstrated that DNA damage that is already present in the DNA of fresh lymphocytes, is maintained throughout the isolation and cryopreservation procedure. Furthermore, a diminished DNA repair capacity of cryopreserved lymphocytes was reported, when exposed to H_2O_2 [33]. These comet assay observations are confirmed by our results, as an increased number of radiation-induced MNi was observed in our cryopreserved PBMCS. Noteworthy, the comet assay was often used in the current literature, however this technique differs from the CBMN assay. The CBMN assay analyses chromosomal fragments resulting from unrepaired or misrepaired DNA DSBs, whereas the comet assay is a straightforward visual method used for the detection of both repairable and unrepairable DNA damage [34]. Further supporting our results, Cheng et al. demonstrated that lymphocytes, from cryopreserved whole blood, were significantly more sensitive to chromatid break induction by γ irradiation, while no significant differences were seen between the baseline levels of chromatid breaks after cryopreservation [35]. In addition, and also worth mentioning, Fowke et al. showed that lymphocytes from cryopreserved whole blood, have a significantly increased probability to suffer from deterioration in terms of viability, apoptosis, and Epstein–Barr virus transformability [36].

Interestingly, Zijno et al. investigated the suitability of cryopreserved PBMCS (18 to 123 w) for the CBMN assay and found no significant differences in MNi counts between cryopreserved PBMCSs and WBC, for both the untreated and irradiated group. However, a direct comparison with our results is not straightforward as different cryopreservation protocols were used and their cryopreserved PBMCS data were compared with mean values of fresh whole blood data from five years earlier [37]. Furthermore, they observed no significant impact of different cryopreservation times, which is in line with our results. In the event that cryopreservation had led to a decrease in damage, this could have been explained by the predominant loss during storage and thawing of more unstable cells [31]. This is further supported by Risom and Knudsen, who stated that cryopreservation of lymphocytes may result in the selective survival of lymphocytes with relatively high DNA repair activity [38].

When performing a radiosensitivity assessment of a patient, it is important to keep in mind that our results indicate a possible effect of the process of cryopreservation on the occurrence of DNA damage. To counter this, we advise to simultaneously process PBMCS of a healthy control sample. Furthermore, as stated by various research groups, care should be taken regarding differences in isolation protocols and storage conditions for all PBMC samples in one study. In addition, it is important to provide a precise description of preanalytical processing and variations [23,32].

Our results indicated that radiosensitivity assessment of patients can be performed using the PBMC CBMN assay. A study of Djuzenova et al. in which PBMCS were used to demonstrate that cancer patients with an adverse skin reaction to radiotherapy displayed increased frequencies of both spontaneous and radiation-induced MN, supports our results [39]. Additional experiments using patients with different genetic defects affecting radiosensitivity, are still needed to fully confirm our hypothesis. The possibility to perform the CBMN assay on cryopreserved PBMCS provides a major advantage as the need for further blood sampling can be prevented. Moreover, we also demonstrated the potential to perform the assay on smaller blood volumes (down to 1 mL), which is especially important for pediatric patients.

Finally, this study showed the ability of the PBMC CBMN assay to be applied to retrospective biological dosimetry, in which the individual absorbed dose after a radiological accident can be estimated.

5. Conclusions

In conclusion, this study presents an optimized, reliable CBMN assay for both fresh and cryopreserved PBMCS. There is a significant difference between the MNi values of WBC and freshly isolated PBMCS. Furthermore, cryopreservation of PBMCS has an impact on the MNi yield. Finally, fresh or cryopreserved PBMCS provide us with a good cell model for CBMN assays in the field of biological dosimetry and radiosensitivity assessments.

Author Contributions: S.S. and K.C. performed the experiments. S.S., A.V. and A.B. wrote the manuscript, revised and prepared the final version. All authors have read and agreed to the published version of the manuscript.

Funding: This research was funded by a grant from the 'Fonds voor Wetenschappelijk Onderzoek' (FWO, G051918N) and by a grant from the 'Bijzonder Onderzoeksfonds starterskrediet' (Ghent University, BOFSTA 20170018).

Acknowledgments: We wish to thank all patients and control donors who participated in this study. In addition, we would like to thank L. Pieters, G. De Smet, J. Aernoudt and E. Bes for technical assistance and E. Duthoo and C. Minaar for editing of the text. Furthermore, we acknowledge E. Duthoo, S. Vermeulen and E. Beyls for their help with MNi scoring.

Conflicts of Interest: The authors declare no conflict of interest.

Abbreviations

CBMN	Cytokinesis-block micronucleus
MNi	Micronuclei
BN	Binucleated
FISH	Fluorescence in situ hybridization
PBMCS	Peripheral blood mononuclear cells
PBS	Phosphate buffered saline
FCS	Fetal calf serum
DMSO	Dimethylsulfoxide
cRPMI	Complete RPMI
PHA-L	Phytohaemagglutanin-L
SARRP	Small animal radiation research platform
NDI	Nuclear division index
CV	Coefficient of variation
WBC	Whole blood cultures
w	Weeks
DSB	Double stranded break

References

1. Collins, A.; Milic, M.; Bonassi, S.; Dusinska, M. The comet assay in human biomonitoring: Technical and epidemiological perspectives. *Mutat. Res* **2019**, *843*, 1–2. [CrossRef] [PubMed]
2. Baeyens, A.; Herd, O.; Francies, F.Z.; Cairns, A.; Katzman, G.; Murdoch, M.; Padiachy, D.; Morford, M.; Vral, A.; Slabbert, J.P. The influence of blood storage time and general anaesthesia on chromosomal radiosensitivity assessment. *Mutagenesis* **2016**, *31*, 181–186. [CrossRef] [PubMed]
3. Sommer, S.; Buraczewska, I.; Kruszewski, M. Micronucleus Assay: The State of Art, and Future Directions. *Int. J. Mol. Sci.* **2020**, *21*, 1534. [CrossRef] [PubMed]
4. Lison, D.; Van Maele-Fabry, G.; Vral, A.; Vermeulen, S.; Bastin, P.; Haufroid, V.; Baeyens, A. Absence of genotoxic impact assessed by micronucleus frequency in circulating lymphocytes of workers exposed to cadmium. *Toxicol. Lett.* **2019**, *303*, 72–77. [CrossRef] [PubMed]
5. Bonassi, S.; Znaor, A.; Ceppi, M.; Lando, C.; Chang, W.P.; Holland, N.; Kirsch-Volders, M.; Zeiger, E.; Ban, S.; Barale, R.; et al. An increased micronucleus frequency in peripheral blood lymphocytes predicts the risk of cancer in humans. *Carcinogenesis* **2007**, *28*, 625–631. [CrossRef]
6. Francies, F.Z.; Wainwright, R.; Poole, J.; De Leeneer, K.; Coene, I.; Wieme, G.; Poirel, H.A.; Brichard, B.; Vermeulen, S.; Vral, A.; et al. Diagnosis of Fanconi Anaemia by ionising radiation- or mitomycin C-induced micronuclei. *DNA Repair* **2018**, *61*, 17–24. [CrossRef]
7. Baeyens, A.; Swanson, R.; Herd, O.; Ainsbury, E.; Mabhengu, T.; Willem, P.; Thierens, H.; Slabbert, J.P.; Vral, A. A semi-automated micronucleus-centromere assay to assess low-dose radiation exposure in human lymphocytes. *Int. J. Radiat. Biol.* **2011**, *87*, 923–931. [CrossRef]
8. Vinnikov, V.; Belyakov, O. Clinical Applications of Biomarkers of Radiation Exposure: Limitations and Possible Solutions through Coordinated Research. *Radiat. Prot. Dosim.* **2019**, *186*, 3–8. [CrossRef]
9. Baselet, B.; Sonveaux, P.; Baatout, S.; Aerts, A. Pathological effects of ionizing radiation: Endothelial activation and dysfunction. *Cell. Mol. Life Sci.* **2019**, *76*, 699–728. [CrossRef]
10. Kazmierczak, U.; Banas, D.; Braziewicz, J.; Buraczewska, I.; Czub, J.; Jaskola, M.; Kazmierczak, L.; Korman, A.; Kruszewski, M.; Lankoff, A.; et al. Investigation of the bystander effect in CHO-K1 cells. *Rep. Pract. Oncol. Radiother.* **2014**, *19*, S37–S41. [CrossRef]
11. Marin, A.; Martin, M.; Linan, O.; Alvarenga, F.; Lopez, M.; Fernandez, L.; Buchser, D.; Cerezo, L. Bystander effects and radiotherapy. *Rep. Pract. Oncol. Radiother.* **2015**, *20*, 12–21. [CrossRef] [PubMed]
12. Silva-Barbosa, I.; Pereira-Magnata, S.; Amaral, A.; Sotero, G.; Melo, H.C. Dose assessment by quantification of chromosome aberrations and micronuclei in peripheral blood lymphocytes from patients exposed to gamma radiation. *Genet. Mol. Biol.* **2005**, *28*, 452–457. [CrossRef]
13. World Health Organization. *Cytogenetic Dosimetry: Applications in Preparedness for and Response to Radiation Emergencies*; International Atomic Energy Agency: Vienna, Austria, 2011.
14. Fenech, M.; Morley, A.A. Measurement of micronuclei in lymphocytes. *Mutat. Res.* **1985**, *147*, 29–36. [CrossRef]
15. Fenech, M. Cytokinesis-block micronucleus cytome assay. *Nat. Protoc.* **2007**, *2*, 1084–1104. [CrossRef] [PubMed]
16. Baeyens, A. Chromosomal radiosensitivity of lymphocytes in South African breast cancer patients of different ethnicity: An indirect measure of cancer susceptibility. *S. Afr. Med. J. Suid-Afrik. Tydskr. Geneeskd.* **2015**, *105*, 675–678. [CrossRef]
17. Baeyens, A.; Vandenbulcke, K.; Philippe, J.; Thierens, H.; De Ridder, L.; Vral, A. The use of IL-2 cultures to measure chromosomal radiosensitivity in breast cancer patients. *Mutagenesis* **2004**, *19*, 493–498. [CrossRef]
18. Bonassi, S.; El-Zein, R.; Bolognesi, C.; Fenech, M. Micronuclei frequency in peripheral blood lymphocytes and cancer risk: Evidence from human studies. *Mutagenesis* **2011**, *26*, 93–100. [CrossRef]
19. Zizza, A.; Grima, P.; Andreassi, M.G.; Tumolo, M.R.; Borghini, A.; de Donno, A.; Negro, P.; Guido, M. HIV infection and frequency of micronucleus in human peripheral blood cells. *J. Prev. Med. Hyg.* **2019**, *60*, E191–E196. [CrossRef]
20. Katic, J.; Cemeli, E.; Baumgartner, A.; Laubenthal, J.; Bassano, I.; Stolevik, S.B.; Granum, B.; Namork, E.; Nygaard, U.C.; Lovik, M.; et al. Evaluation of the genotoxicity of 10 selected dietary/environmental compounds with the in vitro micronucleus cytokinesis-block assay in an interlaboratory comparison. *Food Chem. Toxicol.* **2010**, *48*, 2612–2623. [CrossRef]

21. Odongo, G.A.; Skatchkov, I.; Herz, C.; Lamy, E. Optimization of the alkaline comet assay for easy repair capacity quantification of oxidative DNA damage in PBMC from human volunteers using aphidicolin block. *DNA Repair* **2019**, *77*, 58–64. [CrossRef]
22. Miszczyk, J.; Rawojc, K. Effects of culturing technique on human peripheral blood lymphocytes response to proton and X-ray radiation. *Int. J. Radiat. Biol.* **2020**, *96*, 424–433. [CrossRef] [PubMed]
23. Betsou, F.; Gaignaux, A.; Ammerlaan, W.; Norris, P.J.; Stone, M. Biospecimen Science of Blood for Peripheral Blood Mononuclear Cell (PBMC) Functional Applications. *Curr. Pathobiol. Rep.* **2019**, *7*, 17–27. [CrossRef]
24. Davila, J.A.A.; De Los Rios, A.H. An Overview of Peripheral Blood Mononuclear Cells as a Model for Immunological Research of Toxoplasma gondii and Other Apicomplexan Parasites. *Front. Cell. Infect. Microbiol.* **2019**, *9*. [CrossRef]
25. Mosallaei, M.; Ehtesham, N.; Rahimirad, S.; Saghi, M.; Vatandoost, N.; Khosravi, S. PBMCs: A new source of diagnostic and prognostic biomarkers. *Arch. Physiol. Biochem.* **2020**. [CrossRef]
26. Forkman, J. Estimator and Tests for Common Coefficients of Variation in Normal Distributions. *Commun. Stat. Theory Methods* **2009**, *38*, 233–251. [CrossRef]
27. Zangerle, P.F.; Degroote, D.; Lopez, M.; Meuleman, R.J.; Vrindts, Y.; Fauchet, F.; Dehart, I.; Jadoul, M.; Radoux, D.; Franchimont, P. Direct Stimulation of Cytokines (Il-1-Beta, Tnf-Alpha, Il-6, Il-2, Ifn-Gamma and Gm-Csf) in Whole-Blood: II. Application to Rheumatoid-Arthritis and Osteoarthritis. *Cytokine* **1992**, *4*, 568–575. [CrossRef]
28. Centurione, L.; Aiello, F.B. DnA Repair and Cytokines: TGF-beta, IL-6, and Thrombopoietin as Different Biomarkers of Radioresistance. *Front. Oncol.* **2016**, *6*. [CrossRef]
29. Fenech, M.; Rinaldi, J. A comparison of lymphocyte micronuclei and plasma micronutrients in vegetarians and non-vegetarians. *Carcinogenesis* **1995**, *16*, 223–230. [CrossRef]
30. Odagiri, Y.; Uchida, H. Influence of serum micronutrients on the incidence of kinetochore-positive or -negative micronuclei in human peripheral blood lymphocytes. *Mutat. Res. Genet. Toxicol. Environ.* **1998**, *415*, 35–45. [CrossRef]
31. Ho, C.K.; Choi, S.W.; Siu, P.M.; Benzie, I.F.F. Cryopreservation and Storage Effects on Cell Numbers and DNA Damage in Human Lymphocytes. *Biopreserv. Biobank.* **2011**, *9*, 343–347. [CrossRef]
32. Koppen, G.; De Prins, S.; Jacobs, A.; Nelen, V.; Schoeters, G.; Langie, S.A.S. The comet assay in human biomonitoring: Cryopreservation of whole blood and comparison with isolated mononuclear cells. *Mutagenesis* **2018**, *33*, 41–47. [CrossRef] [PubMed]
33. Duthie, S.J.; Pirie, L.; Jenkinson, A.M.; Narayanan, S. Cryopreserved versus freshly isolated lymphocytes in human biomonitoring: Endogenous and induced DNA damage, antioxidant status and repair capability. *Mutagenesis* **2002**, *17*, 211–214. [CrossRef] [PubMed]
34. He, J.L.; Chen, W.L.; Jin, L.F.; Jin, H.Y. Comparative evaluation of the in vitro micronucleus test and the comet assay for the detection of genotoxic effects of X-ray radiation. *Mutat. Res. Genet. Toxicol. Environ.* **2000**, *469*, 223–231. [CrossRef]
35. Cheng, L.; Wang, L.E.; Spitz, M.R.; Wei, Q. Cryopreserving whole blood for functional assays using viable lymphocytes in molecular epidemiology studies. *Cancer Lett.* **2001**, *166*, 155–163. [CrossRef]
36. Fowke, K.R.; Behnke, J.; Hanson, C.; Shea, K.; Cosentino, M. Apoptosis: A method for evaluating the cryopreservation of whole blood and peripheral blood mononuclear cells. *J. Immunol. Methods* **2000**, *244*, 139–144. [CrossRef]
37. Zijno, A.; Saini, F.; Crebelli, R. Suitability of cryopreserved isolated lymphocytes for the analysis of micronuclei with the cytokinesis-block method. *Mutagenesis* **2007**, *22*, 311–315. [CrossRef]
38. Risom, L.; Knudsen, L.E. Use of cryopreserved peripheral mononuclear blood cells in biomonitoring. *Mutat. Res. Genet. Toxicol. Environ.* **1999**, *440*, 131–138. [CrossRef]
39. Djuzenova, C.S.; Muhl, B.; Fehn, M.; Oppitz, U.; Muller, B.; Flentje, M. Radiosensitivity in breast cancer assessed by the Comet and micronucleus assays. *Br. J. Cancer* **2006**, *94*, 1194–1203. [CrossRef]

Journal of
*Personalized
Medicine*

MDPI

Communication

Comparison of Clonogenic Survival Data Obtained by Pre- and Post-Irradiation Methods

Takahiro Oike [1,2,*], Yuka Hirota [1], Narisa Dewi Maulany Darwis [1,3], Atsushi Shibata [4] and Tatsuya Ohno [1,2]

1 Department of Radiation Oncology, Graduate School of Medicine, Gunma University, 3-39-22, Showa-machi, Maebashi 371-8511, Japan; yukahirota@gunma-u.ac.jp (Y.H.); m1920021@gunma-u.ac.jp (N.D.M.D.); tohno@gunma-u.ac.jp (T.O.)
2 Heavy Ion Medical Center, Gunma University, 3-39-22, Showa-machi, Maebashi 371-8511, Japan
3 Department of Radiation Oncology, Faculty of Medicine Universitas Indonesia—Dr. Cipto Mangunkusumo Hospital, Jl. P. Diponegoro no. 71, Jakarta 10430, Indonesia
4 Initiative for Advanced Research (GIAR), Gunma University, 3-39-22, Showa-machi, Maebashi 371-8511, Japan; shibata.at@gunma-u.ac.jp
* Correspondence: oiketakahiro@gunma-u.ac.jp; Tel.: +81-27-220-8383

Received: 22 September 2020; Accepted: 14 October 2020; Published: 15 October 2020

check for updates

Abstract: Clonogenic assays are the gold standard to measure in vitro radiosensitivity, which use two cell plating methods, before or after irradiation (IR). However, the effect of the plating method on the experimental outcome remains unelucidated. By using common cancer cell lines, here we demonstrate that pre-IR and post-IR plating methods have a negligible effect on the clonogenic assay-derived photon sensitivity as assessed by SF_2, SF_4, SF_6, SF_8, D_{10}, or D_{50} (N.B. SFx indicates the survival at X Gy; Dx indicates the dose providing X% survival). These data provide important biological insight that supports inter-study comparison and integrated analysis of published clonogenic assay data regardless of the plating method used.

Keywords: clonogenic assays; methods; plating; cancer; radiation; radiosensitivity

1. Introduction

Clonogenic assays are the gold standard method for assessing radiosensitivity in vitro [1]. Cancer research studies have reported the radiosensitivity of various cell lines obtained using clonogenic assays [2]. In addition, clonogenic assays are used to determine the relative biological effectiveness (RBE) of carbon ions over photons in clinical carbon ion radiotherapy (CIRT) [3–5].

Recent advances in computer science have enabled the integration of published experimental data into big data platforms. For example, in the field of genomics, published sequencing data are compiled in databases such as the Catalogue of Somatic Mutations in Cancer [6] and Cancer Cell Line Encyclopedia (CCLE) [7]. From this perspective, integration of published radiosensitivity data obtained by clonogenic assays will be a powerful strategy to promote radiation oncology research [8–10]. However, the data integration is difficult because there are two types of clonogenic assays using different cell plating methods; namely, cells are plated before or after irradiation (referred to hereafter as pre-IR plating and post-IR plating, respectively). In pre-IR plating methods, single cells in suspensions are seeded on plates and subjected to a treatment of interest (e.g., drug exposure or irradiation) after additional incubation for a few hours to days that allows cells to attach on the plates. Pre-IR methods are capable of creating multiple technical replicates for a treatment of interest easily; therefore, pre-IR plating methods are predominantly used for cancer research [9]. On the other hand, in post-IR plating methods, plates with subconfluent cells are subjected to a treatment of interest, which is followed by trypsinization, single cell suspension, and seeding for replication. Post-IR plating methods have been utilized in the historical work on the beam design of CIRT [3–5]. This is probably due to the fact that carbon ions are an extremely limited medical resource as there are only 13 institutions available for CIRT across the world as reported on the website of Particle Therapy Co-Operative Group (https://www.ptcog.ch/index.php/facilities-in-operation). We assume that researchers have intended to save precious machine time by avoiding irradiation of all replicates.

In principle, pre-IR and post-IR methods are different in terms of cell condition at the time of irradiation. In post-IR methods, cells are capable of cell-to-cell signal transduction in immediate response to irradiation before being separated from each other, which may affect radiosensitivity. However, the effect of the plating method on the experimental outcomes of clonogenic assays remains unelucidated, which limits progress in radiation oncology research. For example, Amornwichet et al. reported that the RBE of carbon ions in nine *epidermal growth factor receptor (EGFR)*-wild-type non-small cell lung carcinoma (NSCLC) cell lines was 2.6 ± 0.3 at the center of the 6-cm-wide spread-out Bragg peak (SOBP) [11], whereas Kagawa et al. reported that the RBE in human salivary gland (HSG) cells, the cell line used as the reference in the clinical CIRT beam set-up, was 1.8 at the center of the same 6-cm SOBP [5]. Although these data indicate that CIRT is more effective for *EGFR* wild-type NSCLCs, a definitive conclusion cannot be made because the former and latter studies used pre-IR and post-IR plating methods, respectively.

The aim of this study was to elucidate the effect of the clonogenic assay plating method on the experimental outcome of cancer cell radiosensitivity.

2. Materials and Methods

2.1. Cell Line and Cell Culture

A549 (human lung adenocarcinoma cell line) and HSG (human salivary gland tumor cell line) were used in this study. A549 was chosen because this cell line is commonly used for clonogenic assays in general cancer research, which predominantly uses pre-IR plating methods [2,9]. HSG was chosen because this cell line has been used as the reference cell line for CIRT beam set-up, which uses post-IR plating methods [3–5]. Previous studies indicate that both cell lines show intermediate-to-relatively-low sensitivity to photons [11–13]. A549 cells were purchased from ATCC (CCL-185, Manassas, VA, USA). HSG cells were purchased from JCRB Cell Bank (HSGc-C5, JRCB1070, Ibaragi, Japan). Cells were cultured in RPMI-1640 (Sigma-Aldrich, St. Louis, MO, USA) supplemented with 10% fetal bovine serum (Life Technologies, Carlsbad, CA, USA) in a 5% CO_2 incubator at 37 °C. No other additives were used in the media. Cells in the log-phase of growth were used for experiments.

2.2. Clonogenic Assays

Clonogenic assays were performed as described previously [1]. For a given assay, either pre-IR or post-IR plating methods were employed.

For pre-IR plating, cells were detached from culture dishes using trypsin (Sigma-Aldrich) and prepared as single cell suspensions in culture medium. The cells were counted using a hemocytometer under an inverted microscope. The single cell suspensions were subjected to two serial dilutions at 1:10 (i.e., 1:100 dilution in total), and the resulting suspensions were used for plating. The plated cells were incubated for a minimum period to enable cell attachment (approximately 6 h), and were exposed to X-ray irradiation at 2, 4, 6, and 8 Gy, or were sham-irradiated.

For post-IR plating, cells were trypsinized, and 2×10^5 cells were plated on a 3.5-cm dish. After incubation for 48 h, and when the cells reached 80–90% confluency, the cells were exposed to X-ray irradiation at 2, 4, 6, and 8 Gy, or were sham-irradiated. Immediately after irradiation, the cells were trypsinized and prepared as single cell suspensions in culture medium. The cells were counted using a hemocytometer under an inverted microscope. The single cell suspensions were subjected to two serial dilutions at 1:10, and the resulting suspensions were used for plating.

For all experiments, the cells were incubated for an additional 12 days, fixed with methanol, and stained with crystal violet. Colonies comprising ≥50 cells were counted under an inverted microscope. The surviving fraction at a given dose point was calculated by dividing the number of colonies by the number of seeded cells, which was further divided by plating efficiency calculated based on unirradiated controls. The surviving fraction at X Gy is referred to hereafter as SF_X. SF_2, SF_4, SF_6, and SF_8 were fitted to the linear quadratic model [12], from which D_{10} and D_{50} (i.e., the doses decreasing cell survival to 10% and 50%, respectively) were calculated. For both pre-IR and post-IR plating methods and for both cell lines, the number of cells plated per well was unified as 200, 200, 200, 400, and 400 for 0, 2, 4, 6, and 8 Gy, respectively. Experiments were repeated three times. Four samples were used for each experiment.

2.3. Irradiation

X-ray irradiation was performed using an MX-160Labo (160 kVp, 1.06 Gy/min; mediXtec, Matsudo, Japan) [4].

2.4. Statistics

Differences between two groups were examined using the non-parametric two-sided Mann–Whitney U-test. Differences were considered statistically significant at $p < 0.05$. All statistical analyses were performed using Prism8 (GraphPad Software, San Diego, CA, USA).

3. Results

To evaluate the effect of different plating methods on the experimental outcomes of clonogenic assays, we performed clonogenic assays using pre-IR or post-IR plating methods, while keeping the other experimental settings constant. The radiosensitivity endpoints commonly used in this field, i.e., SF_2, SF_4, SF_6, SF_8, D_{10}, and D_{50}, were compared between the two methods [9]. Plating efficiency exceeded 60% in all experiments, with a median of 82%. In the assessment of SF_2, SF_4, SF_6, D_{10}, and D_{50}, the coefficient of variation (CV) among three independent experiments was <20% in all experimental settings (median, 7%; 1–17%); these values were sufficiently low compared with previously published data [2,9]. The CV values for SF_8 were relatively high (median, 27%; 6–47%); nevertheless, these values were still lower than those published by Nuryadi et al., who calculated the CV for SF_8 in A549 cells from 20 repeated experiments using the same protocol in the same laboratory [2]. These data suggest that the experiments in this study were performed in a technically sound manner.

In A549 cells, no statistically significant differences in the outcomes were observed between pre-IR and post-IR plating methods for SF_2, SF_4, SF_6, SF_8, D_{10}, and D_{50} (Figure 1a–b). Survival plots demonstrated a high consistency between the two plating methods (Figure 1c–e). In HSG cells, no statistically significant differences in the outcomes were observed between pre-IR and post-IR plating methods for SF_2, SF_4, SF_6, SF_8, D_{10}, and D_{50} (Figure 2a–b). Survival plots demonstrated a high consistency between the two plating methods (Figure 2c–e). Taken together, these data suggest that the influence of the difference in the plating methods on the outcomes of clonogenic assays is negligible in A549 and HSG cells.

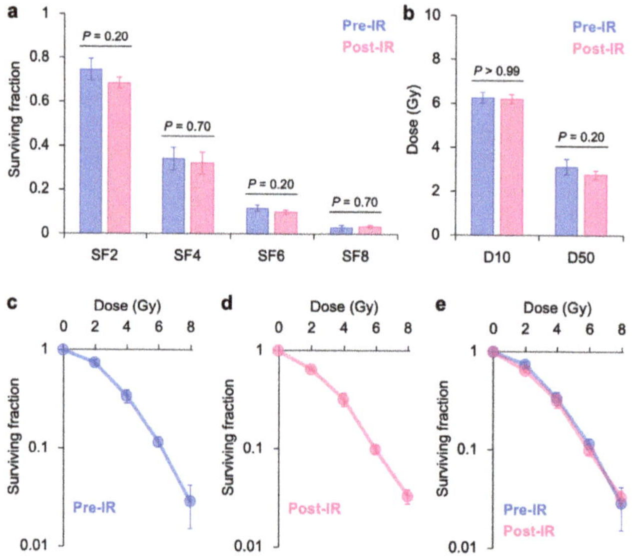

Figure 1. Clonogenic survival of X-ray-irradiated A549 cells assessed using plating methods in which cells are plated before (pre-IR) or after (post-IR) irradiation. (**a**) SF_2, SF_4, SF_6, and SF_8. (**b**) D_{10} and D_{50}. p-values were determined using the Mann–Whitney U-test. (**c**) Survival plots from pre-IR-plated cells. (**d**) Survival plots from post-IR-plated cells. (**e**) Survival plots from pre-IR (blue) or post-IR (violet) plating methods. Graphs are presented in 50% translucent colors; therefore, purple color indicates an overlap between the two plating methods. SFx indicates the survival at X Gy; Dx indicates the dose providing X% survival. Error bars indicate standard deviation.

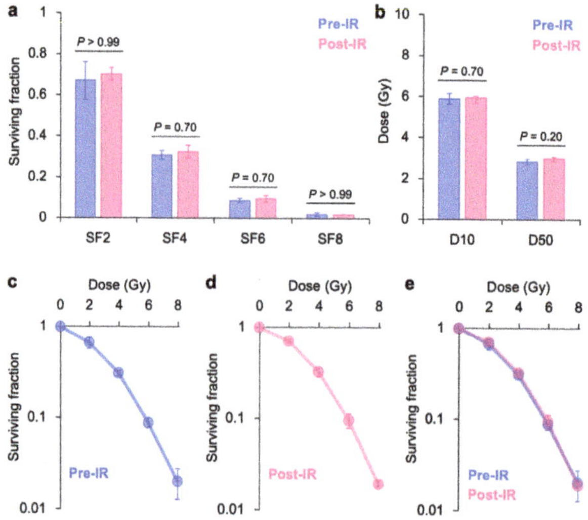

Figure 2. Clonogenic survival of X-ray-irradiated human salivary gland (HSG) cancer cells assessed using pre-IR or post-IR plating methods. (**a**) SF_2, SF_4, SF_6, and SF_8. (**b**) D_{10} and D_{50}. p-values were determined using the Mann–Whitney U-test. (**c**) Survival plots from pre-IR-plated cells. (**d**) Survival plots from post-IR-plated cells. (**e**) Survival plots from pre-IR (blue) or post-IR (violet) plating methods. Graphs are presented in 50% translucent colors; therefore, purple color indicates an overlap between the two plating methods. SFx indicates the survival at X Gy; Dx indicates the dose providing X% survival. Error bars indicate standard deviation.

4. Discussion

To the best of our knowledge, this is the first study to investigate the effect of different plating methods of clonogenic assays on the experimental outcomes. The results provide important insight supporting inter-study comparisons and integrated analysis of published clonogenic assay data regardless of the plating method used, which will contribute the promotion of radiation oncology research in the era of big data science.

The concept of precision medicine, that is optimization of treatment strategy based on genetic information of individual cancers, has become widespread in the field of cancer chemotherapy according to the advancement of next-generation sequencers. For example, if a lung cancer was found to harbor *ret proto-oncogene (RET)* fusions, then the cancer can be efficiently treated with Vandetanib, an inhibitor of RET tyrosine kinase [14]. In the field of radiation oncology on the other hand, the concept of precision medicine has not been applied to the clinic sufficiently. Theoretically, if we could predict the sensitivity of a tumor to radiotherapy at the time of diagnosis, then we can stratify radioresistant cases to the radiotherapy modalities capable of high-dose delivery (e.g., stereotactic body radiotherapy and particle therapies) that are rarer than conventional three-dimensional conformal radiotherapy. To this end, establishment of genetic profiles that predict cancer radioresistance is an urgent need. One of the barriers for the research aiming to meet this need is the absence of the big data pertaining to cancer cell radiosensitivity that can be used for analysis in combination with genomics data. This is in contrast to the situation for chemotherapy, where multiple databases for the sensitivity of cancer cells to anticancer drugs (e.g., CCLE) are open to public [7]. Although we find an enormous number of publications that report on the cancer cell radiosensitivity as assessed by clonogenic assays, the variance in the plating method has prevented us from conducting inter-study comparison and integration of these radiosensitivity data. Our data provide insight in overcoming this issue; using multiple cancer cell lines commonly used in this field, we showed that the difference in the plating method on the clonogenic assay-derived radiosensitivity data is negligibly small in A549 and HSG cells, suggesting that the published clonogenic data can be analyzed in combination regardless of the plating method. In addition, as explained in the Introduction, our data rationalize the inter-translation between genomics-associated radiosensitivity data and carbon-ion RBE data obtained predominantly using pre-IR and post-IR plating methods, respectively. Additionally, we assume that the findings from this study may be applicable to carbon ion experiments, warranting further research.

This study had several limitations. Minor subtypes of plating methods, such as IR in cell suspensions or delayed post-IR plating [9], were not investigated. In addition, cell lines other than A549 and HSG were not included. Research is warranted to further elucidate the influence of the difference in the methods in clonogenic assays on cancer cell radiosensitivity.

5. Conclusions

We showed that SF_2, SF_4, SF_6, SF_8, D_{10}, and D_{50} values obtained using clonogenic assays were highly consistent between pre-IR and post-IR methods in A549 and HSG cells. These data support the strategic robustness of inter-study comparisons and integrated analysis of published clonogenic assay data, regardless of the plating method used. Thus, these data will contribute to promote radiation oncology research in the era of big data science.

Author Contributions: Conceptualization, T.O. (Takahiro Oike); formal analysis, T.O. (Takahiro Oike), N.D.M.D. and Y.H.; writing—original draft preparation, T.O. (Takahiro Oike); writing—review and editing, T.O. (Takahiro Oike); supervision, A.S. and T.O. (Tatsuya Ohno); funding acquisition, T.O. (Tatsuya Ohno). All authors have read and agreed to the published version of the manuscript.

Funding: This research was funded by Grants-in-Aid from the Japan Society for the Promotion of Science for KAKENHI [19K17162]. This work was also supported by Gunma University Heavy Ion Medical Center.

Conflicts of Interest: The authors declare no conflict of interest.

References

1. Franken, N.A.P.; Rodermond, H.M.; Stap, J.; Haveman, J.; Van Bree, C. Clonogenic assay of cells in vitro. *Nat. Protoc.* **2006**, *1*, 2315–2319. [CrossRef] [PubMed]
2. Nuryadi, E.; Permata, T.B.M.; Komatsu, S.; Oike, T.; Nakano, T. Inter-assay precision of clonogenic assays for radiosensitivity in cancer cell line A549. *Oncotarget* **2018**, *9*, 13706–13712. [CrossRef] [PubMed]
3. Kanai, T.; Endo, M.; Minohara, S.; Miyahara, N.; Koyama-Ito, H.; Tomura, H.; Matsufuji, N.; Futami, Y.; Fukumura, A.; Hiraoka, T.; et al. Biophysical characteristics of HIMAC clinical irradiation system for heavy-ion radiation therapy. *Int. J. Radiat. Oncol. Biol. Phys.* **1999**, *44*, 201–210. [CrossRef]
4. Furusawa, Y.; Fukutsu, K.; Aoki, M.; Itsukaichi, H.; Eguchi-Kasai, K.; Ohara, H.; Yatagai, F.; Kanai, T.; Ando, K. Inactivation of aerobic and hypoxic cells from three different cell lines by accelerated (3)He-, (12)C- and (20)Ne-ion beams. *Radiat. Res.* **2000**, *154*, 485–496. [CrossRef]
5. Kagawa, K.; Murakami, M.; Hishikawa, Y.; Abe, M.; Akagi, T.; Yanou, T.; Kagiya, G.; Furusawa, Y.; Ando, K.; Nojima, K.; et al. Preclinical biological assessment of proton and carbon ion beams at Hyogo Ion Beam Medical Center. *Int. J. Radiat. Oncol. Biol. Phys.* **2002**, *54*, 928–938. [CrossRef]
6. COSMIC | Catalogue of Somatic Mutations in Cancer. Available online: https://cancer.sanger.ac.uk/cosmic (accessed on 2 August 2020).
7. Broad Institute Cancer Cell Line Encyclopedia. Available online: https://portals.broadinstitute.org/ccle (accessed on 2 August 2020).
8. Komatsu, S.; Oike, T.; Komatsu, Y.; Kubota, Y.; Sakai, M.; Matsui, T.; Nuryadi, E.; Permata, T.B.M.; Sato, H.; Kawamura, H.; et al. Deep learning-assisted literature mining for in vitro radiosensitivity data. *Radiother. Oncol.* **2019**, *139*, 87–93. [CrossRef] [PubMed]
9. Matsui, T.; Nuryadi, E.; Komatsu, S.; Hirota, Y.; Shibata, A.; Oike, T.; Nakano, T. Robustness of Clonogenic Assays as a Biomarker for Cancer Cell Radiosensitivity. *Int. J. Mol. Sci.* **2019**, *20*, 4148. [CrossRef] [PubMed]
10. Anakura, M.; Nachankar, A.; Kobayashi, D.; Amornwichet, N.; Hirota, Y.; Shibata, A.; Oike, T.; Nakano, T. Radiosensitivity Differences between EGFR Mutant and Wild-Type Lung Cancer Cells are Larger at Lower Doses. *Int. J. Mol. Sci.* **2019**, *20*, 3635. [CrossRef] [PubMed]
11. Amornwichet, N.; Oike, T.; Shibata, A.; Nirodi, C.S.; Ogiwara, H.; Makino, H.; Kimura, Y.; Hirota, Y.; Isono, M.; Yoshida, Y.; et al. The EGFR mutation status affects the relative biological effectiveness of carbon-ion beams in non-small cell lung carcinoma cells. *Sci. Rep.* **2015**, *5*, 11305. [CrossRef] [PubMed]
12. Oike, T.; Ogiwara, H.; Torikai, K.; Nakano, T.; Yokota, J.; Kohno, T. Garcinol, a Histone Acetyltransferase Inhibitor, Radiosensitizes Cancer Cells by Inhibiting Non-Homologous End Joining. *Int. J. Radiat. Oncol. Biol. Phys.* **2012**, *84*, 815–821. [CrossRef] [PubMed]
13. Osu, N.; Kobayashi, D.; Shirai, K.; Musha, A.; Sato, H.; Hirota, Y.; Shibata, A.; Oike, T.; Ohno, T. Relative Biological Effectiveness of Carbon Ions for Head-and-Neck Squamous Cell Carcinomas According to Human Papillomavirus Status. *J. Pers. Med.* **2020**, *10*, 71. [CrossRef] [PubMed]
14. Kohno, T.; Ichikawa, H.; Totoki, Y.; Yasuda, K.; Hiramoto, M.; Nammo, T.; Sakamoto, H.; Tsuta, K.; Furuta, K.; Shimada, Y.; et al. KIF5B-RET fusions in lung adenocarcinoma. *Nat. Med.* **2012**, *18*, 375–377. [CrossRef] [PubMed]

MDPI
St. Alban-Anlage 66
4052 Basel
Switzerland
Tel. +41 61 683 77 34
Fax +41 61 302 89 18
www.mdpi.com

Journal of Personalized Medicine Editorial Office
E-mail: jpm@mdpi.com
www.mdpi.com/journal/jpm

www.ingramcontent.com/pod-product-compliance
Lightning Source LLC
LaVergne TN
LVHW070047120526
838202LV00101B/1507